Statistical DNA Forensics
Theory, Methods and Computation

Wing Kam Fung and Yue-Qing Hu

*Department of Statistics and Actuarial Science, The University
of Hong Kong, Hong Kong*

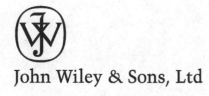

John Wiley & Sons, Ltd

Other Wiley Editorial Offices

John Wiley & Sons Inc., 111 River Street, Hoboken, NJ 07030, USA

Jossey-Bass, 989 Market Street, San Francisco, CA 94103-1741, USA

Wiley-VCH Verlag GmbH, Boschstr. 12, D-69469 Weinheim, Germany

John Wiley & Sons Australia Ltd, 42 McDougall Street, Milton, Queensland 4064, Australia

John Wiley & Sons (Asia) Pte Ltd, 2 Clementi Loop #02-01, Jin Xing Distripark, Singapore 129809

John Wiley & Sons Canada Ltd, 6045 Freemont Blvd, Mississauga, ONT, L5R 4J3

Wiley also publishes its books in a variety of electronic formats. Some content that appears in print may not be
available in electronic books.

British Library Cataloguing in Publication Data

A catalogue record for this book is available from the British Library

ISBN: 978-0-470-06636-2

Typeset in 10/12pt Times by Thomson Digital, India

*To Yuet Siu, Ka Chung and Ka Wing and the
Memory of My Parents Yau Yung and Yiu Fung*

To Tian Shuang and Jia Wen

Contents

Preface

In the early 1990's, one of the authors attended a forensic conference in Arizona, USA and became familiar with DNA profiling. In the meeting, there were heated debates among forensic scientists, statisticians and legal professionals on the pros and cons of the then new forensic DNA technology. These debates began to settle down after the US National Research Council released its second report on the evaluation of forensic DNA evidence in 1996. Currently, the technique is widely employed and accepted in the courtroom due to its high discriminating power and reliability. It is a very powerful tool, not only in the investigation of serious criminal offences including rapes and homicides, but also in voluminous offences such as thefts and burglaries.

Statistics and probability play an important role in the interpretation of forensic DNA. Unlike other areas of forensic science, probability is often needed in assessing the weight of DNA evidence; probabilities in the magnitude of one in millions or one in billions are commonly heard in court cases. A major aim of this book is to introduce the fundamental statistical and probability theory and methods for the evaluation of DNA evidence. The book covers three main applications of DNA profiling, namely identity testing, determination of parentage and kinship, and interpretation of mixed DNA stains. Moreover, we place emphasis on the computational aspects of statistical DNA forensics. Computer programs are available at `http://www.hku.hk/statistics/EasyDNA/` for possible use. Readers can use the software to check the numerical findings of the examples given in the book. This can help readers understand and appreciate the theory and methods behind statistical forensic DNA analysis.

We are most grateful to the following people for their continuous support and assistance: Dart Man Wong and Pui Tsui for introducing the fundamental concepts and sharing their knowledge and experience in DNA forensics; Sze Chung Leung and his forensic laboratory colleagues for encouragement and support; Yuk Ka Chung, Hong Lee and Yan Tsun Choy for computing assistance; John Buckleton for introducing the mixed stain problem; and specifically to Ada Lai for excellent secretarial support and typing the manuscript. We thank the staff at John Wiley for their editorial assistance.

Last but not least, we wish to express our gratitude to our families, Yuet Siu, Ka Chung, Ka Wing, and Tian Shuang, Jia Wen, for their patience and immense support.

W.K. Fung and Y.Q. Hu

Hong Kong

List of tables

1

Introduction

1.1   Statistics, forensic science and the law

Statistics has been playing an important role in forensic science and law. This is very natural, since statistics is the science in dealing with variability and uncertainty, which commonly arise in these two disciplines. In forensic science, data are collected from the crime scene or elsewhere, and statistics is often used to analyze these data. Scientists explain the statistical findings and provide their interpretations to various concerned parties including the client, jury, lawyer and judge. Recently, several books were published on the use of statistics in forensic science and in the courtroom (Aitken and Taroni 2004; Gastwirth 2000; Good 2001; Lucy 2005).

According to (Lucy 2005, p3), a brief inspection of the *Journal of Forensic Sciences* for the years between 1999 and 2002 indicates that about half of the articles have some kind of statistical content. It is noticed that the sort of statistical methods used can vary from the elementary tools such as percentages, means and standard deviations to the more sophisticated techniques including tests of statistical hypotheses, regression and calibration, and classification. An update in glancing through the articles in the *Journal of Forensic Sciences* for the years of 2005 and 2006 indicates that the phenomenon persists, i.e. about half of the articles have some kind of statistical content. Besides those statistical methods mentioned by Lucy (2005), we also find other more complex methods, such as cluster analysis, logistic regression and Fisher's exact test. Moreover, we also notice that about a quarter of the articles are on DNA profiling. Nearly all these DNA articles involve some kind of statistical analyses, ranging from elementary statistical methods to more complicated techniques such as the least-square deconvolution.

1.2   The use of statistics in forensic DNA

DNA profiling has become one of the most commonly used techniques for human identification since its introduction by Jeffreys *et al.* (1985). It is one of the most important tools in forensic science. Nowadays, many forensic laboratories including the Hong Kong Government

Laboratory have the largest teams of scientists working in DNA forensics. DNA can be found in blood, hair/hair root, bone, semen and body fluid such as saliva and sweat. No two persons, except for identical twins, have the same DNA sequence. The current DNA profiling technology uses only a number of genetic markers, and so a unique identification may not be assured. Nevertheless, the technique is widely employed and accepted in courtrooms due to its highly discriminating power and reliability. The US National Research Council (NRC) released two reports on the use of the technique in 1992 and 1996. In NRC II (National Research Council 1996), many discussions were provided on the statistical issues of forensic DNA, and several recommendations related to the proper use of statistics were given. Since NRC II, a few books on the use of statistics in DNA forensics have been published (Balding 2005; Buckleton *et al.* 2005; Evett and Weir 1998).

DNA profiling is not only commonly used in forensic investigation, but also leads to a lot of research in this area. Nowadays, this kind of research constitutes the highest percentage of articles in respectable forensic science journals. In 2007, a daughter journal of Forensic Science International (FSI), *Forensic Science International: Genetics* (*FSI Genetics*), has been newly launched. According to the announcement in the founding issue of *FSI Genetics*, 46% of submissions to *FSI Genetics* fall in the area of forensic genetics, indicating that this discipline can readily support its own journal.

The following quote is taken from the founding volume of *FSI Genetics (2007)*:

> Although forensic genetics is a discipline a century old (the discovery of the ABO group by Karl Landsteiner can be considered the birth of this field), the introduction of DNA profiling to forensic analysis following the development of this technique by Alec Jeffreys and co-workers, 20 years ago, has had a tremendous impact on forensic genetics. The amount of work in this field has increased enormously since 1985, with an increasing number of papers published in this area. This increase shows no signs of slowing down with many new technologies and applications being reported. Major advances in molecular biology and computer technology—allowing DNA samples to be obtained from ever smaller quantities of biological material—are continuously being reported along with new and exciting applications of DNA technology to the analysis of non-human material (crime scene analysis, tracking the illegal trade in endangered species and bioterrorism), or the building and appropriate management of DNA databases is expanding outside of the traditional areas of criminal investigation.

> Forensic genetics is now a reasonably mature field, and generates sufficient high quality content to support a dedicated journal.

> The scope of the new journal would include most of the forensic genetics topics such as (among others):

> - Biostatistical methods in forensic genetics.
>   o Evaluation of DNA evidence in forensic problems (such as paternity or immigration cases, criminal casework, identification), classical and new statistical approaches.

In fact, a high proportion of the papers in forensic genetics has used some sort of statistics. In many situations, simple statistics such as the percentage, mean and standard deviation are sufficient, while in some others, more advanced statistical analyses are needed. The following two articles selected from *FSI 2006* indicate the sorts of advanced techniques used.

Shepard and Herrera (2006) studied allelic frequencies of 15 STR loci from 150 unrelated persons from an Iranian population. Common statistical measures such as the gene diversity index, power of discrimination, power of exclusion and tests for Hardy–Weinberg equilibrium, etc. were constructed. The more advanced statistical techniques–phylogenetic analysis with neighbor-joining trees and multi-dimensional scaling analysis–were performed using F_{st} measures generated from 13 worldwide, geographically targeted populations. Bonferroni adjustment for multiple comparisons and statistical bootstrap analysis were also conducted. Based on the statistical findings, the authors discussed the appropriate choice of databases on which to base forensic calculations for populations located in geographic intersections.

Hammer *et al.* (2006) considered a set of 61 Y-SNPs for a sample of 2517 individuals from 38 populations to infer the geographic origins of Y chromosomes in the United States and to test for paternal admixture. Sophisticated statistical techniques, including hierarchical genetic structuring based on an analysis of molecular variance and multi-dimensional scaling for clustering, were chosen. From the statistical findings, it was inferred that both inter-ethnic admixture and population subdivision might contribute to fine scale Y-STR heterogeneity within US ethnic groups.

Why has statistics attracted more attention in DNA forensics than in other areas of forensic science? Fung *et al.* (2006) have summarized the following, among other possible reasons:

> First, DNA profiling is generally scientifically unambiguous and very powerful. Since the DNA evidence is repeatable, statistical evaluation would then be possible and in most situations objective.

> Second, when there is a match to the DNA evidence, people would like to know how likely there is a random match.

> Third, extremely small probabilities are commonly encountered in DNA profiling, and people are curious about their derivations and interpretations (note: these probabilities are sometimes interpreted incorrectly, e.g. prosecutor's fallacy).

> Fourth, many forensic scientists are not that familiar with statistics, particularly on different approaches of the subject.

> Fifth, some problems such as kinship determinations and DNA mixtures need complex statistical analysis.

It is the fifth point about kinship determinations and assessment of DNA mixtures that requires complex statistical analysis; a major aim of this book is to provide details on the statistical treatment of such problems. In doing so, the other points will also be touched upon.

1.3   Genetic basis of DNA profiling and typing technology

1.3.1   Genetic basis

NRC I and NRC II (National Research Council 1992, 1996) give comprehensive accounts of the general principles of DNA profiling. The following paragraphs on the genetic basis of DNA typing come from Chapter 2 of NRC II.

In higher organisms, the genetic material is organized into microscopic structures called *chromosomes*. A fertilized human egg has 46 chromosomes (23 pairs). A chromosome is a very thin thread of DNA, surrounded by other materials, mainly protein. The DNA thread is actually double – two strands coiled around each other like a twisted rope ladder with stiff wooden steps. The basic chemical unit of DNA is the nucleotide, consisting of a base. There are four kinds of bases, designated A, G, T and C. The total DNA in a genome amounts to about 3 billion nucleotide pairs. A gene is a segment of DNA, ranging from a few thousand to more than a hundred thousand nucleotide pairs. The position on the chromosome at which a particular gene resides is its *locus*.

Alternative forms of a gene are called *alleles*. If the same allele is present in both chromosomes of a pair, then the person is *homozygous*; if the two alleles are different, then the person is *heterozygous*. A person's genetic makeup is the *genotype*. Genotype can refer to a single gene locus with two alleles, A and a, in which case the three possible genotypes are AA, Aa, and aa; or it can be extended to several loci or even to the entire set of genes. In forensic analysis, the genotype for the group of analyzed loci is called the DNA *profile*.

1.3.2   Typing technology

Currently, short tandem repeat (STR) loci are most commonly used for DNA profiling. Usually, about 10 or more unlinked autosomal (the 22 pairs of chromosomes, but not the sex chromosomes) loci are used in practice. After some laboratory procedures, including DNA extraction and the polymerase chain reaction (PCR) process, the STR profiles can then be obtained. For more details on the STR typing technology, interested readers can refer to (Buckleton *et al.* 2005, Chapter 1) and (Balding 2005, Chapter 4).

Figure 1.1 shows the STR profile of a DNA sample from a crime scene obtained by ABI machines and software. Only the three autosomal loci of the yellow panel are shown for illustration. The upper panel corresponds to the allelic ladders of the standard markers. From the figure, we notice that the genotypes at the three loci are respectively 7/11 at locus

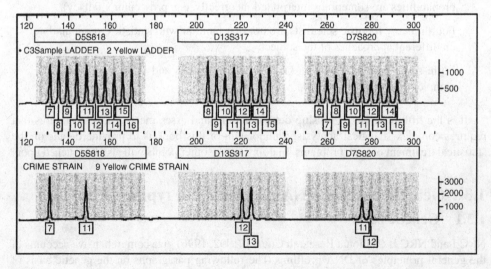

Figure 1.1   An STR profile of a DNA sample from a crime scene, obtained by ABI machines and software.

D5S818 (of chromosome 5), 12/13 at D13S317 (of chromosome 13) and 11/12 at D7S820 (of chromosome 7). The values 7 and 11 at D5S818 may be called allele sizes, which represent the numbers of repeat DNA units in the two alleles. The STR locus has the property that its allele size is discrete and so is easy to interpret and has little ambiguity. The commonly used STR loci usually have slightly below 10 to over 20 alleles, giving a large number of possible genotypes at each locus. In the Hong Kong Chinese population database (Wong *et al.* 2001), it just happens that there are eight different alleles for each of the loci mentioned above, resulting in $8 \times 9/2 = 36$ possible genotypes at each locus.

To show the discriminating power of DNA profiling, we assess the frequency of the DNA profile in Figure 1.1 in the Hong Kong Chinese population. According to Wong *et al.* (2001), the allele frequencies are $p_7 = 0.035$ and $p_{11} = 0.252$ at D5S818; $p_{12} = 0.099$ and $p_{13} = 0.023$ at D13S317; and $p_{11} = 0.376$ and $p_{12} = 0.230$ at D7S820. The frequency of the DNA profile at all three loci may be evaluated as $(2 \times 0.035 \times 0.252) \times (2 \times 0.099 \times 0.023) \times (2 \times 0.376 \times 0.230) = 1.39 \times 10^{-5}$ under Hardy–Weinberg and linkage equilibria (discussion on their validity is given in Chapter 3). In other words, about 1 in 72 000 $[= 1/(1.39 \times 10^{-5})]$ persons in the local Chinese population has such a DNA profile. This shows the highly discriminating power of the technique if a suspect is arrested and his/her genotype is found to match with the crime stain profile.

1.4 About the book

This book aims to introduce the basic statistical theory and methods for the evaluation of DNA evidence. Readers are assumed to have little background knowledge in statistics and probability. Thus, we start by considering simple cases first and then proceed to analyze more complex problems. We illustrate with many examples, so that readers can not only grasp the basic concepts, but also understand the more advanced analyses. The book covers three main applications of DNA profiling, namely identity testing, determination of parentage and kinship, and interpretation of mixed DNA stains. Moreover, we place emphasis on the computational aspects of statistical DNA forensics. Computer programs are available at http://www.hku.hk/statistics/EasyDNA/ for possible use. Readers can use the software to check the numerical findings of the examples given in the book. This can help readers to understand and appreciate the theory and methods behind statistical forensic DNA analysis.

The remainder of the book is organized as follows. Chapter 2 provides the basic probability and statistics that are commonly used in later chapters. Chapter 3 discusses fundamental concepts and introduces some statistical measures in population genetics. The statistical evaluation of single source samples or identity testing, including the theory of subpopulation models and the problems involving relatives, is studied thoroughly. The common parentage identifications are discussed in Chapter 4, while the complex kinship determinations are considered in Chapter 5. The associated computer software can provide a convenient means to analyze those particular paternity and kinship problems. Although the methods and software are illustrated with STR profiles, they can also be applied to analyze single-nucleotide polymorphism (SNP) profiles. Chapters 6 and 7 are on the statistical interpretation of DNA mixture. The associated formulas are often complicated and so the more technical derivations are put in the last section of each chapter. Thus, the reader can focus on the application of the calculating formulas in practical problem without being distracted by the technical derivations. The last chapter (Chapter 8) discusses some other issues in statistical DNA forensics, such as the Y-STR marker, peak information and database search, etc.

2

Probability and statistics

2.1 Probability

Probability is used in situations in which the outcomes occur randomly. It has lots of applications in various disciplines. It plays an important role in evaluating the weight of evidence. Many discussions on the use of probability as well as statistics in the forensic field and the legal profession can be found; see, for example, Aitken and Taroni (2004), Finkelstein and Levin (2001), Gastwirth (2000) and Lucy (2005). In the Second National Research Council Report (NRC II 1996) on the evaluation of forensic DNA evidence, there were a lot of discussions on the probability assessment of forensic DNA; a number of suggestions on the proper use of probability and statistics were provided.

In many situations, we are interested in getting the probability that a particular event occurs. Suppose we have a fair die and consider a single throw of the die. Let E be the event that the outcome is a 2 facing up. Since the die is a fair die with six faces, numbered $1, 2, \ldots, 6$, the probability that the event E occurs is $1/6$. Notionally, we write $P(E) = 1/6$. This fair die example is used below to introduce the three laws of probability.

Let E be any particular event of interest. The *first law of probability* states that

$$0 \leq P(E) \leq 1. \tag{2.1}$$

If event E is certain to occur, then $P(E) = 1$. On the other hand, an impossible event E has zero probability to occur, i.e. $P(E) = 0$.

Consider the event that the die shows the number 2 or below. What is the probability of observing such an event? Most people can provide the correct answer $2/6 = 1/3$, since there are two possibilities out of a total of six possible outcomes. This result can also be obtained from the *second law of probability*, which is provided as follows.

Suppose A and B are two *mutually exclusive* events; then

$$P(A \text{ or } B) = P(A) + P(B). \tag{2.2}$$

This is sometimes called the *additive rule*. The statement 'A or B' is conventionally written as '$A \cup B$'. With reference to the above example, A can be taken as the event that the number shown is a 1 with probability $P(A) = 1/6$, and B be the event that the number shown is a 2 with probability $P(B)$ also being $1/6$. The occurrence of A will preclude the occurrence of B and so the events are called mutually exclusive. Then, according to the second law, the probability that the die will show the number 2 or below is

$$P(A \cup B) = P(A) + P(B) = 1/6 + 1/6 = 1/3.$$

A general form of the second law of probability can be extended to the situation with $k > 2$ *mutually exclusive events* $E_1, E_2, \ldots, E_k$:

$$P(E_1 \cup E_2 \cdots \cup E_k) = P(E_1) + P(E_2) + \cdots + P(E_k). \tag{2.3}$$

It is also common to consider the probability of the occurrence of two (or more) events, say A and B, together. Suppose we throw a fair die twice; what is the probability that the first throw is a 6 and the second is also 6? Before answering this question, we let A denote that a 6 is shown in the first throw, and B denote that a 6 is shown in the second throw. In fact, there are 36 possible outcomes of the two throws of the die, namely $(1, 1), (1, 2), \ldots, (6, 6)$, and they are equally probable. The joint event A and B is $(6, 6)$, which is one of these 36 possibilities, and $P(A \text{ and } B) = 1/36$. If we just consider only event A of the first throw, it is obvious that $P(A) = 1/6$. Similarly, for only the second throw, $P(B) = 1/6$. We arrive at the following result:

$$P(A \text{ and } B) = P(A) \times P(B), \tag{2.4}$$

in which A and B are *independent* events. This is the *third law of probability*, sometimes also called the *product or multiplicative rule*. From here onwards, for brevity, we also write $P(A \text{ and } B)$ as $P(A, B)$, $P(AB)$ or $P(A \cap B)$. The third law can be easily extended to more than two independent events. Suppose $E_1, E_2, \ldots, E_k$ are k *independent* events,

$$P(E_1, E_2, \ldots, E_k) = P(E_1)P(E_2) \cdots P(E_k). \tag{2.5}$$

Let us go back to the second law, Equation (2.2) again. The law considers the probability $P(A \text{ or } B)$ in which the two events A and B are mutually exclusive to each other. In many situations, however, this does not hold true. For example, in a single throw of a fair die, A is the event that the value shown is 3 or below, and B is the event that the value shown is an even number. The occurrence of event A does not preclude the occurrence of event B and vice versa, and so the two events are not mutually exclusive. It is easy to check that $P(A \text{ or } B) = 5/6$, and $P(A) + P(B) = 3/6 + 3/6 = 1$, and they are not equal to each other.

The following *general second law of probability* can be used for the above situation. For any events A and B,

$$P(A \text{ or } B) = P(A) + P(B) - P(A \text{ and } B),$$

or, conventionally,

$$P(A \cup B) = P(A) + P(B) - P(AB). \tag{2.6}$$

With reference to the earlier example, the joint event AB (i.e. A and B) is just the event that the value shown is a 2. Thus, $P(AB) = 1/6$. The right-hand side of Equation (2.6) is $3/6 + 3/6 - 1/6 = 5/6$, which is equal to $P(A \text{ or } B) = 5/6$ that we obtained earlier.

Equation (2.6) can be extended to situations with three events:

$$P(A \cup B \cup C) = P(A) + P(B) + P(C) - P(AB) - P(AC) - P(BC) + P(ABC),$$

or generally with n events $E_1, \ldots, E_n$:

$$P \left(\bigcup_{i=1}^{n} E_i \right) = \sum_{i=1}^{n} P(E_i) - \sum_{i<j} P(E_i E_j) + \sum_{i<j<k} P(E_i E_j E_k) - \cdots$$

$$+ (-1)^{n+1} P \left(\bigcap_{i=1}^{n} E_i \right), \tag{2.7}$$

where the notation $\sum_{i=1}^{k} a_i$ stands for the summation of the terms a_i over the index i from 1 to k, $P \left(\bigcup_{i=1}^{n} E_i \right)$ means $P(E_1 \cup E_2 \cup \cdots \cup E_n)$, and $P \left(\bigcap_{i=1}^{n} E_i \right)$ means $P(E_1 \cap E_2 \cap \cdots \cap E_n)$ or just $P(E_1 E_2 \cdots E_n)$. Equation (2.7) is also called the principle of inclusion and exclusion.

2.2   Dependent events and conditional probability

The third law of probability requires events A and B to be independent. But not all events are independent. Consider one throw of a die with events A and B given earlier, where A is the throwing of a number 3 or below and B is the throwing of an even number. Then, $P(A) = 1/2$, $P(B) = 1/2$, and $P(A, B) = P$(the number shown is a 2) $= 1/6$ which is, however, not equal to $P(A) \times P(B)$. The third law does not hold true here, i.e. $P(A, B) \neq P(A) \times P(B)$, because events A and B are not independent.

The assessment for the probability of the above joint event can also be approached in the following way. Suppose we imagine that event B has already happened, i.e. an even number has been shown and this occurs with a probability $P(B) = 1/2$. Given this situation (event B), what is the probability that the number thrown is 3 or below (event A)? Event B has three outcomes $\{2, 4, 6\}$ and only one of them $\{2\}$ is 3 or below. So, given an even number has been thrown (event B), the probability that it is 3 or below (event A) is $1/3$. In terms of mathematical notation, we write this as $P(A|B) = 1/3$ – the probability that event A occurs *given* or *on condition* that event B has occurred is $1/3$. In the above example, we notice that $P(A, B) = 1/6 = P(A|B)P(B) = 1/3 \times 1/2$.

Generally, we can write

$$P(A, B) = P(A|B)P(B). \tag{2.8}$$

This is sometimes known as the *third law of probability for dependent events*. If A and B are independent events, then the *conditional probability* $P(A|B)$ becomes $P(A)$, i.e. the probability that A occurs does not depend on whether event B has occurred or not.

It is clear that the order of events A and B in Equation (2.8) is irrelevant, and so it is also true to have

$$P(A, B) = P(B|A)P(A). \tag{2.9}$$

The extended version of the third law Equation (2.8) or (2.9) applies to any two events A and B, and is not restricted to the specific example given above. It can be applied to a general situation and is commonly employed in evidence evaluation. Furthermore, the above Equations (2.8) and (2.9) can be generalized to deal with problems having more than two events.

Suppose that there are three events A, B, C of interest. Can we get an equation for evaluating the probability of the joint event A, B and C, $P(A, B, C)$, like Equation (2.8), in terms of the conditional probabilities? To achieve our purpose, let us first denote $E = (B, C)$. Then, from Equation (2.9), we obtain

$$P(A, E) = P(E|A)P(A).$$

Putting back E as (B, C), the equation becomes

$$P(A, B, C) = P(B, C|A)P(A). \tag{2.10}$$

Now, applying Equation (2.9) to $P(B, C|A)$ gives

$$P(B, C|A) = P(C|A, B)P(B|A). \tag{2.11}$$

Substituting Equation (2.11) into Equation (2.10), we get

$$P(A, B, C) = P(C|A, B)P(B|A)P(A). \tag{2.12}$$

Suppose we are interested in four events A, B, C and D. Using a similar derivation to the above, we can obtain

$$P(A, B, C, D) = P(B, C, D|A)P(A), \tag{2.13}$$

$$P(B, C, D|A) = P(C, D|A, B)P(B|A), \tag{2.14}$$

$$P(B, C, D|A) = P(D|A, B, C)P(B, C|A), \tag{2.15}$$

$$P(C, D|A, B) = P(D|A, B, C)P(C|A, B), \tag{2.16}$$

$$P(A, B, C, D) = P(D|A, B, C)P(C|A, B)P(B|A)P(A). \tag{2.17}$$

There are many applications of these formulas in the later part of this book.

2.3   Law of total probability

Consider one throw of a fair die. Let B_1 and B_2 be the events for the throwing of an odd number and an even number, respectively. These two events are mutually exclusive because the occurrence of one event precludes the occurrence of the other, and they are exhaustive because they exhaust all possibilities, since the throwing can only be an odd or an even number. They are called *mutually exclusive and exhaustive events*, and have the property that

$$P(B_1 \text{ or } B_2) = P(B_1) + P(B_2) = 1.$$

Consider the event A that the number thrown is 3 or below. The probability $P(A)$ is obviously $1/2$. The events 'A and B_1' and 'A and B_2' are mutually exclusive, since they cannot both occur. The outcomes for 'A and B_1' are $\{1, 3\}$, and the outcome for 'A and B_2' is $\{2\}$. So, the event 'A and B_1' or 'A and B_2' is $\{1, 2, 3\}$, which are just the outcomes for event A. Thus,

$$P(A) = P(\text{'}A \text{ and } B_1\text{' or '}A \text{ and } B_2\text{'})$$

$$= P(A \text{ and } B_1) + P(A \text{ and } B_2)$$

$$= P(A|B_1)P(B_1) + P(A|B_2)P(B_2).$$

The last equality results from the third law of probability for dependent events [see Equation (2.8)].

An extension of the argument to any number of mutually exclusive and exhaustive events is given as follows: If $B_1, B_2, \ldots$, and B_k are k *mutually exclusive and exhaustive events*, then, for any event A,

$$P(A) = P(A|B_1)P(B_1) + \cdots + P(A|B_k)P(B_k)$$

$$= \sum_{i=1}^{k} P(A|B_i)P(B_i), \tag{2.18}$$

$$= \sum_{i=1}^{k} P(A, B_i). \tag{2.19}$$

This is called the *law of total probability* or the *rule of elimination*.

2.4 Bayes' Theorem

Bayes' Theorem is an important result for the evaluation of probability. It was introduced by Thomas Bayes in the 18th century, and could be regarded as a useful means to assess the weight of evidence.

Consider the third law of probability for dependent events in Equation (2.8):

$$P(A, B) = P(A|B)P(B).$$

The law can also be expressed as in Equation (2.9):

$$P(A, B) = P(B|A)P(A).$$

Thus,

$$P(B|A)P(A) = P(A|B)P(B). \tag{2.20}$$

If $P(A) \neq 0$, we write

$$P(B|A) = \frac{P(A|B)P(B)}{P(A)}. \tag{2.21}$$

This is called *Bayes' Theorem*, and it relates the conditional probabilities to unconditional probabilities.

Consider two mutually exclusive and exhaustive events B and $\bar{B}$, where $\bar{B}$ is a complementary event of B, i.e. not B. Using the law of total probability for $P(A)$, Equation (2.21) can be rewritten as

$$P(B|A) = \frac{P(A|B)P(B)}{P(A|B)P(B) + P(A|\bar{B})P(\bar{B})}. \tag{2.22}$$

Generally, let $B_1, B_2, \ldots, B_k$ denote k mutually exclusive and exhaustive events. Then, for any event A with $P(A) \neq 0$, the general form of Bayes' Theorem is given as

$$P(B_i|A) = \frac{P(A|B_i)(B_i)}{\sum_{j=1}^{k} P(A|B_j)P(B_j)}, \quad i = 1, \ldots, k. \tag{2.23}$$

Bayes' Theorem is a fundamental theorem in probability. It has lots of applications in forensic science, law and other disciplines. The application of the theorem to parentage testing, say, can be referred to in Section 4.1.3.

2.5   Binomial probability distribution

Probability distribution is commonly employed in the study of probability. One popular probability distribution is the binomial distribution. Suppose a fair die is thrown three times; what is the probability that two 4s are observed? To answer this question, we may first consider the possible outcome in each throw, which is 1, 2, ..., or 6. However, we are interested in whether 4 occurs or not. In that connection, we can consider the outcome as being a 4, or not a 4, and they are denoted as 4 and $\bar{4}$ respectively. For each of the throws, $P(4) = 1/6$ and $P(\bar{4}) = 5/6$.

In calculating the probability that two 4s are shown in three throws of a die, one simple way is to use the tree diagram provided in Figure 2.1.

There are three ways of getting two 4s, namely $44\bar{4}$, $4\bar{4}4$ and $\bar{4}44$, and each corresponds to a probability $(1/6)^2(5/6)$, resulting in the overall probability of $3(1/6)^2(5/6)$. The probabilities for observing various numbers of 4s in Figure 2.1 are summarized in Table 2.1.

This problem can also be tackled without using the tree diagram to enumerate all possible outcomes. Let X be the number of occurrences of a 4 in three throws of a die. Then, in this case, X takes a particular value from the set of $\{0, 1, 2, 3\}$. Denote this particular value by x.

In a single throw of the die, the probability of throwing a 4 is $1/6$; the probability of not throwing a 4 is $5/6$. The probability of getting x 4s in three throws of the die is

$$P(X = x) = \binom{3}{x}\left(\frac{1}{6}\right)^x\left(\frac{5}{6}\right)^{3-x}, \quad x = 0, 1, 2, 3.$$

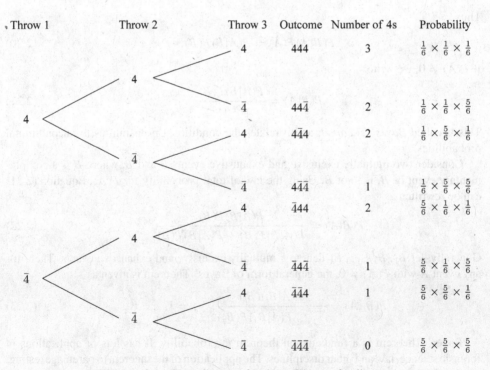

Figure 2.1   Tree diagram for three throws of a die.

Table 2.1   Probabilities for observing the number of 4s for three throws of a die.

Number of 4s	0	1	2	3
Probability	$\left(\dfrac{5}{6}\right)^3$	$3\left(\dfrac{1}{6}\right)\left(\dfrac{5}{6}\right)^2$	$3\left(\dfrac{1}{6}\right)^2\left(\dfrac{5}{6}\right)$	$\left(\dfrac{1}{6}\right)^3$

The term $\binom{3}{x}$ is the binomial coefficient which evaluates the number of ways in which x 4s can be selected from three throws of a die. It is denoted as:

$$\binom{3}{x} = \frac{3!}{x!(3-x)!},$$

where $x! = x(x-1)(x-2)\cdots 1$, known as x-factorial, with $0! = 1$. When $x = 2$, we have

$$P(X = 2) = \binom{3}{2}\left(\frac{1}{6}\right)^2\left(\frac{5}{6}\right)^1$$

$$= \frac{3!}{2!1!}\left(\frac{1}{6}\right)^2\left(\frac{5}{6}\right)$$

$$= 3\left(\frac{1}{6}\right)^2\left(\frac{5}{6}\right),$$

which is the same as that observed in Table 2.1. The probabilities for other x values can be obtained similarly and they coincide with those listed in Table 2.1.

The above derivation is a special case of the *binomial probability*, which is given as:

$$P(X = x) = \binom{n}{x}p^x(1-p)^{n-x}, \quad x = 0, 1, \ldots, n, \tag{2.24}$$

where

n = number of trials; it is three in the case above;

x = the number of occurrences of the event or value which is of particular interest in our problem;

p = the probability of observing that particular event or value in a single trial;

$$\binom{n}{x} = \frac{n!}{x!(n-x)!}.$$

Conventionally, we write $X \sim Bin(n, p)$. It is obvious that the application of the *binomial distribution* is not restricted to the throw of a die.

2.6   Multinomial distribution

Suppose a die is thrown n times; what is the probability that 1 appears x_1 times, 2 appears x_2 times, ..., and 6 appears x_6 times, where $x_1 + x_2 + \cdots + x_6 = n$? Using a similar argument as in deriving the binomial distribution, the resulting probability can be obtained based on the *multinomial distribution* given below:

$$P(X_1 = x_1, X_2 = x_2, \ldots, X_k = x_k) = \frac{n!}{x_1! x_2! \cdots x_k!} p_1^{x_1} p_2^{x_2} \cdots p_k^{x_k};$$

$$0 \le p_i \le 1; \; p_1 + p_2 + \cdots + p_k = 1; \; x_1 + x_2 + \cdots + x_k = n, \qquad (2.25)$$

where p_i is the probability that the value i is observed in a single trial. Notice that for the multinomial distribution, there are no restrictions on p_i's, except $0 \le p_i \le 1$ and $p_1 + p_2 + \cdots + p_k = 1$, and so p_i's need not be equal to one another. For a fair die situation, we have $k = 6$, $p_1 = p_2 = \cdots = p_6 = 1/6$. The binomial distribution is just a particular case of the multinomial distribution with $k = 2$.

To illustrate the use of the multinomial probability formula, we take $n = 5$ and like to evaluate the probability of having $(x_1, x_2, \ldots, x_6)$ being $(1, 2, 1, 0, 0, 1)$. From Equation (2.25), this probability is equal to

$$\frac{5!}{1! 2! 1! 0! 0! 1!} \left(\frac{1}{6}\right)^1 \left(\frac{1}{6}\right)^2 \left(\frac{1}{6}\right)^1 \left(\frac{1}{6}\right)^0 \left(\frac{1}{6}\right)^0 \left(\frac{1}{6}\right)^1 = \frac{60}{6^5} = \frac{5}{648}.$$

2.7   Poisson distribution

The Poisson distribution is another popular discrete distribution. Suppose we are interested in modeling the number of car accidents in a highway on a particular day, and the Poisson distribution is commonly used for such a purpose. In assessing the probability using the Poisson distribution, a parameter λ representing the mean or average number of occurrences has to be specified. The probability of x occurrences is evaluated as

$$P(X = x) = \frac{e^{-\lambda} \lambda^x}{x!}, \quad x = 0, 1, 2, \ldots. \qquad (2.26)$$

To illustrate the use of the Poisson distribution, we take, for example, the daily average number of car accidents in a highway as $\lambda = 1.4$. The probability that, on a particular day, there are three accidents is

$$P(X = 3) = \frac{e^{-1.4} 1.4^3}{3!} = 0.113.$$

Note that, unlike the binomial distribution, the number of cars (n) riding on the highway on that particular day is not needed for the Poisson distribution.

2.8   Normal distribution

The probability distributions–binomial, multinomial and Poisson–that we discussed earlier are discrete distributions. The random variables of interest–X and X_i in Equations (2.24)–(2.26)–take discrete values of $0, 1, 2, \ldots$. There is another kind of probability distribution, called the continuous distribution, in which the random variable of interest X is continuous. Many measurements, such as the height of a person and the length of the femur of a female adult (Lucy 2005), are continuous in nature.

A continuous distribution is often characterized by its probability density function and/or its parameter values. One of the most commonly used continuous distributions is the normal distribution. The distribution is characterized by the parameters mean μ and variance σ^2. The

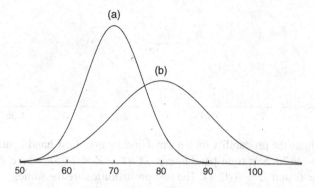

Figure 2.2   Normal density curves; (a) $X \sim N(70, 6^2)$ and (b) $X \sim N(80, 10^2)$.

square root of variance is called the standard deviation σ. The mean and the standard deviation measure the central location and the spread of the random variable, respectively.

Let X be the random variable, which is normally distributed with mean μ and variance σ^2; we write $X \sim N(\mu, \sigma^2)$.[1] Suppose we are interested in the weights of Chinese male adults in Hong Kong; the weight X is regarded as normally distributed with mean $\mu = 70$kg and variance $\sigma^2 = 6^2$ kg^2, i.e. $N(70, 6^2)$. The probability density function of this particular distribution is shown as curve (a) in Figure 2.2. The central location of the curve is at $\mu = 70$. Notice that a normal distribution is always symmetric about its mean μ. If we also consider the weights of Caucasian male adults in Hong Kong and assume that it is normally distributed with mean $\mu = 80$ and variance $\sigma^2 = 10^2$, i.e. $N(80, 10^2)$, then the density function is shown as curve (b) in Figure 2.2. Comparing the two curves, we notice that the Caucasian not only has a higher mean μ, but also a larger dispersion σ^2 in the weights. It is observed from the figure that the normal distribution is characterized by its mean and variance parameter values.

Unlike in the discrete case, a continuous random variable X has the property that $P(X = x)$ is always equal to 0 for any value of x. Instead, we often evaluate the probability for X lying inside an interval such as $P(a < X < b)$. Unlike in the discrete probability case, there is no simple analytical formula for obtaining the probability for the normal distribution. Instead, in evaluating such a probability, we often consider the transformation $Z = (X - \mu)/\sigma$. It can be shown that

$$\text{when} \quad X \sim N(\mu, \sigma^2), \quad \text{then} \quad Z = \frac{X - \mu}{\sigma} \sim N(0, 1),$$

which is a normal distribution with mean 0 and variance 1. The particular $N(0, 1)$ distribution is called the standard normal distribution. We consider the evaluation of $P(64 < X < 78.1)$ when $X \sim N(70, 6^2)$. In principle, according to probability theory, we need to evaluate the area at values 64 and 78.1 under the probability density curve (note that the total area under any density curve is 1). Graphically, this area is shown on the left-hand side of Figure 2.3.

---

[1]The probability density function (pdf) for a normal distribution, $X \sim N(\mu, \sigma^2)$, is
$$f(x) = \left(\sqrt{2\pi}\sigma\right)^{-1} \exp[-(x - \mu)^2/(2\sigma^2)], \quad -\infty < x < \infty.$$

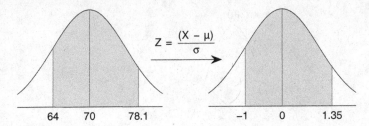

Figure 2.3   Evaluate the probability for a normal distribution. Left-hand figure: $P(64 < X < 78.1)$, where $X \sim N(70, 6^2)$; right-hand figure: $P(-1 < Z < 1.35)$, where $Z = (X - \mu)/\sigma$ with $\mu = 70, \sigma = 6$, and $Z \sim N(0, 1)$. The two probabilities are the same.

In practice, we consider the transformation $Z = (X - \mu)/\sigma$ for probability evaluation in the following way:

$$P(64 < X < 78.1)$$

$$= P\left(\frac{64 - 70}{6} < \frac{X - 70}{6} < \frac{78.1 - 70}{6}\right)$$

$$= P(-1 < Z < 1.35).$$

Thus, the probability $P(64 < X < 78.1)$, where $X \sim N(70, 6^2)$, can be equivalently evaluated as $P(-1 < Z < 1.35)$, where $Z \sim N(0, 1)$. Graphically, this equivalence is shown in Figure 2.3. To evaluate the latter probability, we can write

$$P(-1 < Z < 1.35)$$

$$= P(-1 < Z < 0) + P(0 \leq Z < 1.35)$$

$$= 0.3413 + 0.4115$$

$$= 0.7528.$$

Both probabilities 0.3413 and 0.4115 are obtained from the standard normal probability table given in Appendix A. The first probability $P(-1 < Z < 0)$ is obtained based on the fact that the standard normal distribution is symmetric about its mean 0.

2.9   Likelihood ratio

Consider a blood donation center in which every donor is required to have a screening blood test for a particular kind of disease. Suppose a person has had the test and the result is positive. In this situation, two propositions or explanations may be considered:

H_0: the person is a carrier of the disease;
H_1: the person is not a carrier of the disease.

These propositions are rival or mutually exclusive to each other. They are called the null and alternative hypotheses in statistics.

The statistical hypotheses testing framework fits very well in the legal setting, in which two propositions are also considered. The propositions often come from the prosecution as well as the defense sides. Suppose that there was a murder case, and a blood stain from the perpetrator was found at the crime scene; a suspect was later arrested and, serologically, his blood type was found to match with that found at the crime scene. Two competing propositions or explanations are considered:

H_p: the blood stain came from the suspect;
H_d: the blood stain did not come from the suspect.

In assessing the weight of the *evidence* which, in this case, is the blood type of the crime stain and that of the suspect, the likelihood ratio (LR) is often used:

$$LR = \frac{P(\text{evidence}|H_p)}{P(\text{evidence}|H_d)}. \tag{2.27}$$

The ratio evaluates the relative size for the probability of observing the evidence if H_p is true to the probability if H_d is true (or, equivalently, if H_p is not true). As can be seen here, the likelihood ratio approach assesses the evidence by considering explanations from both the prosecution and defense sides. This is consistent with the situation in common court cases. This likelihood ratio approach is the main tool that we adopt in this book for assessing the weight of DNA evidence. In fact, the likelihood ratio is the major tool used in assessing the weight of evidence numerically, not only in DNA forensics (Balding 2005; Buckleton *et al.* 2005; Evett and Weir 1998; National Research Council 1996), but also in other kinds of scientific evidence, such as fibers and glass fragments, etc. (Aitken and Taroni 2004; Lucy 2005).

2.10 Statistical inference

2.10.1 Test of hypothesis

Hypothesis testing is commonly used for statistical inference. In previous discussions, we assumed that the die is a fair die and then made the probability calculations accordingly. But is the die really a fair die? How can we test the assumption that it is a fair die?

In answering this question, we can conduct an experiment by throwing the die repeatedly for n times and count the number of times that value 1, 2, ..., or 6 appears. Table 2.2 presents the summarized findings of one such experiment with $n = 120$. The null and alternative hypotheses of interest are

H_0: the die is a fair die;
H_1: the die is not a fair die.

If the die is a fair one, i.e. under the null hypothesis H_0, then the probability of getting the value i in a single throw is $p_i = 1/6$, $i = 1, 2, \ldots, 6$. Under H_0, we expect to have $E_i = n \times p_i = 120 \times 1/6 = 20$ times that value i will appear. If there are large discrepancies

Table 2.2 The observed frequencies of observing value i, $i = 1, \ldots, 6$, in throwing a die 120 times.

Value i	1	2	3	4	5	6
Observed frequency O_i	25	18	19	23	14	21

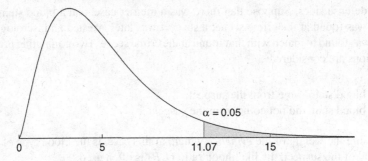

Figure 2.4   A chi-square distribution with $v = 5$ degrees of freedom. The value 11.07 corresponds to the upper 5% point of the distribution.

between the observed and expected frequencies O_i and E_i, we may doubt whether H_0 holds or not. The chi-square *goodness-of-fit test* is a commonly used test statistic to measure the overall discrepancy. The test statistic is denoted as T, where

$$T = \sum_{i=1}^{k} \frac{(O_i - E_i)^2}{E_i}. \tag{2.28}$$

When H_0 is true, with a large n, this statistic has a (approximately) *chi-square χ^2 distribution* with $k - 1$ degrees of freedom (df), where k is equal to 6 for the above example. A usual rule of thumb is to have each $E_i, i = 1, \ldots, k$ being greater than 5, in giving a good approximation of the chi-square distribution for the test statistic. The chi-square distribution is a continuous distribution, commonly used for goodness-of-fit tests. As we can see from Equation (2.28), if there are large discrepancies between O_i and E_i, then the test statistic T would be large and it casts doubt on whether the null hypothesis is true. Statistical hypothesis testing theory suggests that the null hypothesis H_0 be rejected if T is greater than a certain critical value obtained from the chi-square table given in Appendix B.

It can be shown that when H_0 is true, the statistic T is distributed as a chi-square distribution with the degrees of freedom given by

$$df = \text{number of cells} - 1 - \text{number of independent parameters fitted}, \tag{2.29}$$

which determines the location and shape of the distribution. For the above example, there are no independent parameters fitted and so $df = 6 - 1 = 5$. The probability density function of the chi-square distribution with five degrees of freedom[2] is plotted in Figure 2.4. As can be observed from the figure, the value of the statistic T is normally smaller than 11.07 (with 95% chance, or 5% chance that $T > 11.07$; see Appendix B) when the null hypothesis H_0 is true.

---

[2] The probability density function for a χ^2 distribution with v degrees of freedom is

$$f(t) = [2^{v/2} \Gamma(v/2)]^{-1} t^{(v-2)/2} e^{-t/2}, \quad t > 0,$$

where $\Gamma(u)$ is the gamma function with properties $\Gamma(u) = (u - 1)\Gamma(u - 1)$, $\Gamma(1) = 1$ and $\Gamma(1/2) = \sqrt{\pi}$.

For the example given in Table 2.2, the test statistic is evaluated as

$$T = \sum_{i=1}^{k} \frac{(O_i - E_i)^2}{E_i}$$

$$= \frac{(25 - 20)^2}{20} + \frac{(18 - 20)^2}{20} + \cdots + \frac{(21 - 20)^2}{20}$$

$$= (25 + 4 + 1 + 9 + 36 + 1)/20$$

$$= 3.8,$$

which is smaller than the 5% critical value 11.07 obtained from the table in Appendix B. Thus, we conclude that the null hypothesis is not rejected (or is accepted) at the 5% level of significance.

The goodness-of-fit test is easy to understand and construct. Sometimes, it may not be the most powerful method. The Fisher (1935) exact test can be more powerful, but is more difficult to construct. More details of Fisher's exact test will be discussed in Chapter 3.

2.10.2 Estimation and testing

Estimation is another important procedure for statistical inference. Suppose we are interested in estimating the mean height of the Chinese male adults in Hong Kong. A random sample of n male adults is taken and their heights are recorded as $X_1, X_2, \ldots, X_n$. The sample mean $\bar{X} = \sum_{i=1}^{n} X_i/n$ is commonly used to estimate the population mean μ. This quantity is called a point estimator. The point estimator itself, however, does not tell you how accurate the estimator is.

Suppose that X_i follows a normal distribution with mean μ and variance σ^2, i.e. $X_i \sim N(\mu, \sigma^2)$, $i = 1, \ldots, n$, and the X_i's are statistically independent of one another. It can be proved that the random quantity $\bar{X}$ is also normally distributed, having mean μ and variance $\sigma_{\bar{X}}^2$, i.e.

$$\bar{X} \sim N\left(\mu, \sigma_{\bar{X}}^2\right), \tag{2.30}$$

where $\sigma_{\bar{X}}^2 = \sigma^2/n$ is the (sampling) variance of $\bar{X}$. We call $N(\mu, \sigma_{\bar{X}}^2)$ the *sampling distribution* of $\bar{X}$. The standard deviation of $\bar{X}$ is $\sigma_{\bar{X}} = \sigma/\sqrt{n}$, which is also called the *standard error* of $\bar{X}$. According to the normal distribution theory given in Section 2.8, we know that

$$Z = \frac{\bar{X} - \mu}{\sigma_{\bar{X}}} \sim N(0, 1).$$

From the normal probability table in Appendix A, we have

$$P(-1.96 < Z < 1.96) = 0.95.$$

Plug in $Z = (\bar{X} - \mu)/\sigma_{\bar{X}}$, and, after rearranging the terms, then we obtain

$$P(\bar{X} - 1.96\sigma_{\bar{X}} < \mu < \bar{X} + 1.96\sigma_{\bar{X}}) = 0.95.$$

We call

$$(\bar{X} - 1.96\sigma_{\bar{X}}, \ \bar{X} + 1.96\sigma_{\bar{X}}) \tag{2.31}$$

the 95% *confidence interval* for the mean μ of the population. The coefficient 1.96 is sometimes replaced by 2 for simplicity for an approximate 95% confidence interval:

$$(\bar{X} - 2\sigma_{\bar{X}},\ \bar{X} + 2\sigma_{\bar{X}}) \quad \text{or} \quad (\bar{X} - 2SE,\ \bar{X} + 2SE), \tag{2.32}$$

where SE stands for the standard error of the estimator $\bar{X}$. Notice that when σ^2 is unknown, the parameter σ in the standard error $\sigma_{\bar{X}} = \sigma/\sqrt{n}$ can be replaced by the sample estimate $\hat{\sigma} = \left[\sum_{i=1}^{n}(X_i - \bar{X})^2/(n-1)\right]^{1/2}$. The 95% interval is the most commonly used interval, though the 90 and 99% intervals, etc. are also employed.

Let us consider the estimation of a parameter for a discrete distribution. Suppose that we are interested in estimating the probability of observing a head, p, in a toss of an unfair/loaded coin. In doing so, an experiment is constructed as follows. The coin is tossed n times and the number of heads X is counted. Then, $X \sim Bin(n, p)$. The sample proportion $\hat{p} = X/n$ can be used to estimate p.

Since the quantity X is random, so the estimator $\hat{p} = X/n$ is random too. It can be shown that when n is large, the sampling distribution of $\hat{p}$ is approximately normally distributed, i.e.

$$\hat{p} \sim N(\mu_{\hat{p}}, \sigma_{\hat{p}}^2) \quad \text{approximately}, \tag{2.33}$$

where $\mu_{\hat{p}} = p$ and $\sigma_{\hat{p}}^2 = p(1-p)/n$. The standard error of $\hat{p}$ is $SE = \sigma_{\hat{p}} = \sqrt{p(1-p)/n}$. Using a similar derivation for the normal case, the (approximate) 95% confidence interval for the parameter p is

$$(\hat{p} - 2\sigma_{\hat{p}},\ \hat{p} + 2\sigma_{\hat{p}}) \quad \text{or} \quad (\hat{p} - 2SE,\ \hat{p} + 2SE), \tag{2.34}$$

in which the value p in $\sigma_{\hat{p}}$ or SE is replaced by its estimator $\hat{p}$.

Although the above procedure is used for estimation of unknown parameters, it may also be employed for hypothesis testing. For example, suppose we want to test whether a coin is a fair one, i.e. $H_0 : p = 0.5$. If the hypothesized value $p = 0.5$ lies outside the interval in Equation (2.34), then we reject the null hypothesis H_0 at the 5% level of significance.

2.11 Problems

1. Suppose A, B, C are three events with $P(A) = 0.2$, $P(B) = 0.3$ and $P(C) = 0.4$, respectively. Furthermore, $P(AB) = P(AC) = 0.1$, $P(BC) = 0$. Find

   (a) $P(A \cup B)$ (b) $P(B|A)$ and $P(A|C)$ (c) $P(A \cup B \cup C)$.

2. A box contains eight red balls together with four yellow balls. Now two balls are sequentially drawn at random without replacement. Find

   (a) the probability that the two balls are of different colors;

   (b) the probability that the second ball drawn is red;

   (c) the conditional probability that the first ball drawn is red given that the second one is red.

3. Find the probability that four of six persons will recur after operation if we can assume independence and the probability is 0.1 that any one of them will recur after operation.

4. At a diallelic locus, the three genotype frequencies of AA, Aa and aa are, respectively, 0.09, 0.42 and 0.49. Find the probability that among seven randomly chosen persons, one will be of AA, two will be of Aa, and four will be of aa.

5. Let $X \sim N(4, 10^2)$. Find

   (a) $P(X > 6)$;

   (b) $P(-2 < X < 8)$;

   (c) the value of x such that $P(X > x) = 0.025$.

6. Test at the 0.05 level of significance whether a coin is balanced if we flip it 300 times and find a head 145 times.

7. A random sample of nine observations is drawn from a normal population: 9.75, 6.13, 15.26, 2.12, 29.83, 6.64, 9.14, 18.67, 8.60. Construct a 95% confidence interval for the population mean μ. Construct the 99% confidence interval, too.

3

Population genetics

In Chapter 2, various probability models, including binomial, multinomial and normal models, were introduced. Based on these models, we are able to make statistical and probability calculations for the problems that we are interested in. A model can be employed for practical use if it can capture the main features of the real problems. A good statistical or probability model may sometimes simplify the numerical calculations a lot for some problems and make the calculations feasible for others. Although it is difficult to prove that a model is correct philosophically or scientifically (Box 1980), we may use the statistical hypothesis testing theory to test whether a model is acceptable and consistent with the observed data.

In this chapter, we are going to introduce some population genetic models that are commonly used in DNA profiling. Based on the models, we can show that DNA profiling is highly discriminating. For a test battery of 12 STR loci, the probability of identify, i.e. the probability that two unrelated persons have the same genotype, can be less than one in a trillion, resulting in an extremely high power of discrimination (see Section 3.3.2). However, like other kinds of models, genetic models are obtained under various assumptions and restrictions. In the following, we are going to examine the validity of the assumptions and the applicability of these models to DNA profiling.

3.1 Hardy–Weinberg equilibrium

One of the main tasks in the statistical assessment of forensic DNA is to evaluate the match probability of a DNA profile. This evaluation may be taken in the situation in which the population is in Hardy–Weinberg equilibrium (HWE). In genetics, if the population is in HWE, the two alleles of a genotype at a particular locus are statistically independent of each other, thus greatly simplifying the calculations.

To demonstrate the Hardy–Weinberg law, we consider random mating between members in an infinite population. For simplicity, an autosomal locus with only two alleles A_1 and A_2 is taken. The three possible genotypes are denoted as A_1A_1, A_1A_2 and A_2A_2. Let the genotype

Statistical DNA Forensics: Theory, Methods and Computation   Wing Kam Fung and Yue-Qing Hu
© 2008 John Wiley & Sons, Ltd

Table 3.1   Outcomes for random mating in a parental generation with an infinite population size.

Parental generation			Offspring generation		
Father	Mother	Probability	A_1A_1	A_1A_2	A_2A_2
A_1A_1	A_1A_1	P_{11}^2	1	0	0
	A_1A_2	$P_{11}P_{12}$	1/2	1/2	0
	A_2A_2	$P_{11}P_{22}$	0	1	0
A_1A_2	A_1A_1	$P_{12}P_{11}$	1/2	1/2	0
	A_1A_2	P_{12}^2	1/4	1/2	1/4
	A_2A_2	$P_{12}P_{22}$	0	1/2	1/2
A_2A_2	A_1A_1	$P_{22}P_{11}$	0	1	0
	A_1A_2	$P_{22}P_{12}$	0	1/2	1/2
	A_2A_2	P_{22}^2	0	0	1

proportions be P_{11}, P_{12} and P_{22}, respectively. Then, the frequencies for alleles A_1 and A_2 would, respectively, be

$$p_1 = P_{11} + P_{12}/2; \quad p_2 = P_{22} + P_{12}/2. \tag{3.1}$$

Table 3.1 shows the outcomes of random mating in an infinite population. Let P_{11}^*, P_{12}^* and P_{22}^*, respectively, be the proportions of genotypes A_1A_1, A_1A_2 and A_2A_2 among the offspring of the second generation. From Table 3.1, we can obtain these proportions based on the genotype proportions of the parental generation. For example,

$$P_{11}^* = (1)P_{11} \times P_{11} + (1/2)P_{11} \times P_{12} + (1/2)P_{12} \times P_{11} + (1/4)P_{12} \times P_{12}$$

$$= (P_{11} + P_{12}/2)^2.$$

According to Equation (3.1), this proportion can also be expressed as

$$P_{11}^* = p_1^2.$$

For the proportion of genotype A_1A_2 of the offspring, we have

$$P_{12}^* = (1/2)P_{11} \times P_{12} + (1)P_{11} \times P_{22} + (1/2)P_{12} \times P_{11} + (1/2)P_{12} \times P_{12}$$

$$+ (1/2)P_{12} \times P_{22} + (1)P_{22} \times P_{11} + (1/2)P_{22} \times P_{12}$$

$$= 2(P_{11} + P_{12}/2)(P_{22} + P_{12}/2)$$

$$= 2p_1p_2.$$

Similarly, we can obtain the proportion of A_2A_2 among the offspring, which is equal to $P_{22}^* = p_1^2$. In summary, we have

$$P_{11}^* = p_1^2, \quad P_{12}^* = 2p_1p_2 \quad \text{and} \quad P_{22}^* = p_2^2. \tag{3.2}$$

The offspring genotype proportions can be completely determined by the parental allele proportions.

Based on Equation (3.1), we can also express the proportions of alleles A_1 and A_2 in the second generation as –

$$p_1^* = P_{11}^* + P_{12}^*/2$$
$$= p_1^2 + 2p_1p_2/2$$
$$= p_1(p_1 + p_2)$$
$$= p_1,$$

and $p_2^* = 1 - p_1^* = 1 - p_1 = p_2$. In other words, the following equations hold for the relationship amongst the genotype and allele proportions of the offspring in the second generation:

$$P_{11}^* = p_1^{*2}, \quad P_{12}^* = 2p_1^*p_2^* \quad \text{and} \quad P_{22}^* = p_2^{*2}. \tag{3.3}$$

This demonstrates the Hardy–Weinberg law; the genotype proportions can be completely determined by the allele proportions using the product rule. As we can see that the second generation is in Hardy–Weinberg equilibrium when there is random mating for the parental generation which has an infinite population size, there is no requirement that the parental population is in Hardy–Weinberg equilibrium.

The Hardy–Weinberg law plays an important role in genetic studies, including DNA profiling. Besides the random mating and infinite population size assumptions, the mathematical model for the establishment of the Hardy–Weinberg law also relies on other assumptions, including no selection, no migration and no mutation. Readers interested in the Hardy–Weinberg law and the violation of the assumptions for the law can refer to Nei (1987), Hartl and Clark (1989) and Evett and Weir (1998), among many others.

3.2   Test for Hardy–Weinberg equilibrium

Let the alleles of a particular locus be denoted as $A_1, A_2, \ldots, A_k$, and the associated allele frequencies be $p_1, p_2, \ldots, p_k$, respectively. Also let A_iA_j, $i, j = 1, \ldots, k$ be a genotype. When the population is in Hardy–Weinberg equilibrium, the genotype probability can be evaluated as

$$p_{ij} \equiv P(A_iA_j) = \begin{cases} p_i^2, & i = j, \\ 2p_ip_j, & i \neq j, \end{cases} \tag{3.4}$$

i.e. the genotype probability can be expressed as a simple product of the allele probabilities. The result in Equation (3.4) is often called the product rule in DNA forensics. This rule basically regards the alleles being statistically independent of each other. The term '2' in Equation (3.4) accounts for the two possibilities of having the genotype combination, i.e. one allele being A_i and the other being A_j, or vice versa.

Since Hardy–Weinberg equilibrium is commonly employed in DNA profiling, it is important to check how valid it is for a particular population. Some common methods for testing for Hardy–Weinberg equilibrium are introduced in the following sections.

3.2.1   Observed and expected heterozygosities

Consider the STR locus TPOX for the Hong Kong Chinese population (Wong *et al.* 2001). A sample of $n = 275$ individuals was taken and their DNA profiles were obtained. There are a total of $k = 5$ alleles at this locus. Table 3.2 summarizes the genotyping results and provides the number of individuals n_{ij}, $i \leq j$, $i, j = 1, \ldots, k$, having genotype A_iA_j at that locus. The

Table 3.2   The count n_{ij} for genotype A_iA_j at locus TPOX for a population database of $n = 275$ Hong Kong Chinese. The values in brackets are corresponding proportions, i.e. $\hat{p}_{ij} = n_{ij}/n$.

		A_j			
A_i	8	9	10	11	12
8	85 (0.309)	30 (0.109)	6 (0.022)	87 (0.316)	7 (0.025)
9		4 (0.015)	1 (0.004)	16 (0.058)	0 (0)
10			0 (0)	5 (0.018)	0 (0)
11				30 (0.109)	4 (0.015)
12					0 (0)

genotype proportions $\hat{p}_{ij} = n_{ij}/n$ are shown in brackets. When the alleles are of interest, Table 3.3 lists the allele count n_i of allele A_i, where

$$n_i = 2n_{ii} + \sum_{j=1}^{i-1} n_{ji} + \sum_{j=i+1}^{k} n_{ij}, \tag{3.5}$$

and the total number of alleles is $\sum_{i=1}^{k} n_i = 2n = 550$. By the counting method, the frequency for allele A_i can be estimated by $\hat{p}_i = n_i/(2n)$, and these frequencies are listed in the last row of Table 3.3.

The following hypotheses for the TPOX locus are considered:

H_0 :   population is in Hardy–Weinberg equilibrium;

H_1 :   population is not in Hardy–Weinberg equilibrium.   (3.6)

To examine whether H_0 holds for TPOX, one simple way is to compare whether the observed heterozygosity is consistent with the expected heterozygosity obtained under Hardy–Weinberg equilibrium, where heterozygosity refers to the proportion of heterozygous genotypes. The observed heterozygosity is obtained as

$$OH = 1 - \sum_{i=1}^{k} \hat{p}_{ii},$$

which, in this case, is evaluated as

$$OH = 1 - 0.309 - 0.015 - 0 - 0.109 - 0$$

$$= 0.567.$$

Table 3.3   The count n_i for allele A_i at locus TPOX for a population database of $n = 275$ Hong Kong Chinese.

Allele A_i	8	9	10	11	12
Count n_i	300	55	12	172	11
Allele frequency $\hat{p}_i$	0.545	0.100	0.022	0.313	0.020

When H_0 is true, based on Equation (3.4), the frequency for the homozygous genotype $A_i A_i$ can be evaluated by $\hat{p}_i^2$. Thus, the expected heterozygosity can be obtained as

$$EH = 1 - \sum_{i=1}^{k} \hat{p}_i^2.$$

For locus TPOX, this quantity is equal to

$$EH = 1 - 0.545^2 - 0.100^2 - 0.022^2 - 0.313^2 - 0.020^2$$
$$= 0.594.$$

This expected heterozygosity is only an estimate under H_0. The standard error of this estimate is equal to (Nei and Roychoudhury 1974)

$$SE = \left[\frac{EH(1 - EH)}{n}\right]^{1/2} = \left[\frac{0.594(1 - 0.594)}{275}\right]^{1/2} = 0.030.$$

The observed heterozygosity $OH = 0.567$ which is within 2 standard errors of the expected heterozygosity $EH = 0.594$. Thus, according to the theory of statistical inference (Section 2.10), with the 5% level of significance, we do not have strong statistical evidence to reject the null hypothesis that the population is in Hardy–Weinberg equilibrium at locus TPOX.

3.2.2   Chi-square test

The chi-square test is commonly used for testing for statistical independence of row and column factors of a contingency table (Conover 1980). This test can be found in many statistical texts such as Miller and Miller (2004). However, the table as shown in Table 3.2 is a special kind of contingency table; the row and column factors correspond to the two alleles A_i and A_j of a genotype where genotypes $A_i A_j$ and $A_j A_i$ are indistinguishable. Thus, the standard chi-square test for independence in a contingency table cannot be applied here.

To construct an appropriate chi-square test for independence, we let n_{ij} denote the observed counts for genotype $A_i A_j, i \leq j, i, j = 1, \ldots, k$ at a particular locus in a population database of n individuals. The allele count n_i of allele A_i is defined in the same way as in Section 3.2.1 [see also Equation (3.5)]. When the null hypothesis H_0 of Hardy–Weinberg equilibrium in Equation (3.6) holds, according to Equation (3.4), the probability for genotype $A_i A_j$ can be obtained as $p_{ij} = p_i^2$ if $i = j$, and $p_{ij} = 2p_i p_j$ otherwise. The probability of allele A_i is estimated using $\hat{p}_i = n_i/(2n)$. Thus, when H_0 is true, we can estimate the expected count for genotype $A_i A_j$ in a sample of n individuals as

$$E_{ij} = \begin{cases} n\,\hat{p}_i^2, & i = j, \\ 2n\hat{p}_i\hat{p}_j, & i \neq j. \end{cases} \tag{3.7}$$

The chi-square test for the null hypothesis of Hardy–Weinberg equilibrium is constructed as (Geisser and Johnson 1992, 1995; Weir 1993)

$$T = \sum_{i=1}^{k} \sum_{j=i}^{k} \frac{(n_{ij} - E_{ij})^2}{E_{ij}}. \tag{3.8}$$

This test is shown to be χ^2 distributed when n is large. Since there are $k - 1$ independent parameters, $p_1, p_2, \ldots, p_{k-1}$, (as $p_k = 1 - p_1 - \cdots - p_{k-1}$) fitted, so the number of degrees

Table 3.4 The observed and expected counts (in brackets) for genotype $A_i A_j$ at locus TPOX for a database of 275 Hong Kong Chinese.

		A_j			
A_i	8	9	10	11	12
8	85 (81.8)	30 (30.0)	6 (6.54)	87 (93.8)	7 (6.00)
9		4 (2.75)	1 (1.20)	16 (17.2)	0 (1.10)
10			0 (0.13)	5 (3.75)	0 (0.24)
11				30 (26.9)	4 (3.44)
12					0 (0.11)

of freedom of the chi-square distribution as given in Equation (2.29) is obtained as $df = k(k + 1)/2 - 1 - (k - 1) = k(k - 1)/2$. Notice that the rule of thumb to use this chi-square test is that the expected counts E_{ij}'s have to be greater than 5. If this is not the case, then one suggestion is to merge adjacent alleles with small expected counts until the rule is satisfied.

Table 3.4 lists the observed and expected genotype counts at locus TPOX. As we can see that some of the expected counts are below 5, we can merge some adjacent alleles having small expected counts. We can start by merging alleles 11 and 12 to form a new allele 11*. Some expected counts are still below 5. So we have a new allele 9* by merging alleles 9 and 10. Table 3.5 presents the observed counts having the newly defined genotypes. The frequencies of the new set of alleles are $\hat{p}_8 = 0.545$, $\hat{p}_{9*} = (36 + 5 \times 2 + 21)/550 = 0.122 = \hat{p}_9 + \hat{p}_{10}$ and $\hat{p}_{11*} = 0.333 = \hat{p}_{11} + \hat{p}_{12}$. Based on Equation (3.7), the expected counts can be obtained and they are shown in brackets in Table 3.5.

The chi-square statistic can then be evaluated as

$$T = \frac{(85 - 81.8)^2}{81.8} + \frac{(36 - 36.5)^2}{36.5} + \frac{(94 - 99.8)^2}{99.8}$$
$$+ \frac{(5 - 4.08)^2}{4.08} + \frac{(21 - 22.3)^2}{22.3} + \frac{(34 - 30.4)^2}{30.4}$$
$$= 1.17.$$

The 5% critical value for a χ^2 distribution with $3(3 - 1)/2 = 3$ degrees of freedom is 7.81 (Appendix B), which is larger than the test statistic $T = 1.17$. Thus, we do not have strong evidence to reject the null hypothesis of Hardy–Weinberg equilibrium at TPOX. Notice that there is an expected count (4.08) smaller than 5. However, the rule of 5 is often too conservative

Table 3.5 The observed and expected counts (in brackets) for genotype $A_i A_j$ at locus TPOX for a database of 275 Hong Kong Chinese. The new alleles 9* and 11* are obtained by merging original alleles 9 and 10, and 11 and 12, respectively.

		A_j	
A_i	8	9*	11*
8	85 (81.8)	36 (36.5)	94 (99.8)
9*		5 (4.08)	21 (22.3)
11*			34 (30.4)

(Fienberg 1979) and the chi-square test can still be used even when some of the expected counts are smaller than 5–say, about 3 or so. Nevertheless, if there is a substantial deviation from the rule of 5, then the approximation of the χ^2 distribution can be rather poor in some situations.

3.2.3   Fisher's exact test

Consider a diallelic locus with two alleles a and b. Let n_a and n_b denote the allele counts, and n_{aa}, n_{ab}, n_{bb} denote the genotype counts in a sample of n individuals. The population allele proportions are denoted as p_a and p_b. Under the hypothesis of Hardy–Weinberg equilibrium, the probability of obtaining the genotype counts conditional on the allele counts is

$$P(n_{aa}, n_{ab}, n_{bb}|n_a, n_b) = \frac{n!n_a!n_b!2^{n_{ab}}}{(2n)!n_{aa}!n_{ab}!n_{bb}!}. \tag{3.9}$$

Fisher's (1935) exact test evaluates the summation of the probabilities for all outcomes that are as probable as or less probable than the observed outcome (Evett and Weir 1998). Consider a simple example with $n = 30$, $n_{aa} = 15$, $n_{ab} = 8$ and $n_{bb} = 7$ (see Table 3.6). The allele counts are $n_a = 38$ and $n_b = 22$. Given these allele counts, the probability for observing those genotype counts, according to Equation (3.9), is

$$P(n_{aa} = 15, n_{ab} = 8, n_{bb} = 7|n_a = 38, n_b = 22)$$

$$= \frac{30!38!22!2^8}{60!15!8!7!}$$

$$= 0.0181.$$

The probabilities of observing all possible genotype outcomes given the allele counts are listed in Table 3.7. Only five of these probabilities are less than or equal to the observed probability 0.0181. The sum of these figures, 0.0219 ($= 0 + 0 + 0.0001 + 0.0020 + 0.0181 + 0.0017$), is the probability ($p$-) value of the Fisher's exact test under the null hypothesis of Hardy–Weinberg equilibrium. Since the p-value is less than 5%, we reject the hypothesis that Hardy–Weinberg equilibrium holds for this diallelic locus.

The Fisher's exact test can also be applied to loci with more than two alleles. In such situations, the evaluation of all the probabilities in order to obtain the p-value of the Fisher's exact test is cumbersome, especially when the sample size is large. Guo and Thompson (1992) described two methods to approximate the p-value [see also Zaykin et al. (1995)]. The bootstrap resampling methods (Efron and Tibshirani 1993) can also be employed to obtain the p-value.

Table 3.6   Genotype counts for a diallelic locus.

Allele	Allele	
	a	b
a	15	8
b		7

Table 3.7   Calculations for probabilities for Fisher's exact test for the data set given in Table 3.6.

n_{aa}	n_{ab}	n_{bb}	Probability
19	0	11	0.0000
18	2	10	0.0000
17	4	9	0.0001
16	6	8	0.0020
15	8	7	0.0181
14	10	6	0.0843
13	12	5	0.2145
12	14	4	0.3064
11	16	3	0.2451
10	18	2	0.1057
9	20	1	0.0223
8	22	0	0.0017
			1.0000

3.2.4   Computer software

Although the ideas in Sections 3.2.1–3.2.3 for testing for Hardy–Weinberg equilibrium are rather simple, the statistics there may not be found in standard statistical packages. We have developed a computer software called EasyDNA_PopuData that can give the allele frequencies and some common statistics, including those mentioned earlier for a population database. The software can be found at http://www.hku.hk/statistics/EasyDNA/. What we need to do is to click the *Calculate* button after loading the population data. All those statistics, except the Fisher's exact test result, could come up very quickly. Fisher's exact test, however, requires the resampling procedure to approximate the p-value, and so a longer time is taken. The statistical results can then be saved by clicking the *Save* button. Figure 3.1 gives the captured screen for running the program in the analysis of the Hong Kong Chinese population database of 12 loci (Wong *et al.* 2001).

Table 3.8 gives the summarized statistics including the observed heterozygosity (OH), estimate of the expected heterozygosity (EH) and its standard error (SE), the chi-square test (T) and the p-value of the Fisher's exact test (pFE) for each of the 12 loci of the Hong Kong Chinese population data. None, except the one at FGA, of the OH/EH pairs differs by more than two standard errors. If we look at the chi-square test and the Fisher's exact test, none of the results at all 12 loci is found to be statistically significant when the 5% level of significance is taken. In summary, based on these findings, we do not have strong statistical evidence to reject the assumption of Hardy–Weinberg equilibrium for the Hong Kong Chinese population data. This is in line with the conclusion of the NRC II Report (National Research Council 1996, p109) that in the large databases of the major races, the populations are quite close to Hardy–Weinberg equilibrium.

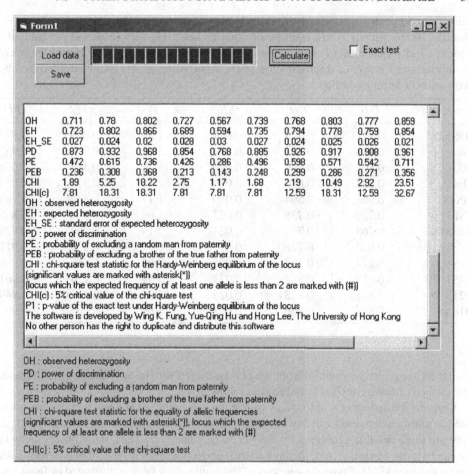

Figure 3.1   Captured screen for running the EasyDNA_PopuData software for the Hong Kong Chinese population database.

3.3   Other statistics for analysis of a population database

3.3.1   Linkage equilibrium

Hardy–Weinberg equilibrium allows us to use the product rule and multiply allele frequencies to assess the probability of a genotype within a locus. The two alleles of a genotype within a locus are statistically independent when the Hardy–Weinberg law is satisfied. As we know, in practice, many (STR) loci are used for DNA profiling. If all the loci are in linkage equilibrium, then the alleles and genotypes amongst different loci are statistically independent from one another. In that regard, the probability of a DNA profile (at all loci) can then be obtained by multiplying the probabilities of genotypes across all loci.

Chi-square tests (Geisser and Johnson 1995; Weir 1993) have been constructed for testing for linkage equilibrium. Fung (1997) also proposed tests for linkage equilibrium, and for jointly Hardy–Weinberg and linkage equilibria, for a pair of loci. These tests come from

Table 3.8   Summary statistics for the Hong Kong Chinese population database: observed heterozygosity (OH), estimate of expected heterozygosity (EH) and its standard error (SE), chi-square test (T) and p-value of Fisher's exact test (pFE) for Hardy-Weinberg equilibrium, and power of discrimination (PD), from Wong *et al.* (2001). (Reproduced by permission of Springer-Verlag.)

Locus	OH	EH	SE	T	pFE	PD
D3S1358	0.711	0.723	0.027	1.89	0.853	0.873
vWA	0.780	0.802	0.024	5.25	0.999	0.932
FGA	0.802	0.866	0.020	18.22	0.572	0.968
THO1	0.727	0.689	0.028	2.75	0.377	0.854
TPOX	0.567	0.594	0.030	1.17	0.832	0.768
CSF1PO	0.739	0.735	0.027	1.68	0.968	0.885
D5S818	0.768	0.794	0.024	2.19	0.993	0.926
D13S317	0.803	0.778	0.025	10.49	0.505	0.917
D7S820	0.777	0.759	0.026	2.92	0.860	0.908
D8S1179	0.859	0.854	0.021	23.51	0.224	0.961
D21S11	0.851	0.828	0.023	16.99	0.912	0.949
D18S51	0.848	0.866	0.021	11.69	0.205	0.968

similar ideas and are generalized from the chi-square test for Hardy–Weinberg equilibrium. The method of Fung (1997) is introduced as follows.

Consider a database of n individuals with genotypes collected at a few loci. We are interested in testing independence at any two loci, each of which is diallelic. At locus k, $k = 1, 2$, there are three possible genotypes, namely $G_{11}^{(k)}$, $G_{12}^{(k)}$ and $G_{22}^{(k)}$. Thus, the n observations in the database can be categorized, for any two loci, into a contingency table of two factors, each having the three kinds of possible genotypes. The contingency table is illustrated in Table 3.9. A chi-square test for independence between the two loci can be constructed.

Let $n_{ij,\ell m}$ be the count of people having genotype $G_{ij}^{(1)}$ at locus 1 and genotype $G_{\ell m}^{(2)}$ at locus 2, $i \leq j$, $\ell \leq m$. Let $p_{ij,\ell m}$ denote the associated probability for that particular set of

Table 3.9   Illustration of genotype counts n's and probabilities p's (in brackets) for a pair of diallelic loci.

Locus 1's genotype	Locus 2's genotype			Sum
	$G_{11}^{(2)}$	$G_{12}^{(2)}$	$G_{22}^{(2)}$	
$G_{11}^{(1)}$	$n_{11,11}$ $(p_{11,11})$	$n_{11,12}$ $(p_{11,12})$	$n_{11,22}$ $(p_{11,22})$	$n_{11}^{(1)}$ $(p_{11}^{(1)})$
$G_{12}^{(1)}$	$n_{12,11}$ $(p_{12,11})$	$n_{12,12}$ $(p_{12,12})$	$n_{12,22}$ $(p_{12,22})$	$n_{12}^{(1)}$ $(p_{12}^{(1)})$
$G_{22}^{(1)}$	$n_{22,11}$ $(p_{22,11})$	$n_{22,12}$ $(p_{22,12})$	$n_{22,22}$ $(p_{22,22})$	$n_{22}^{(1)}$ $(p_{22}^{(1)})$
Sum	$n_{11}^{(2)}$ $(p_{11}^{(2)})$	$n_{12}^{(2)}$ $(p_{12}^{(2)})$	$n_{22}^{(2)}$ $(p_{22}^{(2)})$	n (1)

genotypes $(G_{ij}^{(1)}, G_{\ell m}^{(2)})$. Referring to Table 3.9, we define the sums of $n_{ij,\ell m}$ and $p_{ij,\ell m}$ over the rows and over the columns.

The hypothesis of linkage equilibrium that the genotypes at the two loci are independent can be formulated mathematically as

$$H_0 : p_{ij,\ell m} = p_{ij}^{(1)} p_{\ell m}^{(2)} \quad \text{for all} \quad i \leq j, \quad \ell \leq m.$$

The probabilities are estimated as $\hat{p}_{ij}^{(1)} = n_{ij}^{(1)}/n$ and $\hat{p}_{\ell m}^{(2)} = n_{\ell m}^{(2)}/n$, which can be obtained from the marginals $n_{ij}^{(1)}$ and $n_{\ell m}^{(2)}$ in the contingency table as given in Table 3.9. Under the null hypothesis H_0, the expected count for $n_{ij,\ell m}$ is estimated as $n \hat{p}_{ij}^{(1)} \hat{p}_{\ell m}^{(2)}$. Thus, given the marginals, the usual chi-square test for independence can be employed for testing linkage equilibrium:

$$T_L = \sum_{i \leq j} \sum_{\ell \leq m} \frac{\left(n_{ij,\ell m} - n \hat{p}_{ij}^{(1)} \hat{p}_{\ell m}^{(2)}\right)^2}{n \hat{p}_{ij}^{(1)} \hat{p}_{\ell m}^{(2)}},$$

which is χ^2 distributed when n is large. The degrees of freedom of the χ^2 distribution would be $(L_1 - 1)(L_2 - 1)$, as in ordinary contingency table testing, where $L_i = k_i(k_i + 1)/2$ is the number of possible genotypes for locus i having k_i alleles, $i = 1, 2$. Notice that the test T_L can be applied for loci with more than two alleles, although the illustration of notations in Table 3.9 only applies to diallelic loci.

As in testing for Hardy–Weinberg equilibrium, Fisher's exact test can also be employed for testing for linkage equilibrium. Zaykin *et al.* (1995) have developed the software for such a purpose. The permutation resampling procedure is used to approximate the p-value for testing for linkage equilibrium.

Table 3.10 presents such p-values for paired loci for the Hong Kong Chinese population data (Wong *et al.* 2001). Five pairs of loci, namely 1 and 3 (D3S1358 and FGA), 1 and 12 (D3S1358 and D18S51), 2 and 3 (vWA and FGA), 3 and 6 (FGA and CSF1PO), and 3 and 12 (FGA and D18S51), indicate some degrees of linkage disequilibrium. However, the associated p-values 2.8, 4.9, 2.4, 1.3 and 2.2%, respectively, are not too small. Other combinations of any two loci seem to be in linkage equilibrium. Statistically, when the 5% significance rule is adopted, it is not unusual to have five significant results for a total of 78 tests, even in a situation of total independence. Furthermore, none of the results was found to be significant if the 1% level was taken.

The main cause of linkage disequilibrium is incomplete mixing of different ancestral populations (National Research Council 1996). The findings in Table 3.10 do not indicate strong deviations from linkage equilibrium. This is in line with NRC II's conclusion (National Research Council 1996, p109) that major race populations are close to linkage equilibrium.

The chi-square and Fisher's exact tests can, in theory, be extended to situations with more than two loci. However, since most STR population databases are of sizes of only a few hundred individuals, the resulting contingency tables are sparse, with many small or zero counts, which would give rise to a low power for the statistical tests. Hence, testing for linkage equilibrium for three or more loci is normally not recommended (Fung 2003a).

3.3.2 Power of discrimination

DNA profiling is commonly used for human identification and it is important to have loci which give high discriminating power. The power of discrimination (Jones 1972; Sensabaugh 1982) is one such measure that can be used for showing the discriminating power of a locus.

Table 3.10   *P*-values of the exact tests for linkage equilibrium for pairs of 12 loci
(1: D3S1358, 2: vWA, 3: FGA, 4: THO1, 5: TPOX, 6: CSF1PO, 7: D5S818, 8: D13S317,
9: D7S820, 10: D8S1179, 11: D21S11, 12: D18S51), from Wong *et al.* (2001).
(Reproduced by permission of Springer-Verlag.)

Loci pair	*P*-value	Loci pair	*P*-value	Loci pair	*P*-value
1/2	0.280	3/5	0.557	5/12	0.497
1/3	0.028*	3/6	0.013*	6/7	0.994
1/4	0.442	3/7	0.168	6/8	0.663
1/5	0.774	3/8	0.248	6/9	0.954
1/6	0.396	3/9	0.526	6/10	0.464
1/7	0.376	3/10	0.104	6/11	0.979
1/8	0.798	3/11	0.428	6/12	0.218
1/9	0.690	3/12	0.022*	7/8	0.861
1/10	0.108	4/5	0.284	7/9	0.753
1/11	0.708	4/6	0.512	7/10	0.663
1/12	0.049*	4/7	0.162	7/11	0.570
2/3	0.024*	4/8	0.551	7/12	0.063
2/4	0.867	4/9	0.696	8/9	0.948
2/5	0.807	4/10	0.672	8/10	0.675
2/6	0.556	4/11	0.297	8/11	0.793
2/7	0.706	4/12	0.463	8/12	0.220
2/8	0.401	5/6	0.758	9/10	0.783
2/9	0.961	5/7	0.338	9/11	0.998
2/10	0.696	5/8	0.169	9/12	0.641
2/11	0.579	5/9	0.476	10/11	0.629
2/12	0.079	5/10	0.203	10/12	0.449
3/4	0.584	5/11	0.685	11/12	0.280

* Significant value

Suppose a blood stain is typed with DNA profile X at a particular locus having possible
alleles $A_1, A_2, \ldots, A_k$. A random person is typed with profile Y at that locus. The person will
not be discriminated as the possible source of the blood stain if Y and X are the same. The
profile X can take any possible genotype $A_i A_j$, $i \leq j$, $i, j = 1, \ldots, k$, and the probability of
identity, i.e. $P(X = Y)$, is

$$PI = \sum_{i \leq j} P(X = A_i A_j, Y = A_i A_j)$$

$$= \sum_{i \leq j} P(X = A_i A_j) P(Y = A_i A_j)$$

for X and Y coming from two unrelated individuals. Assuming Hardy–Weinberg equilibrium,
the probability of identity is

$$PI = \sum_{i=1}^{k} p_i^2 \times p_i^2 + \sum_{i < j} (2 p_i p_j)(2 p_i p_j).$$

Using TPOX in Table 3.3 as an example, this probability is evaluated as

$$PI = 0.545^4 + \cdots + 0.02^4 + (2 \times 0.545 \times 0.1)^2 + \cdots + (2 \times 0.313 \times 0.02)^2$$

$$= 0.232.$$

The power of discrimination is obtained as

$$PD = 1 - PI$$

$$= 1 - 0.232$$

$$= 0.768.$$

This figure suggests that TPOX has 76.8% power of discriminating a random individual as being not the source of the stain.

The powers of discrimination for other loci of the Hong Kong Chinese population database can be obtained similarly, and they are shown in the last column of Table 3.8. The power of discrimination ranges from 0.768 to 0.968. The combined probability of identity for the battery of 12 loci is $\prod_{\ell=1}^{12} PI_\ell = 4.1 \times 10^{-14}$, giving the overall power of discrimination of $1 - 4.1 \times 10^{-14}$, which is extremely discriminating.

3.4 DNA profiling

Suppose that a crime scene DNA sample was recovered; two suspects were later arrested. The DNA profiles of the crime stain, suspect 1, suspect 2 and the victim were typed. Figure 3.2 shows the DNA profiles of a CTT triplex at three STR loci–CSF1PO, THO1 and TPOX– obtained using ABI proprietary machines and software. As can be seen from the figure, the stain did not come from the victim; nor did it belong to suspect 2, who would then be released.

Suspect 1, however, has genotypes 9/9, 8/9 and 9/12 at loci THO1, TPOX and CSF1PO, respectively, which match with the crime scene profile. This suspect is not excluded from the pool of possible perpetrators. Either this suspect or someone else left the crime stain. This is called the single source or identity testing problem. We want to assess the probability of finding the profile in the 'someone else' case (National Research Council 1996).

That 'someone else' person is assumed to be a random person, unrelated to the suspects, in the population of possible suspects. So, we would like to evaluate the probability that a person other than the suspect, randomly selected from the population, will have the profile. This probability is often called the random-match probability or match probability, which sometimes may also be interpreted as the frequency of the profile in the population.

Suppose the DNA profiles of the crime stain and the suspect are denoted as $C = A_i A_j$ and $S = A_i A_j$. Under the Hardy–Weinberg law, the match probability given that a random person other than the suspect is the perpetrator is evaluated as

$$P(C = A_i A_j | S = A_i A_j) = \begin{cases} p_i^2, & i = j, \\ 2p_i p_j, & i \neq j. \end{cases} \tag{3.10}$$

Another popular way to deal with this problem is by means of the likelihood ratio approach. We first consider the prosecution and defense propositions,

$$
\begin{aligned}
&H_p: \quad \text{the suspect left the crime stain;} \\
&H_d: \quad \text{a random person other than the suspect left the crime stain.}
\end{aligned}
\tag{3.11}
$$

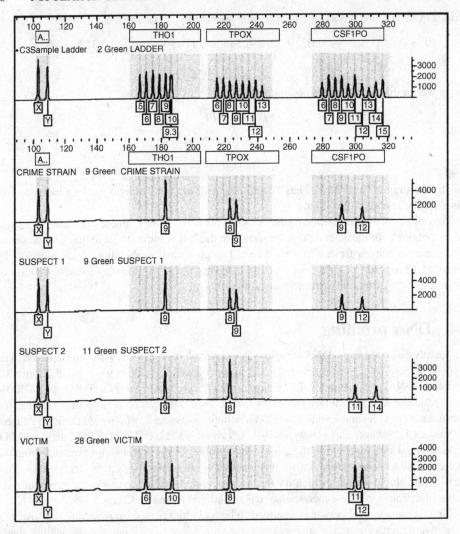

Figure 3.2   DNA profiles of the crime stain, suspects 1 and 2 and the victim at three STR loci–THO1, TPOX and CSF1PO–obtained using ABI proprietary machines and software.

The likelihood ratio formula as given in Equation (2.27) is

$$LR = \frac{P(\text{evidence} \mid H_p)}{P(\text{evidence} \mid H_d)},\tag{3.12}$$

where the evidence in this case is $C = A_i A_j$ and $S = A_i A_j$. The likelihood ratio is thus evaluated as

$$LR = \frac{P(C = A_i A_j, S = A_i A_j \mid H_p)}{P(C = A_i A_j, S = A_i A_j \mid H_d)}$$

$$= \frac{P(C = A_i A_j \mid S = A_i A_j, H_p)}{P(C = A_i A_j \mid S = A_i A_j, H_d)} \frac{P(S = A_i A_j \mid H_p)}{P(S = A_i A_j \mid H_d)},$$

which is obtained based on the conditional probability formula in Equation (2.11). The two probabilities corresponding to the latter ratio are the same, since the probability that the suspect has genotype $A_i A_j$ is independent of whether he is (i.e. H_p) or he is not (i.e. H_d) the source of the crime stain. Thus, we have

$$LR = \frac{P(C = A_i A_j | S = A_i A_j, H_p)}{P(C = A_i A_j | S = A_i A_j, H_d)}.$$

The numerator is equal to 1 unless an error has occurred in the DNA typing. When Hardy–Weinberg equilibrium holds, the denominator is p_i^2 if $i = j$, or $2p_i p_j$ otherwise. So

$$LR = \begin{cases} 1/p_i^2, & i = j, \\ 1/(2p_i p_j), & i \neq j. \end{cases} \tag{3.13}$$

The likelihood ratio is just the reciprocal of the match probability.

The allele frequencies p's are needed to evaluate the likelihood ratio. There are different ways of estimating the p's. In the examples that we consider in this book, the observed allele proportions in the population database are taken to estimate the p's for simplicity. Of course, other estimates such as the Bayesian or some conservative estimates can also be used [see Buckleton *et al.* (2005), among others].

We are going to evaluate the match probability and likelihood ratio for the CTT triplex case example as shown in Figure 3.2. The genotypes of the crime stain are 9/9 at THO1, 8/9 at TPOX and 9/12 at CSF1PO. The allele frequencies for the triplex of the Hong Kong Chinese (Law *et al.* 2001; Wong *et al.* 2001) are shown in Table 3.11. The match probabilities or the genotype frequencies are then estimated as $0.440^2 = 0.1936$ at THO1, $2 \times 0.545 \times 0.100 = 0.109$ at TPOX, and $2 \times 0.037 \times 0.362 = 0.0268$ at CSF1PO. The overall match probability is $0.1936 \times 0.109 \times 0.0268 = 5.655 \times 10^{-4}$. That is, the probability that the genotype of a random person other than the suspect will match the DNA sample in the crime scene at the CTT triplex is 5.655×10^{-4}, or 1 in 1768.

The likelihood ratio for the pair of propositions (3.11) can be evaluated based on Equation (3.13), which is obtained as $1/(5.655 \times 10^{-4}) = 1768$. We can have the following interpretation for this figure: the CTT triplex profile is 1768 times as likely to be observed were the crime stain to have come from the suspect than were it to have come from a random unrelated person in the population.

It is to be noticed that various assumptions, including Hardy–Weinberg and linkage equilibrium, have been employed in the above calculations. Having these assumptions seems a rather widely acceptable simplification (Aitken and Taroni 2004; Evett and Weir 1998; National Research Council 1996). Nevertheless, these assumptions are unlikely to be exactly correct. In the next section, we are using the subpopulation models to account for possible departure from Hardy–Weinberg equilibrium.

3.5   Subpopulation models

In the previous section, the population was assumed to be in Hardy–Weinberg equilibrium. However, the Hardy–Weinberg law is hardly exactly correct, since the conditions for equilibrium are seldom met. Nevertheless, the match probabilities are easily calculated under the Hardy–Weinberg law and these values provide good ideas about the order of magnitude of the probabilities. When the population under consideration comprises various subpopulations, the population is no longer homogeneous and the Hardy–Weinberg law would then be violated. This situation happens quite often. For example, the Chinese population in Hong Kong

Table 3.11   Allele frequencies for the CTT triplex at loci THO1, TPOX and CSF1PO for Hong Kong Chinese, from Wong *et al.* (2001). (Reproduced by permission of Springer-Verlag.)

Locus	Allele	Frequency
THO1	6	0.100
	7	0.316
	8	0.053
	9	0.440
	9.3	0.029
	10	0.060
	11	0.002
TPOX	8	0.545
	9	0.100
	10	0.022
	11	0.313
	12	0.020
CSF1PO	7	0.009
	8	0.002
	9	0.037
	10	0.239
	11	0.261
	12	0.362
	13	0.082
	14	0.006
	15	0.002

comprises various Chinese subpopulations from southern China, northern China, different minority ethnic groups in China, and overseas (total tens of millions of overseas Chinese), etc. Notable differences in frequencies for some alleles across subpopulations could be found. Different subpopulation models have been proposed to correct for Hardy-Weinberg disequilibrium and to take into account the variation in subpopulation allele frequencies. The following model, which is rather commonly accepted in the forensic field, is considered.

Suppose that the population under consideration has reached the state of evolutionary equilibrium; then, allele proportions are found to follow the Dirichlet distribution (Wright 1951). This distribution is written in the form

$$P(\{p_i\}) = \frac{\Gamma(\gamma)}{\prod_i \Gamma(\gamma_i)} \prod_i p_i^{\gamma_i - 1},$$

where

$$\gamma_i = (1 - \theta)p_i/\theta, \quad \gamma = \sum_i \gamma_i = (1 - \theta)/\theta,$$

$\prod_i a_i$ stands for the product of the terms a_i over the indices i's, $\Gamma(x)$ is a gamma function with the property that $\Gamma(x + 1) = x\Gamma(x)$, p_i is the proportion of allele A_i averaged over subpopulations, and θ, which is taken to be positive here, can be regarded as a measure of the variation in subpopulation allele proportions. The Dirichlet distribution is a continuous probability distribution commonly used to model proportions or frequencies [see Johnson and Kotz (1972)]. A specific Dirichlet distribution is the Beta distribution, which is more well known to scientists. The symbol F_{st}, which has a similar meaning to θ, was originally used by Wright (1951), while θ is more commonly employed in forensic science. The coefficient F_{st} or θ may be called the inbreeding coefficient, which can also measure the relatedness between people in the subpopulations as well as the degree of population subdivision (Balding 2005; Balding and Nichols 1994; Buckleton *et al.* 2005; Evett and Weir 1998; National Research Council 1996).

Given the proportions p's, in a set of random sample of m alleles, allele A_i occurring m_i times is taken to follow a multinomial distribution (Section 2.6), i.e.

$$P\left(\prod_i A_i^{m_i}|\{p_i\}\right) = \frac{(\sum_i m_i)!}{\prod_i (m_i)!}\prod_i p_i^{m_i}.$$

The marginal probability is then evaluated as

$$P\left(\prod_i A_i^{m_i}\right) = \int_{p_is} P\left(\prod_i A_i^{m_i}|\{p_i\}\right) P(\{p_i\})\prod_i dp_i.$$

After integration and simplification, this probability can be expressed in the following form, i.e. the probability that a set of m alleles has m_i copies of A_i is (Evett and Weir 1998)

$$P\left(\prod_i A_i^{m_i}\right) = \frac{\Gamma(\gamma)}{\Gamma(\gamma + m)}\prod_i \frac{\Gamma(\gamma_i + m_i)}{\Gamma(\gamma_i)}. \tag{3.14}$$

For a single allele A_i, the equation gives

$$P(A_i) = \frac{\Gamma(\gamma)}{\Gamma(\gamma + 1)}\frac{\Gamma(\gamma_i + 1)}{\Gamma(\gamma_i)} = \frac{\gamma_i}{\gamma} = p_i.$$

For a homozygous pair $A_i A_i$,

$$P(A_i A_i) = \frac{\Gamma(\gamma)}{\Gamma(\gamma + 2)}\frac{\Gamma(\gamma_i + 2)}{\Gamma(\gamma_i)}$$

$$= \frac{\gamma_i(\gamma_i + 1)}{\gamma(\gamma + 1)},$$

$$= p_i[(1 - \theta)p_i + \theta]$$

$$= p_i^2 + p_i(1 - p_i)\theta.$$

When the allele pair is $A_i A_j$, $i \neq j$, we have

$$P(A_i A_j) = \frac{\Gamma(\gamma)}{\Gamma(\gamma + 2)}\frac{\Gamma(\gamma_i + 1)}{\Gamma(\gamma_i)}\frac{\Gamma(\gamma_j + 1)}{\Gamma(\gamma_j)}$$

$$= \frac{\gamma_i\gamma_j}{\gamma(\gamma + 1)}$$

$$= p_i p_j(1 - \theta).$$

It is noticed that the probability for the genotype $A_i A_j$ is twice the above probability due to the two allele orders $A_i A_j$ and $A_j A_i$.

As noticed from these formulas, the probabilities for homozygotes are inflated while those for heterozygotes are deflated. For conservativeness, the Hardy–Weinberg relation for heterozygotes is used by NRC II (National Research Council 1996). Thus, NRC II recommends in its Recommendation 4.1 the following formulas for evaluating the genotype frequency for systems in which exact genotypes can be determined (e.g. STR loci):

$$P(A_i A_j) = \begin{cases} p_i^2 + p_i(1 - p_i)\theta, & i = j, \\ 2p_i p_j, & i \neq j. \end{cases} \tag{3.15}$$

Besides this genotype frequency assessment, there is another approach which evaluates the conditional probability of the genotype of the suspect given that of the perpetrator (National Research Council 1996, p114). Various formulas have been proposed under different assumptions and methods of derivation but they agree very well with one another for common values of θ (Balding and Nichols 1994, 1995; Crow and Denniston 1993; Morton 1992; National Research Council 1996; Roeder 1994; Weir 1994). The following match probability formulas were given by Balding and Nichols (1994, 1995):

$$P_{ij} = \begin{cases} \dfrac{[2\theta + (1 - \theta)p_i][3\theta + (1 - \theta)p_i]}{(1 + \theta)(1 + 2\theta)}, & i = j, \\ \dfrac{2[\theta + (1 - \theta)p_i][\theta + (1 - \theta)p_j]}{(1 + \theta)(1 + 2\theta)}, & i \neq j. \end{cases} \tag{3.16}$$

These formulas appeared as Equation (4.10) in NRC II. They are essentially conditional probabilities and were obtained by Balding and Nichols on the basis of genetic and statistical justification [see also Lindley (1990)], which were further explained by Balding and Nichols (1995). The derivations of these two formulas are provided below (Evett and Weir 1998).

From Equation (3.14), we can derive the following conditional probability formula:

$$P(A_i \mid y \; A_i \text{ alleles among } n \text{ alleles}) = \frac{y\theta + (1 - \theta)p_i}{1 + (n - 1)\theta}. \tag{3.17}$$

The equation was also obtained by Balding and Nichols (1994) based on alternate derivations. This formula is handy and easy to use. It will be employed in the later part of this book in the evaluation of match probabilities in subdivided or structured populations. To illustrate its use, we consider whether a random person other than the suspect (S) is the source of the crime stain (C) and the evaluation of the match probability $P(S = A_i A_j | C = A_i A_j)$ is, for $i = j$,

$$P_{ii} = P(A_i A_i | A_i A_i)$$

$$= P(A_i | A_i A_i) P(A_i | A_i A_i A_i)$$

$$= \left[\frac{2\theta + (1 - \theta)p_i}{1 + (2 - 1)\theta}\right] \left[\frac{3\theta + (1 - \theta)p_i}{1 + (3 - 1)\theta}\right]$$

$$= \frac{[2\theta + (1 - \theta)p_i][3\theta + (1 - \theta)p_i]}{(1 + \theta)(1 + 2\theta)},$$

and for $i \neq j$,

$$
\begin{aligned}
P_{ij} &= 2P(A_iA_j|A_iA_j) \\
&= 2P(A_i|A_iA_j)P(A_j|A_iA_iA_j) \\
&= 2\left[\frac{\theta + (1-\theta)p_i}{1 + (2-1)\theta}\right]\left[\frac{\theta + (1-\theta)p_j}{1 + (3-1)\theta}\right] \\
&= \frac{2[\theta + (1-\theta)p_i][\theta + (1-\theta)p_j]}{(1+\theta)(1+2\theta)}.
\end{aligned}
$$

The value 2 appears because of the two possible allele orders A_iA_j and A_jA_i. The formulas given in Equation (3.16) are thus derived.

NRC II suggests that, in general, Equation (3.15) should be used for the calculation of the profile frequency or match probability for each locus (NRC II Recommendation 4.1). When the allele frequencies for the subpopulation are not available, it is suggested that the calculation should use the population-structure Equation (3.16) (NRC II Equation 4.10, Recommendation 4.2). For either approach, the multiplication of the resulting results across loci is suggested. NRC II (National Research Council 1996, p122) proposes to adopt the degree of subdivision $\theta = 0.01$–a conservative value for the US population; the value 0.03 may be more appropriate for some small isolated populations. Empirical studies from various authors (e.g. Budowle and Chakraborty 2001; Budowle *et al.* 2001; Law *et al.* 2001; Roeder 1994; Weir 1994) find that the values of θ are (much) smaller than 0.01 for major ethnic populations, including African Americans, US Caucasians, Hispanics, Asians and Europeans.

NRC II Recommendation 4.1 is adopted by some forensic laboratories, especially those in the US. Buckleton *et al.* (2005, p87) comment that this recommendation is a logical way of correcting for Hardy–Weinberg disequilibrium, but makes no attempt to correct for linkage equilibrium; hence, this approach may have a very mild tendency to underestimate multilocus genotype probabilities (see also Curran *et al.* 2003). Some researchers, including Ayres (2000), Balding and Nichols (1997), Buckleton and Triggs (2005), Curran *et al.* (1999) and Evett and Weir (1998), suggested the calculation of conditional match probabilities based on Equation (3.16). As we have seen earlier, both Equations (3.15) and (3.16) are obtained based on the Dirichlet distribution under the assumption that the population has reached the state of evolutionary equilibrium. The match probability evaluated based on Equation (3.16) is often more conservative, i.e. larger than that evaluated according to Equation (3.15). In the following, we use an example to illustrate the difference between the two approaches.

Table 3.12 gives the match probabilities for the crime scene CTT triplex profile as shown in Figure 3.2, evaluated under Equations (3.15) and (3.16) using $\theta = 0.01$ and 0.03. We notice that the match probability based on Equation (3.16) increases with θ. This is also true for Equation (3.15) with homozygous genotypes. When $\theta = 0.01$, the overall match probability based on Equation (3.16) is 39% higher than that based on Equation (3.15) which is slightly (1%) higher than the probability 5.655×10^{-4} obtained under the Hardy–Weinberg law. When $\theta = 0.03$, the difference is more pronounced; the probability obtained by Equation (3.16) is more than double that obtained by Equation (3.15). When we have a full profile of 10 loci or more, the match probabilities are frequently smaller than 10^{-10}, no matter which equation we are using. The match probabilities based on Equation (3.16) could be one or two orders of magnitude higher but are still extremely small. These small probabilities are often very unfavorable to the defendants, irrespective of which equation is adopted.

Table 3.12   Match probabilities for the crime scene CTT triplex profile as shown in Figure 3.2 evaluated under Equations (3.15) and (3.16) using $\theta = 0.01$ and 0.03.

Locus	Genotype	Equation (3.15)		Equation (3.16)	
		$\theta = 0.01$	0.03	0.01	0.03
THO1	9/9	0.1961	0.2010	0.2059	0.2304.
TPOX	8/9	0.109	0.109	0.1163	0.1300
CSF1PO	9/12	0.0268	0.0268	0.0333	0.0460
Overall		5.73×10^{-4}	5.87×10^{-4}	7.97×10^{-4}	1.38×10^{-3}

3.6   Relatives

Suppose that the DNA sample of the crime stain is $C = A_i A_j$. A suspect is arrested and found to have the same genotype, $S = A_i A_j$. It is possible that a close relative of the suspect is the source of the crime stain (Balding and Donnelly 1994; Evett 1992; Lempert 1991; National Research Council 1996). The following proposition may be posed by the defendant:

H_d : a relative of the suspect is the source of the crime stain.

In this situation, we may have to evaluate the match probability $P(C = A_i A_j | S = A_i A_j)$ under such particular H_d.

For two persons X and Y, define the relatedness coefficients $(k_0, 2k_1, k_2)$ as

$$k_0 = P \text{ (neither allele of } X \text{ is identical by descent to alleles of } Y);$$

$$2k_1 = P \text{ (one or the other of the alleles of } X \text{ is ibd to one of the alleles of } Y,$$
$$\text{but the second allele is not); and} \tag{3.18}$$

$$k_2 = P \text{ (both alleles of } X \text{ are ibd to those of } Y).$$

Note that two alleles are said to be identical by descent (ibd) if the two alleles come from the same ancestor.

Values of the relatedness coefficients for some common relationships are listed in Table 3.13. Using the law of total probability, the match probability can be written as

$$P(A_i A_j | A_i A_j) = \sum_{t=0}^{2} P(A_i A_j | A_i A_j, \ t \text{ ibd alleles}) P(t \text{ ibd alleles}), \tag{3.19}$$

which is evaluated as

$$P(A_i A_j | A_i A_j) = 2 p_i p_j (k_0) + [p_i(1/2) + p_j(1/2)](2k_1) + 1(k_2), \tag{3.20}$$

under the Hardy–Weinberg law.

Suppose we denote the kinship coefficient F between two individuals X and Y as

$$F = P \text{ (two alleles, one randomly taken from each of the two individuals, are ibd).} \tag{3.21}$$

It is noticed that $k_1 + k_2 = 2F$. For noninbred unilineal relatives (relatives who have at most one ibd allele; siblings are not unilineal), $k_2 = 0$, and so giving $k_1 = 2F$ and $k_0 = 1 - 2k_1 = 1 - 4F$. Thus, the match probability for unilineal relatives can then be expressed as

$$2 p_i p_j (1 - 4F) + (p_i + p_j) 2F = 2 p_i p_j + 2(p_i + p_j - 4 p_i p_j) F. \tag{3.22}$$

Table 3.13   Relatedness coefficients (k_0, $2k_1$, k_2) for some common relationships between two persons.

Relationship	k_0	$2k_1$	k_2
Parent–child	0	1	0
Full siblings	1/4	1/2	1/4
Half siblings	1/2	1/2	0
Grandparent–grandchild	1/2	1/2	0
Uncle–nephew	1/2	1/2	0
First cousins	3/4	1/4	0
Second cousins	15/16	1/16	0

Siblings are bilineal rather than unilineal and so require different formulas. The match probability for heterozygous genotypes can be obtained based on Equation (3.20). For homozygous genotypes, we can do something similar to Equation (3.19). Table 3.14 lists the match probabilities under the proposition H_d that a relative of the suspect is the source of the crime sample. Some common kinship coefficients for relatives are: $F = 1/4$ for parent–child; $1/8$ for half siblings, grandparent–grandchild and uncle–nephew; $1/16$ for first cousins.

For subpopulation models having the degree of subdivision θ, Equation (3.19) can still be employed. The probability can be evaluated using Equation (3.17) as

$$P(A_iA_j|A_iA_j) = P(A_iA_j|A_iA_j, \text{ no ibd alleles})k_0$$
$$+ P(A_iA_j|A_iA_j, \text{ one ibd allele})(2k_1)$$
$$+ P(A_iA_j|A_iA_j, \text{ two ibd allele})k_2$$
$$= 2P(A_i|A_iA_j)P(A_j|A_iA_iA_j)k_0$$
$$+ \left[(1/2)P(A_i|A_iA_j) + (1/2)P(A_j|A_iA_j)\right](2k_1)$$
$$+ 1 \times k_2$$
$$= 2\left[\frac{\theta + (1-\theta)p_i}{1 + (2-1)\theta}\right]\left[\frac{\theta + (1-\theta)p_j}{1 + (3-1)\theta}\right]k_0$$

Table 3.14   Match probability for the genotypes of the crime stain and suspect under the proposition H_d that a relative of the suspect is the source of the crime stain.

Relationship	Genotype	Match probability
Full siblings	A_iA_i	$(1 + 2p_i + p_i^2)/4$
	A_iA_j	$(1 + p_i + p_j + 2p_ip_j)/4$
Unilineal[a]	A_iA_i	$p_i^2 + 4p_i(1 - p_i)F$
	A_iA_j	$2p_ip_j + 2(p_i + p_j - 4p_ip_j)F$

[a]For parent–child, $F = 1/4$; for half siblings, grandparent–grandchild and uncle–nephew, $F = 1/8$; for first cousins, $F = 1/16$

Table 3.15 Match probability for crime stain genotypes in a subdivided population under the proposition H_d that a relative of the suspect is the source of the stain.

Relationship	Match probability
Homozygotes $A_i A_i$	
Parent–child	$\dfrac{2\theta + (1-\theta)p_i}{1+\theta}$
Full siblings	$\dfrac{1}{4} + \dfrac{1}{4}\left[\dfrac{2\theta + (1-\theta)p_i}{1+\theta}\right]\left[2 + \dfrac{3\theta + (1-\theta)p_i}{1+2\theta}\right]$
Half siblings[a]	$\dfrac{1}{2}\left[\dfrac{2\theta + (1-\theta)p_i}{1+\theta}\right]\left[1 + \dfrac{3\theta + (1-\theta)p_i}{1+2\theta}\right]$
First cousins	$\dfrac{1}{4}\left[\dfrac{2\theta + (1-\theta)p_i}{1+\theta}\right]\left[1 + \dfrac{3\{3\theta + (1-\theta)p_i\}}{1+2\theta}\right]$
Heterozygotes $A_i A_j$	
Parent–child	$\dfrac{2\theta + (1-\theta)(p_i + p_j)}{2(1+\theta)}$
Full siblings	$\dfrac{1}{4} + \dfrac{2\theta + (1-\theta)(p_i + p_j)}{4(1+\theta)} + \dfrac{[\theta + (1-\theta)p_i][\theta + (1-\theta)p_j]}{2(1+\theta)(1+2\theta)}$
Half siblings[a]	$\dfrac{2\theta + (1-\theta)(p_i + p_j)}{4(1+\theta)} + \dfrac{[\theta + (1-\theta)p_i][\theta + (1-\theta)p_j]}{(1+\theta)(1+2\theta)}$
First cousins	$\dfrac{2\theta + (1-\theta)(p_i + p_j)}{8(1+\theta)} + \dfrac{3[\theta + (1-\theta)p_i][\theta + (1-\theta)p_j]}{2(1+\theta)(1+2\theta)}$

[a]Grandparent–grandchild and uncle–nephew have the same match probability

$$+ \left[\frac{\theta + (1-\theta)p_i}{1 + (2-1)\theta} + \frac{\theta + (1-\theta)p_j}{1 + (2-1)\theta}\right]k_1 + k_2$$

$$= \frac{2k_0[\theta + (1-\theta)p_i][\theta + (1-\theta)p_j]}{(1+\theta)(1+2\theta)}$$

$$+ \frac{k_1[2\theta + (1-\theta)(p_i + p_j)]}{1+\theta} + k_2. \qquad (3.23)$$

The match probability for a homozygous genotype is obtained similarly as

$$P(A_i A_i | A_i A_i) = \left[\frac{2\theta + (1-\theta)p_i}{1+\theta}\right]\left[\frac{\{3\theta + (1-\theta)p_i\}k_0}{1+2\theta} + 2k_1\right] + k_2. \qquad (3.24)$$

Based on Equations (3.23) and (3.24) and taking appropriate relatedness coefficients $(k_0, 2k_1, k_2)$, we can obtain the crime stain genotype probabilities for a subdivided population for some common relationships under the proposition that a relative of the suspect is the source of the stain. These probabilities are listed in Table 3.15 [see also Weir (2003) and Buckleton *et al.* (2005)].

Table 3.16   Match probabilities for the CTT triplex genotypes of the crime stain and suspect 1 as shown in Figure 3.2 evaluated under the defense propositions H_{d1}: a random man is the source of the stain, and H_{d2}: a half sib of the suspect is the source of the stain.

Locus	Genotype	H_{d1}		H_{d2}	
		$\theta = 0$	0.03	0	0.03
THO1	9/9	0.1936	0.2304	0.3168	0.3515
TPOX	8/9	0.1090	0.1300	0.2158	0.2314
CSF1PO	9/12	0.0268	0.0460	0.1131	0.1315
Overall		5.66×10^{-4}	1.38×10^{-3}	7.73×10^{-3}	0.0107

As an illustration, we consider the CTT triplex genotypes of the crime stain and the suspect as shown in Figure 3.2. The following two defense propositions are studied:

H_{d1} : a man unrelated to the suspect is the source of the stain, and

H_{d2} : a half sib of the suspect is the source of the stain,

with $\theta = 0$ and 0.03. The results are shown in Table 3.16. The overall match probability under H_{d2} is about 10 times the probability under H_{d1}, indicating that the defense proposition can have a substantial effect on the size of the match probability. The closer the relationship (e.g. father–child; full siblings), the larger the increase for the match probability. The degree of population subdivision also affects the match probability but with a much smaller magnitude.

3.7   Problems

1. Suppose a sample of 30 individuals is randomly selected from a population and they are typed at a locus with two alleles A and a. Eighteen of them are of genotype AA, eight are Aa and four are aa.

   (a) Find the frequency estimates for alleles A and a.

   (b) Find the observed heterozygosity and estimate of expected heterozygosity.

   (c) Employ the chi-square test to test whether the population is in Hardy–Weinberg equilibrium at the locus. Use the 5% level of significance.

   (d) Obtain the standard error for the estimate of expected heterozygosity. Based on this and the results you obtain in (b), test for Hardy–Weinberg at the locus.

2. The following genotype counts are obtained for a tri-allelic locus:

   $$n_{11} = 14, \quad n_{12} = 18, \quad n_{13} = 22, \quad n_{22} = 12, \quad n_{23} = 20, \quad n_{33} = 14.$$

   Find the power of discrimination of the locus assuming Hardy–Weinberg equilibrium.

3. In a criminal offence, a blood stain was found at the crime scene; a suspect was later arrested. Suppose the DNA profiles of the crime stain and the suspect are $C = 8/8$ and $S = 8/8$ at locus THO1, and are $C = 8/9$ and $S = 8/9$ at locus TPOX.

Let

$$H_p : \text{the suspect left the crime stain;}$$

$$H_d : \text{a random man left the crime stain.}$$

(a) Find the likelihood ratios for the above hypotheses under (i) Hardy–Weinberg equilibrium, and (ii) a subdivided population with the degree of subdivision θ; the conditional probability framework is used here.

(b) Evaluate the likelihood ratios for (i) and for (ii) with $\theta = 0$ and $\theta = 0.03$ based on the allele frequencies given in Table 3.11.

4. Obtain Equation (3.17) using Equation (3.14).

5. Observe that the genotypes of the victim (V) and the suspect (S) are, respectively, 6/6 and 6/7 at locus THO1, and 8/9 and 9/10 at locus TPOX. Find the joint genotype probability $P(V, S)$ if they come from a subdivided population with the degree of subdivision θ.

6. Show that the relatedness coefficients ($k_0, 2k_1, k_2$) between two full siblings are $(1/4, 1/2, 1/4)$.

7. Show that the kinship coefficient F between parent and child is $1/4$.

8. Find the relationship between the kinship coefficient F and the relatedness coefficients $(k_0, 2k_1, k_2)$.

9. Prove that the match probability $P(A_i A_i | A_i A_i)$ in Equation (3.24) for DNA samples of the crime stain $C = A_i A_i$ and the suspect $S = A_i A_i$, under the defense proposition H_d : a relative of the suspect is the source of the stain, is

$$P(A_i A_i | A_i A_i) = \left[\frac{2\theta + (1 - \theta) p_i}{1 + \theta} \right] \left[\frac{\{3\theta + (1 - \theta) p_i\} k_0}{1 + 2\theta} + 2k_1 \right] + k_2,$$

where $(k_0, 2k_1, k_2)$ are the relatedness coefficients between the suspect and his relative.

4

Parentage testing

DNA profiling has proven to be a powerful technique for human identification. Besides its usual application in criminal offences for identifying the contributor of a crime stain, the technique is also frequently used in parentage and kinship determinations. Common parentage problems include standard trio cases and motherless cases, etc. (Clayton *et al.* 2002; Evett and Weir 1998; Lee *et al.* 2000; Thomson *et al.* 1999); others include complex kinship determinations having more than three or four typed persons. The former problems are investigated in this chapter, while the latter ones are studied in the next chapter.

4.1 Standard trio

4.1.1 Paternity index

The standard trio problem is commonly encountered in paternity testing. The DNA profiles of the mother, child and alleged father are obtained. The mother, alleged father and biological father of the child are taken as unrelated to one another. The mother and biological father belong to the same ethnic population. This population is taken to be in Hardy–Weinberg equilibrium (HWE) in this chapter unless otherwise stated. Moreover, we also assume no mutation unless we state otherwise. The two competing hypotheses for the standard trio problem are given as:

H_p : the alleged father is the biological father of the child;
H_d : the true father is a random unrelated man. (4.1)

Let M, C and AF be the genotypes of the mother, her child and the alleged father, respectively. So, the DNA evidence constitutes the sets of genotypes M, C and AF. The likelihood ratio (LR) that we mentioned in Equation (2.2) is the most commonly used measure in paternity testing. In fact, the paternity index used in the field is actually a likelihood ratio, which can be evaluated as

$$PI = LR = \frac{P(\text{evidence}|H_p)}{P(\text{evidence}|H_d)}$$

Statistical DNA Forensics: Theory, Methods and Computation Wing Kam Fung and Yue-Qing Hu
© 2008 John Wiley & Sons, Ltd

$$= \frac{P(C, M, AF|H_p)}{P(C, M, AF|H_d)}$$

$$= \frac{P(C|M, AF, H_p)}{P(C|M, AF, H_d)} \frac{P(M, AF|H_p)}{P(M, AF|H_d)}. \qquad (4.2)$$

The last equality is due to the conditional probability result given in Equation (2.15). The two probabilities $P(M, AF|H_p)$ and $P(M, AF|H_d)$ are the same, since the probability of the genotypes of the mother and the alleged father does not depend on whether the alleged father is the true father or not (H_p or H_d). Thus,

$$PI = \frac{P(C|M, AF, H_p)}{P(C|M, AF, H_d)}. \qquad (4.3)$$

Given H_d that the alleged father is not the true father of the child, $P(C|M, AF, H_d)$ can also be written as $P(C|M, H_d)$, thus giving

$$PI = \frac{P(C|M, AF, H_p)}{P(C|M, H_d)}. \qquad (4.4)$$

Consider an example that the genotypes of the child, mother and alleged father at a particular locus are obtained as $C = A_i A_j$, $M = A_i A_k$ and $AF = A_j A_l$. In this situation, the numerator of PI is $(1/2)(1/2)$, since there is a $1/2$ chance that the mother transmits the allele A_i to the child, and similarly a $1/2$ chance that the alleged father who is the biological father under H_p transmits A_j to the child. For the denominator, under H_d, there is still a $1/2$ chance that the mother transmits the allele A_i. However, under H_d, the alleged father is not the biological father of the child and hence the probability that the child has an A_j for the other allele is p_j. Thus, the denominator is just $(1/2)p_j$, and so $PI = (1/4)/(p_j/2) = 1/(2p_j)$.

There are other genotype combinations for the mother, child and alleged father. The PI's can be obtained in similar ways, and they are listed in the fourth column of Table 4.1. Notice that in this book, the subscripts $i, j, k, \ldots$ of alleles A_i, A_j, A_k, etc. are taken as different among themselves unless otherwise stated.

4.1.2   An example

Here, we consider an example for the standard trio problem. For illustration, only genotypes for three loci are considered. Table 4.2 gives the genotypes of the mother, child and alleged father at loci D3S1358, vWA and FGA. The allele frequencies at these loci for the Hong Kong Chinese population (Wong et al. 2001) are listed in Table 4.3. Based on the formulas given in the fourth column of Table 4.1, the paternity indices are obtained as

$$\text{D3S1358} : PI = 1/(2p_{17}) = 1/(2 \times 0.239) = 2.09,$$

$$\text{vWA} : PI = 1/p_{18} = 1/0.16 = 6.25,$$

$$\text{FGA} : PI = 1/[2(p_{20} + p_{21})] = 1/[2(0.044 + 0.131)] = 2.86.$$

If there is linkage equilibrium among loci, then the paternity index for the whole profile is the product of the indices for individual loci, which is $2.09 \times 6.25 \times 2.86 = 37.36$. Thus, the profile is 37.36 times as likely to be observed were the alleged father to be the biological father of the child than were an unrelated random man to be the biological father.

Table 4.1 Paternity index (PI) for a standard trio case. The LR^0 is evaluated under H_p: the alleged father is the biological father of the child versus H_d: a relative of the alleged father is the true father of the child. F is the kinship coefficient of the alleged father and his relative who is the true father under H_d.

C	M	AF	PI	LR^0
A_iA_i	A_iA_i	A_iA_i	$1/p_i$	$1/[2F + (1-2F)p_i]$
		A_iA_j	$1/(2p_i)$	$1/[2F + 2(1-2F)p_i]$
	A_iA_j	A_iA_i	$1/p_i$	$1/[2F + (1-2F)p_i]$
		A_iA_j	$1/(2p_i)$	$1/[2F + 2(1-2F)p_i]$
		A_iA_k	$1/(2p_i)$	$1/[2F + 2(1-2F)p_i]$
A_iA_j	A_iA_i	A_iA_j	$1/(2p_j)$	$1/[2F + 2(1-2F)p_j]$
		A_jA_j	$1/p_j$	$1/[2F + (1-2F)p_j]$
		A_jA_k	$1/(2p_j)$	$1/[2F + 2(1-2F)p_j]$
	A_iA_j	A_iA_i	$1/(p_i + p_j)$	$1/[2F + (1-2F)(p_i + p_j)]$
		A_iA_j	$1/(p_i + p_j)$	$1/[2F + (1-2F)(p_i + p_j)]$
		A_iA_k	$1/[2(p_i + p_j)]$	$1/[2F + 2(1-2F)(p_i + p_j)]$
	A_iA_k	A_iA_j	$1/(2p_j)$	$1/[2F + 2(1-2F)p_j]$
		A_jA_j	$1/p_j$	$1/[2F + (1-2F)p_j]$
		A_jA_k	$1/(2p_j)$	$1/[2F + 2(1-2F)p_j]$
		A_jA_l	$1/(2p_j)$	$1/[2F + 2(1-2F)p_j]$

Subscripts $i, j, k, \ldots$ are all different

Table 4.2 Genotype data of the mother, child and alleged father at loci D3S1358, vWA and FGA.

Locus	C	M	AF
D3S1358	15/17	15/16	17/18
vWA	18/18	18/19	18/18
FGA	20/21	20/21	19/20

4.1.3 Posterior odds and probability of paternity

Another way of evaluating the strength of genetic evidence is by means of the posterior odds. Based on Equation (2.20) in Chapter 2, by Bayes' Theorem, we have

$$\frac{P(H_p|\text{evidence})}{P(H_d|\text{evidence})} = \frac{P(\text{evidence}|H_p)}{P(\text{evidence}|H_d)} \frac{P(H_p)}{P(H_d)},$$

Table 4.3   Allele frequencies for D3S1358, vWA and FGA for Hong Kong Chinese, from Wong *et al.* (2001). (Reproduced by permission of Springer-Verlag.)

Locus	Allele	Relative frequency
D3S1358	13	0.002
	14	0.033
	15	0.331
	16	0.326
	17	0.239
	18	0.056
	19	0.011
	20	0.002
vWA	13	0.004
	14	0.254
	15	0.035
	16	0.156
	17	0.266
	18	0.160
	19	0.106
	20	0.020
FGA	17	0.002
	18	0.025
	19	0.065
	20	0.044
	21	0.131
	21.2	0.004
	22	0.178
	22.2	0.004
	23	0.189
	23.2	0.004
	24	0.166
	24.2	0.007
	25	0.110
	25.2	0.007
	26	0.048
	26.2	0.005
	27	0.011
	28	0.002

where $P(H_p)$ and $P(H_d)$ are called prior probabilities, $P(H_p|\text{evidence})$ and $P(H_d|\text{evidence})$ are called posterior probabilities, and $P(H_p)/P(H_d)$ and $P(H_p|\text{evidence})/P(H_d|\text{evidence})$ are the prior odds and posterior odds, respectively. So

$$\text{posterior odds} = LR \times \text{prior odds.} \qquad (4.5)$$

The posterior odds are directly proportional to the prior odds. In practice, it is often nontrivial or even controversial to choose suitable prior odds. Sometimes, some people may take a convenient choice of the value 1. This choice, however, may be subject to criticism, since it assumes a priori probability of a half that the alleged father is the true father of the child, i.e. $P(H_p) = 1/2 = P(H_d)$. In fact, the prior probability may depend on a number of factors, such as the number of sexual partners that the mother has. Moreover, the form of the alternative hypothesis H_d also affects the choice of the prior probability $[$note $: P(H_p) = 1 - P(H_d)]$. For example, we may expect a different $P(H_p)$ or prior odds if the alternative explanation H_d is changed from a random unrelated man to the brother of the alleged father being the true father of the child. The evaluation of the likelihood ratio for such scenario can be found in the later section of this chapter.

Instead of just taking a single prior probability of $1/2$ for $P(H_p)$, some people like to report the posterior odds having different prior probability values for $P(H_p)$, e.g. 0.1 and 0.9, etc. Moreover, some researchers may like to provide the posterior probability as well. This probability can be derived from Equation (4.5) as

$$P(H_p|\text{evidence}) = \text{posterior odds}/(1 + \text{posterior odds}), \qquad (4.6)$$

since $P(H_p|\text{evidence}) + P(H_d|\text{evidence}) = 1$. The quantity $P(H_p|\text{evidence})$ is sometimes called the probability of paternity. Equations (4.5) and (4.6) show that the larger the likelihood ratio, the larger the possibility of H_p occurring, given the evidence.

Consider the example given in Section 4.1.2; the overall likelihood ratio is 37.36. We take the prior probability $P(H_p)$ as being 0.1, 0.5 and 0.9. The associated posterior odds and probabilities of paternity are shown in Table 4.4. As can be seen from the table, for this particular example, the posterior odds can be very different for different prior probabilities. This phenomenon is also found for the posterior probability.

It is to be noticed that the above evaluation is based on Bayes' Theorem, in which the specification of the prior probability is needed. Some researchers and paternity laboratories, however, prefer to use the likelihood ratio approach and report the paternity index only, since there is subjectiveness in the assignment of the prior probability. Nevertheless, the choice of the prior probability has to be made carefully. In this book, we are mainly using the likelihood ratio approach, which evaluates the weight of genetic evidence in a scientific manner. The assignment of the prior probability is left to individuals, researchers or jurors, and may have to be determined on a case-by-case basis.

Table 4.4   The posterior odds and probability of paternity $P(H_p|\text{evidence})$ for various values of the prior probability $P(H_p)$ for the standard trio example given in Section 4.1.2.

Prior probability $P(H_p)$	Prior odds	Posterior odds	Probability of paternity $P(H_p|\text{evidence})$
0.1	0.111	4.15	0.806
0.5	1	37.36	0.974
0.9	9	336.24	0.997

4.2   Paternity computer software

4.2.1   Steps in running the software

The authors have written computer software to deal with various paternity problems. The software EasyDNA_Trio deals with standard trio problems under Hardy–Weinberg equilibrium. The computer program is run in a window mode. It consists of the following steps:

Steps in running the EasyDNA_Trio software

1 Click the *Load frequency file* button after loading the EasyDNA program, then select the appropriate file

2 Choose the allele pairs at the locus for C, M and Z

3a Choose the appropriate paternal relation between C and Z under H_p (which is, in this standard trio case, *Child–parent*)

3b Choose the appropriate paternal relation between C and Z under H_d (which is, in this standard trio case, *Unrelated*)

4 Click the *Calculate* button

5 Repeat steps 2 and 4 for each of the remaining loci; step 3 (3a–3b) is blocked, since it is no longer needed for the remaining loci.

The software can be found at http://www.hku.hk/statistics/EasyDNA/.

Notice that Z in the software stands for the alleged father in the standard trio problem. Also, after the first run, step 3 is prohibited, since the relation between C and Z under H_p and that under H_d are already fixed and so no more input is needed. The likelihood ratio for each locus is obtained in step 4. After finishing calculations for all the loci, the findings can be saved to an output file by clicking the *Save* button.

Let us see how the software deals with the paternity example given in the earlier section. In step 1, we select the appropriate allele frequencies file with filename AlleleFreqAll, which is essentially in the same form as Table 4.3. Then, in step 2, we choose the allele pairs 15/16, 15/17 and 17/18 for the genotypes of M, C and Z at locus D3S1358. After running step 3, we click the *Calculate* button in step 4; the likelihood ratio 2.09 is obtained and shown in the screen. Then, do the same for the other loci, and the likelihood ratios are obtained as 6.25 at vWA and 2.86 at FGA, giving an overall likelihood ratio of 37.36, which is the same as that obtained earlier by formulas. The above procedure can be summarized in the captured screen shown in Figure 4.1. As can be seen from the figure, the procedure is simple and easy to follow.

The output findings can then be saved to a file by clicking the *Save* button. The output file is screen captured and presented in Figure 4.2. The file can be used for checking to avoid any possible manual inputting errors, as well as for reporting purpose.

4.2.2   The software to deal with an incest case

When the alleged father and the mother are closely related, the paternity issue becomes an incest case, which is a criminal offence. In many places, the relationships that are prohibited by law correspond to kinship coefficients greater than 1/16 (Evett and Weir 1998). These

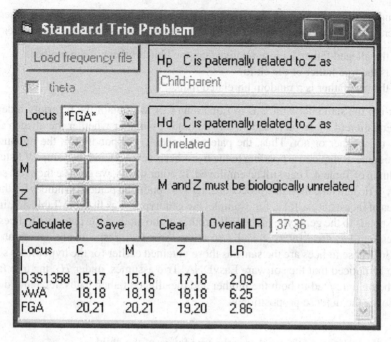

Figure 4.1 Captured screen for running the EasyDNA_Trio software for a standard trio problem with genotype data given in Table 4.2.

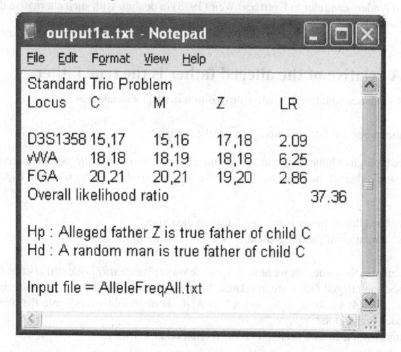

Figure 4.2 Captured screen for the output file of a standard trio problem with genotype data given in Table 4.2.

relationships include the alleged father being the father, the brother or the half-brother, etc. of the mother. In this situation, the prosecution and defense propositions are formulated as

H_p :   the alleged father, a close relative (say the half-brother) of the mother,
           is the true father of the child;   (4.7)
H_d :   the true father is a random unrelated man.

Following the same derivation as in Equation (4.2), we obtain the paternity index PI as given in Equation (4.3). In fact, Equation (4.3) holds no matter whether the alleged father is related to the mother or not. Thus, the paternity index corresponding to the hypothesis set (4.1) is the same as that corresponding to the hypothesis set (4.7), i.e. the same PI listed in the fourth column of Table 4.1 can still be employed. In other words, we can use the same software EasyDNA_Trio and take the same procedure steps to obtain the paternity indices for the above hypotheses of incest cases. Take, for example, the genotype set as listed in Table 4.2, in which AF corresponds to the genotype of the half-brother of the mother, the paternity indices for the hypotheses set (4.7) are 2.09, 6.25 and 2.86 at the three loci, respectively, giving an overall PI of 37.36. These indices are the same as those obtained earlier for the hypotheses set (4.1).

It is to be noticed that the software EasyDNA_Trio assumes, under H_d, the true father of the child being unrelated to both the mother and the alleged father. Thus, it cannot deal with the situation if the defense proposition is

H_d : another relative of the mother is the true father of the child.

Interested readers can refer to Evett and Weir (1998) in dealing with such alternative defense explanations.

4.3   A relative of the alleged father is the true father

In the previous section, the alternative proposition in (4.1) was taken as

H_d : the biological father is a random unrelated man,

where the biological father was unrelated to the alleged father. If the alleged father argues that he is not the father of the child but his relative, say his brother, is, the resultant hypotheses become

H_p :   the alleged father is the true father of the child;
H_d^0 :   a relative of the alleged father is the true father of the child.   (4.8)

The H_p remains the same, but we have a new defense explanation H_d^0. We still assume that the mother and the alleged father are unrelated. Suppose we consider the same set of genotypes as before: $C = A_i A_j$, $M = A_i A_k$ and $AF = A_j A_l$. How should we evaluate the likelihood ratio in such a situation?

We start from the basic principle of the likelihood ratio formula

$$LR^0 = \frac{P(\text{evidence}|H_p)}{P(\text{evidence}|H_d^0)} = \frac{P(C, M, AF|H_p)}{P(C, M, AF|H_d^0)}.$$

The numerator is

$$P(C = A_iA_j, M = A_iA_k, AF = A_jA_l|H_p)$$

$$= P(C = A_iA_j|M = A_iA_k, AF = A_jA_l, H_p)P(M = A_iA_k, AF = A_jA_l|H_p)$$

$$= [(1/2) \times (1/2)] (2p_ip_k \times 2p_jp_l)$$

$$= p_ip_jp_kp_l.$$

The first equality is due to the conditional probability formula in Equation (2.15).

For the denominator, we write the child's genotype $C = A_iA_j$ as $C_M = A_i$ and $C_P = A_j$, where C_M and C_P stand for the maternal and paternal alleles of the child, respectively. Thus,

$$P(C = A_iA_j, M = A_iA_k, AF = A_jA_l|H_d^0)$$

$$= P(M = A_iA_k, C_M = A_i, C_P = A_j, AF = A_jA_l|H_d^0)$$

$$= P(M = A_iA_k, C_M = A_i|H_d^0)P(C_P = A_j, AF = A_jA_l|H_d^0). \qquad (4.9)$$

The first probability is equal to $(2p_ip_k) \times (1/2)$, and the second one can be evaluated using the law of total probability in Equation (2.19):

$$P(C_P = A_j, AF = A_jA_l|H_d^0)$$

$$= \sum_{t=0}^{2} P\left(C_P = A_j, AF = A_jA_l|H_d^0, \text{ child and alleged father have } t \text{ ibd alleles}\right)$$

$$\times P\left(\text{child and alleged father have } t \text{ ibd alleles } |H_d^0\right)$$

$$= (p_j \times 2p_jp_l)k_0 + [(1/2) \times 2p_jp_l] (2k_1), \qquad (4.10)$$

where the k's are the relatedness coefficients [see Equation (3.18) in Section 3.6 for details] of the child and alleged father. Notice that $k_2 = 0$ in this case, since the alleged father and the mother are unrelated and so the probability that the alleged father and the child share two ibd alleles is zero. Substituting Equation (4.10) into Equation (4.9), we obtain

$$P(C = A_iA_j, M = A_iA_k, AF = A_jA_l|H_d^0)$$

$$= (2p_ip_k)(1/2) (p_j \times 2p_jp_l \times k_0 + p_jp_l \times 2k_1)$$

$$= p_ip_jp_kp_l(2k_1 + 2k_0p_j).$$

Thus, the likelihood ratio for the competing hypotheses H_p versus H_d^0 in (4.8) becomes

$$LR^0 = \frac{p_ip_jp_kp_l}{p_ip_jp_kp_l(2k_1 + 2k_0p_j)}$$

$$= 1/(2k_1 + 2k_0p_j)$$

$$= 1/[2k_1 + 2(1 - 2k_1)p_j]. \qquad (4.11)$$

The latter equality is due to the fact that $k_0 + 2k_1 + k_2 = 1$, in which $k_2 = 0$ in this particular case.

Suppose we denote the kinship coefficient [see Equation (3.21) in Section 3.6 for details] between the alleged father and his relative who is the true father by F. The coefficient is just the probability that two alleles, one taken at random from each of the alleged father and true father, are ibd. Since each of the two alleles of the true father is equally likely to be transmitted to the child, F and k_1 are equivalent. So, the likelihood ratio for $C = A_i A_j$, $M = A_i A_k$ and $AF = A_j A_l$ [Equation (4.11)], can also be expressed as

$$LR^0 = 1/[2F + 2(1 - 2F)p_j].$$

The likelihood ratios for other combinations of genotypes for C, M and AF under hypotheses set (4.8) can be similarly derived. They are all shown in the last column of Table 4.1 [see also Fung and Hu (2005)].

Now, we consider the example that we gave earlier (see Table 4.2 for genotypes). The hypotheses of interest are taken as

H_p : the alleged father is the true father of the child;
H_d^0 : a brother of the alleged father is the true father of the child.

The kinship coefficient for brothers is $F = 1/4 = 0.25$. Based on the formulas of the last column of Table 4.1 and the allele frequencies given in Table 4.3, we obtain the following likelihood ratios for individual loci:

$$\text{D3S1358} : \quad LR = 1/[2F + 2(1 - 2F)p_{17}]$$
$$= 1/[2 \times 0.25 + 2(1 - 2 \times 0.25) \times 0.239] = 1.35,$$

$$\text{vWA} : \quad LR = 1/[2F + (1 - 2F)p_{18}]$$
$$= 1/[2 \times 0.25 + (1 - 2 \times 0.25) \times 0.16] = 1.72,$$

$$\text{FGA} : \quad LR = 1/[2F + 2(1 - 2F)(p_{20} + p_{21})]$$
$$= 1/[2 \times 0.25 + 2(1 - 2 \times 0.25) \times (0.044 + 0.131)] = 1.48.$$

The overall likelihood ratio is

$$1.35 \times 1.72 \times 1.48 = 3.44.$$

Is it possible to obtain the likelihood ratio using the computer software? Yes, the procedure is actually very simple. In Section 4.2, we used the EasyDNA_Trio program to evaluate the likelihood ratio for the standard trio problem. Only a few steps are needed in running the program. In fact, the program is not restricted to standard trio problems, but can also be applied to other situations, such as the one that is of interest here, i.e. the defense hypothesis that a brother, or, in general, a relative, of the alleged father is the true father of the child. In doing so, what we need to do is to follow the same procedure steps listed in Section 4.2 except for a change in the following one:

Step 3b   Choose the appropriate paternal relation between C and Z under H_d (which is, in this case, *Nephew–uncle*).

The software is designed in such a way that a relation between C and the alleged father Z needs to be specified under both H_p and H_d. Under H_d that the brother of the alleged father is the father of the child is equivalent to saying that C and Z are *Nephew–uncle*.

The running of the computer program for this particular problem can be summarized in the captured screen which is shown in Figure 4.3. The procedure is almost the same as that shown in Figure 4.1 except for the box under H_d. The likelihood ratios for individual loci are

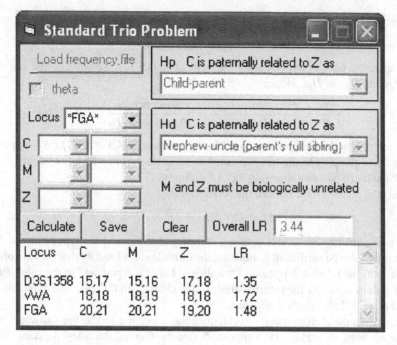

Figure 4.3 Captured screen for paternity testing for a trio problem where H_d: a brother of the alleged father Z is the true father of the child C.

1.35, 1.72 and 1.48, with the overall likelihood ratio being 3.44, which are the same as those obtained using the formulas given in Table 4.1.

4.4 Alleged father unavailable but his relative is

On some occasions, the alleged father may not be available for genotyping, for example dead, but typing is possible for his relative R. This problem has been considered by Morris *et al.* (1988) and Evett and Weir (1998). In this situation, the following set of hypotheses is of interest:

H_p : a relative of R is the true father of the child;
H_d : the true father is a random unrelated man. $\qquad\qquad$ (4.12)

The mother and R are taken to be unrelated.

This problem has been studied by Morris *et al.* (1988). They called the likelihood ratio for this particular problem the 'avuncular index' (AI) as an alternative to paternity index. This terminology is also adopted for this particular scenario in this book for convenience.

So far in this chapter, three sets of hypotheses besides the incest case have been considered for paternity analysis. They are given in Equations (4.1), (4.8) and (4.12). For simplicity, we write the associated pairs of null and alternative hypotheses as H_{p1} and H_{d1}; H_{p2} and H_{d2}; and H_{p3} and H_{d3}, respectively. The corresponding likelihood ratios are evaluated as

$$ PI = \frac{P(\text{evidence}|H_{p1})}{P(\text{evidence}|H_{d1})}, \quad LR^0 = \frac{P(\text{evidence}|H_{p2})}{P(\text{evidence}|H_{d2})} $$

and

$$AI = \frac{P(\text{evidence}|H_{p3})}{P(\text{evidence}|H_{d3})}.$$

If we compare the pairs of hypotheses in (4.1), (4.8) and (4.12), we observe that $H_{p1} \equiv H_{p2}$, $H_{d1} \equiv H_{d3}$ and $H_{d2} \equiv H_{p3}$. Hence,

$$\frac{PI}{LR^0} = \frac{P(\text{evidence}|H_{d2})}{P(\text{evidence}|H_{d1})} = \frac{P(\text{evidence}|H_{p3})}{P(\text{evidence}|H_{d3})} = AI.$$

Thus, we can obtain the likelihood ratio AI for hypotheses in (4.12) as PI/LR^0–a ratio of the quantities corresponding to the last two columns of Table 4.1, in which the genotypes of the relative R are listed as those shown in the AF column.

Morris *et al.* (1988) have noticed the relationship

$$AI = (1 - 2F) + 2F \times PI,$$

where F is the kinship coefficient between the alleged father and the typed relative R. This relationship can also be verified by comparing the formulas of AI and PI that we have obtained. Notice that now the relative R instead of the alleged father is typed, and so the value PI could be zero if R does not carry the paternal allele of the child C. In this case, the avuncular index AI would be $(1 - 2F)$, which is non-zero.

Besides using the above formula to calculate the avuncular index, our software provides an alternative way of evaluation. Suppose R is a brother of the alleged father. We take the same procedure steps as those listed in Section 4.2, except for the following modification:

Step 3a   Choose the appropriate paternal relation between C and Z under H_p (which is, in this case, *Nephew–uncle*).

Notice that Z in the software stands for the relative R in this case. The likelihood ratios are evaluated as 1.55, 3.62 and 1.93, respectively, for the three loci, with an overall likelihood ratio of 10.83.

4.5   Motherless case

4.5.1   Paternity index

In some paternity problems, the mother is unavailable for genotyping. Nevertheless, the following hypotheses are still of interest:

H_p: the alleged father is the true father of the child;
H_d: the true father is a random unrelated man.

The mother and the alleged father are taken as unrelated.

The paternity index for such a motherless case is evaluated as

$$PI = \frac{P(\text{evidence}|H_p)}{P(\text{evidence}|H_d)}$$

$$= \frac{P(C, AF|H_p)}{P(C, AF|H_d)}$$

Table 4.5 Paternity index (PI) for a motherless case. The LR^0 is evaluated under H_p: the alleged father is the true father of the child versus H_d: a relative of the alleged father is the true father of the child. F is the kinship coefficient of the alleged father and his relative.

C	AF	PI	LR^0
A_iA_i	A_iA_i	$1/p_i$	$1/[2F + (1 - 2F)p_i]$
A_iA_i	A_iA_j	$1/(2p_i)$	$1/[2F + 2(1 - 2F)p_i]$
A_iA_j	A_iA_i	$1/(2p_i)$	$1/[2F + 2(1 - 2F)p_i]$
A_iA_j	A_iA_j	$(p_i + p_j)/(4p_ip_j)$	$1/[2F + 4(1 - 2F)p_ip_j/(p_i + p_j)]$
A_iA_j	A_iA_k	$1/(4p_i)$	$1/[2F + 4(1 - 2F)p_i]$

$$= \frac{P(C|AF, H_p)}{P(C|AF, H_d)} \frac{P(AF|H_p)}{P(AF|H_d)}$$

$$= \frac{P(C|AF, H_p)}{P(C|AF, H_d)}$$

$$= \frac{P(C|AF, H_p)}{P(C|H_d)}.$$

The penultimate equality is due to the fact that the probability of the alleged father's genotype does not depend on whether the alleged father is the true father of the child or not. Suppose the genotypes of the child and the alleged father are $C = A_iA_j$ and $AF = A_iA_k$, respectively. The paternity index is

$$PI = \frac{P(C = A_iA_j|AF = A_iA_k, H_p)}{P(C = A_iA_j|H_d)}.$$

The numerator of PI takes the form of $(1/2)p_j$, since the alleged father who is the true father under H_p has a $1/2$ chance of transmitting allele A_i to the child and the chance that the child has an A_j for the other allele is p_j. The denominator, however, is just $2p_ip_j$. Thus, the index becomes

$$PI = \frac{(1/2)p_j}{2p_ip_j} = \frac{1}{4p_i}.$$

This quantity is shown at the last row of Table 4.5. The paternity indices for the other genotype combinations of C and AF can be obtained in similar ways. They are also shown in Table 4.5.

4.5.2 Computer software and example

Let us use the same data set listed in Table 4.2 for illustration. The mother of the child is, however, not available for typing. In other words, the genotypes of the child and the alleged father are provided; they are D3S1358: $C = 15/17$, $AF = 17/18$; vWA: $C = 18/18$, $AF = 18/18$; and FGA: $C = 20/21$, $AF = 19/20$. Based on the formulas given in Table 4.5, the paternity indices are evaluated as

$$D3S1358 : PI = 1/(4 \times p_{17}) = 1/(4 \times 0.239) = 1.05,$$

$$vWA : PI = 1/p_{18} = 1/0.160 = 6.25,$$

$$FGA \; : \; PI = 1/(4 \times p_{20}) = 1/(4 \times 0.044) = 5.68.$$

The overall PI is $1.05 \times 6.25 \times 5.68 = 37.28$, which is (slightly) less than the overall PI 37.36 for the standard trio case and this is generally true. The genotype of the mother in the standard trio case provides more genetic evidence for evaluation when the null hypothesis H_p holds true.

The computer software EasyDNA_Motherless developed by the authors deals with the motherless case under Hardy–Weinberg equilibrium. The steps in running the program are essentially the same as those listed in Section 4.2 for EasyDNA_Trio of the trio case, except that we do not need to input the mother's genotypes, which are unavailable.

Steps in running the EasyDNA_Motherless software

1 Click the *Load frequency file* button after loading the EasyDNA program, then select the appropriate file

2 Choose the allele pairs at the locus for C and Z

3a Choose the appropriate paternal relation between C and Z under H_p (which is, in this case, *Child–parent*)

3b Choose the appropriate paternal relation between C and Z under H_d (which is, in this case, *Unrelated*)

4 Click the *Calculate* button

5 Repeat steps 2 and 4 for each of the remaining loci; step 3 (3a–3b) is blocked, since it is no longer needed for the remaining loci.

The procedure steps are straightforward and readers can easily get familiar with the process after trying it a few times.

The motherless case example is analyzed by the software. Figure 4.4 summarizes the findings of the analysis. As can be seen from the figure, the interface of the EasyDNA_Motherless is more concise than the EasyDNA_Trio software. The overall PI obtained by the software is 37.28.

4.6 Motherless case: relatives involved

4.6.1 A relative of the alleged father is the true father

As in the trio situation, the alleged father in the motherless case might have argued with the following defense explanation:

$$H_d^0 : \text{ a relative of the alleged father is the true father of the child,} \tag{4.13}$$

while the prosecution proposition H_p remains as that the alleged father is the true father of the child.

The likelihood ratio, for $C = A_i A_j$ and $AF = A_i A_k$, is evaluated as

$$LR^0 = \frac{P(C = A_i A_j, \, AF = A_i A_k | H_p)}{P(C = A_i A_j, \, AF = A_i A_k | H_d^0)}.$$

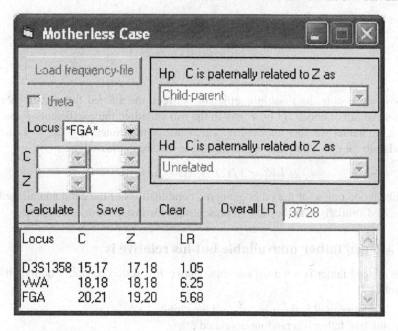

Figure 4.4   Captured screen for running the EasyDNA_Motherless software for a motherless case with genotype data of the child C and alleged father AF given in Table 4.2.

The numerator

$$P(C = A_i A_j, AF = A_i A_k | H_p)$$
$$= P(C = A_i A_j | AF = A_i A_k, H_p) P(AF = A_i A_k | H_p)$$
$$= (p_j \times 1/2)(2 p_i p_k)$$
$$= p_i p_j p_k.$$

The denominator, with the genotype of the child partitioned maternally and paternally, becomes

$$P(C = A_i A_j, AF = A_i A_k | H_d^0)$$
$$= P(C_M{=}A_i, C_P{=}A_j, AF{=}A_i A_k | H_d^0) + P(C_M{=}A_j, C_P = A_i, AF = A_i A_k | H_d^0)$$
$$= P(C_M = A_i) P(C_P = A_j, AF = A_i A_k | H_d^0)$$
$$\quad + P(C_M = A_j) P(C_P = A_i, AF = A_i A_k | H_d^0)$$
$$= p_i P(C_P = A_j, AF = A_i A_k | H_d^0) + p_j P(C_P = A_i, AF = A_i A_k | H_d^0)$$
$$= p_i \times k_0 p_j \times 2 p_i p_k + p_j [k_0 p_i \times 2 p_i p_k + (2k_1) p_i p_k]$$
$$= p_i p_j p_k (4 k_0 p_i + 2 k_1),$$

where k_j's are the relatedness coefficients between the child and alleged father under H_d^0. The penultimate equality is obtained in a similar way to that in Equation (4.10). Thus, the likelihood ratio is obtained as

$$LR^0 = \frac{p_i p_j p_k}{p_i p_j p_k (4k_0 p_i + 2k_1)}$$

$$= 1/(2k_1 + 4k_0 p_i).$$

Suppose we denote the kinship coefficient between the alleged father and his relative who is the true father under H_d^0 by F. As in the trio situation, the coefficients F and k_1 are equivalent, no matter whether the mother is available or not. Since $k_0 + 2k_1 = 1$, the above likelihood ratio for $C = A_i A_j$ and $AF = A_i A_k$ can also be expressed as

$$LR^0 = 1/[2F + 4(1 - 2F)p_i].$$

The likelihood ratios for the other genotype combinations of the child and alleged father can be derived similarly, and they are all presented in the last column of Table 4.5.

4.6.2   Alleged father unavailable but his relative is

When the alleged father is not available, his relative R is tested instead. The hypotheses of interest are

H_p :   a relative of R is the true father of the child;

H_d :   the true father is a random unrelated man.   (4.14)

Using a similar argument as that for the trio case, we are able to derive the relationship for the avuncular index for the motherless case as

$$AI = \frac{PI}{LR^0},$$ (4.15)

where PI and LR^0 refer to Table 4.5, in which the genotypes of the relative R are listed as those shown in the AF column.

It can also be easily verified that the finding of Morris *et al.* (1988) also holds for the motherless case, i.e.

$$AI = (1 - 2F) + 2F \times PI,$$ (4.16)

where F is the kinship coefficient between the alleged father and the typed relative R. For other combinations of genotypes of C and R (i.e. column AF) not listed in Table 4.5, their PI values are zeros, thus giving the avuncular index $AI = (1 - 2F)$, which is non-zero.

4.6.3   Computer software and example

The software EasyDNA_Motherless can easily deal with the special paternity problems involving relatives, in which the mother is not available. The steps in running the program are the same as those listed in Section 4.5 except for an appropriate choice of paternal relation between C and Z in step 3a or 3b. The choice of this relationship is the same as that in the trio case and can be referred to in Sections 4.3 and 4.4.

We analyze the illustrative example that has been given earlier for the motherless case with genotypes, namely D3S1358: $C = 15/17$, $AF = 17/18$; vWA: $C = 18/18$, $AF = 18/18$; and FGA: $C = 20/21$, $AF = 19/20$. The likelihood ratios for the prosecution hypothesis H_p that the alleged father is the true father of the child versus the defense explanation (4.13) H_d^0 that the brother of the alleged father is the true father of the child are 1.02, 1.72 and

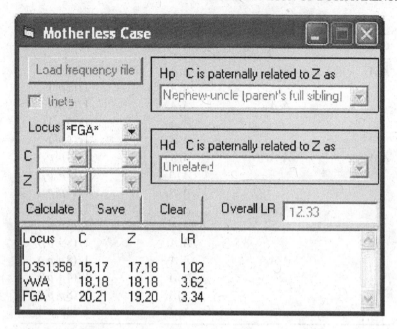

Figure 4.5   Captured screen for paternity testing for a motherless case where H_p: a brother of Z is the true father of the child C versus H_d: the true father is a random unrelated man.

1.70 for loci D3S1358, vWA and FGA, respectively, with an overall likelihood ratio of 2.98. These figures can easily be checked manually by calculator using the LR^0 formulas listed in Table 4.5 or by running the EasyDNA_Motherless software.

If the pair of hypotheses (4.14) is of interest and suppose a relative R, the brother of the alleged father, instead of the alleged father himself, is typed, then we run the EasyDNA_ Motherless following the same steps as listed in Section 4.5, except with the modification of

> Step 3a   Choose the appropriate paternal relation between C and Z under H_p (which is, in this case, *Nephew–uncle*).

Notice that Z in the software stands for the relative R in this case. The child C and the relative R who is the brother of the alleged father are *nephew and uncle* under H_p. Based on the EasyDNA_Motherless software, the avuncular indices (likelihood ratios) are 1.02, 3.62 and 3.34 at D3S1358, vWA and FGA, respectively, giving an overall avuncular index or likelihood ratio of 12.33. The running of the software is shown in the captured screen given in Figure 4.5. The indices can also be obtained from formulas given in Equations (4.15) and (4.16).

4.7   Determination of both parents

In May 1993, a newborn baby girl was stolen from a local hospital in Hong Kong. An abandoned infant of unknown identity was found on a street two days later. The parents of the missing baby girl thought that the abandoned baby was their missing child. DNA profiling

Table 4.6   Likelihood ratio (LR) for determination of both parents.

C	AM	AF	LR
A_iA_i	A_iA_i	A_iA_i	$1/p_i^2$
		A_iA_j	$1/(2p_i^2)$
	A_iA_j	A_iA_i	$1/(2p_i^2)$
		A_iA_j	$1/(4p_i^2)$
		A_iA_k	$1/(4p_i^2)$
A_iA_j	A_iA_i	A_iA_j	$1/(4p_ip_j)$
		A_jA_j	$1/(2p_ip_j)$
		A_jA_k	$1/(4p_ip_j)$
	A_iA_j	A_iA_i	$1/(4p_ip_j)$
		A_iA_j	$1/(4p_ip_j)$
		A_iA_k	$1/(8p_ip_j)$
	A_iA_k	A_iA_j	$1/(8p_ip_j)$
		A_jA_j	$1/(4p_ip_j)$
		A_jA_k	$1/(8p_ip_j)$
		A_jA_l	$1/(8p_ip_j)$

tests based on restriction fragment length polymorphism (RFLP) were performed. Details of the test results can be found in Fung *et al.* (1996).

The null and alternative propositions for such problems can be formulated as follows:

H_p :   the alleged parents are true parents of the child;

H_d :   a random unrelated couple are true parents of the child.

(4.17)

Let AF and AM denote the genotypes of the alleged father and alleged mother, respectively. The likelihood ratio can be determined as

$$
\begin{aligned}
LR &= \frac{P(\text{evidence}|H_p)}{P(\text{evidence}|H_d)} \\
&= \frac{P(C, AF, AM|H_p)}{P(C, AF, AM|H_d)} \\
&= \frac{P(C|AF, AM, H_p)}{P(C|AF, AM, H_d)} \times \frac{P(AF, AM|H_p)}{P(AF, AM|H_d)} \\
&= \frac{P(C|AF, AM, H_p)}{P(C|AF, AM, H_d)} \\
&= \frac{P(C|AF, AM, H_p)}{P(C)}.
\end{aligned}
$$

Suppose that $C = A_iA_j$, $AM = A_iA_k$ and $AF = A_jA_l$. The likelihood ratio is

$$
LR = \frac{(1/2)(1/2)}{2p_ip_j} = \frac{1}{8p_ip_j}.
$$

Table 4.7   Genotype data of the alleged couple (alleged mother and alleged father) and child.

Locus	C	AM	AF
D3S1358	17/17	17/18	17/17
vWA	14/18	14/18	14/17
FGA	23/25	23/24	25/25

The likelihood ratios for other genotype combinations can be obtained similarly. These ratios are all shown in Table 4.6. More details on the derivation can be referred to in Fung *et al.* (1996).

Table 4.7 gives an example with genotypes at three loci from the alleged couple and child for parentage determination of both parents. Based on the formulas listed in Table 4.6, the likelihood ratios at the loci are

$$D3S1358 \; : \; LR = 1/(2p_{17}^2) = 1/(2 \times 0.239^2) = 8.75,$$

$$vWA \; : \; LR = 1/(8p_{14}p_{18}) = 1/(8 \times 0.254 \times 0.160) = 3.08,$$

$$FGA \; : \; LR = 1/(4p_{23}p_{25}) = 1/(4 \times 0.189 \times 0.110) = 12.03.$$

The overall likelihood ratio is $8.75 \times 3.08 \times 12.03 = 324.21$.

We have developed the software EasyDNA_BothParents primarily for the purpose of determination of both parents. The steps in running the EasyDNA_BothParents software are

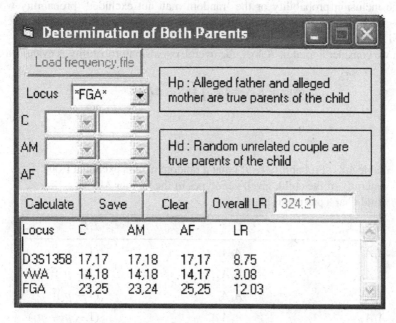

Figure 4.6   Captured screen for running the EasyDNA_BothParents software for determination of both parents with genotype data given in Table 4.7.

essentially the same as those in running the EasyDNA_Trio, except that the former software does not need steps 3a and 3b and is thus simpler. The program is run to analyze the example given in Table 4.7. The findings are shown in the captured screen in Figure 4.6.

In theory, there are variations of hypotheses given in Equation (4.17). These variations, however, are not that common in practice and so are not included in this book.

4.8 Probability of excluding a random man from paternity

Besides the paternity index (i.e. the likelihood ratio) and the probability of paternity (i.e. the posterior probability), the probability of excluding a random man from paternity is another quantity that may be used by some scientists and paternity laboratories. Given the genotypes of a child C and the mother M, the exclusion probability (EP) for a particular mother–child genotype combination is the proportion of random men that can be excluded from being the father of this child, based on genotypes C and M (Fung et al. 2002). Unlike the paternity index, the exclusion probability can be calculated even before the collection of the genotype of the alleged father, and it gives the proportion of random men in the population to be excluded from paternity of the child.

Suppose that the mother and the child have genotypes $M = A_i A_j$ and $C = A_i A_k$ at a particular locus l, respectively. A man without allele A_k (i.e. both of his alleles are not A_k) will be excluded as the true father of the child. Thus, the probability that a random individual in the male population is excluded from paternity in this case is $(1 - p_k)^2$. This exclusion probability at locus l is

$$EP_l = (1 - p_k)^2,$$

and so the inclusion probability or the 'random man not excluded' probability would be $IP_l = 1 - EP_l$. The EP_l's for various combinations of genotypes of the mother and child can be derived similarly and are given in Table 4.8.

When we consider a total of K loci, the overall exclusion probability is evaluated as

$$\text{overall } EP = 1 - \prod_{l=1}^{K}(1 - EP_l). \tag{4.18}$$

Table 4.8 Probability (EP_l) that a random man is excluded from paternity of the child, given genotypes of the mother M and child C at a particular locus l.

M	C	EP_l
$A_i A_i$	$A_i A_i$	$(1 - p_i)^2$
$A_i A_i$	$A_i A_j$	$(1 - p_j)^2$
$A_i A_j$	$A_i A_i$	$(1 - p_i)^2$
$A_i A_j$	$A_i A_j$	$(1 - p_i - p_j)^2$
$A_i A_j$	$A_i A_k$	$(1 - p_k)^2$

Consider the standard trio example we provided earlier in Table 4.2. Using the exclusion probability formulas, we obtain the probabilities at

locus 1,   D3S1358 : $EP_1 = (1 - p_{17})^2 = (1 - 0.239)^2 = 0.5791,$

locus 2,   vWA : $EP_2 = (1 - p_{18})^2 = (1 - 0.160)^2 = 0.7056,$

locus 3,   FGA : $EP_3 = (1 - p_{20} - p_{21})^2 = (1 - 0.044 - 0.131)^2 = 0.6806,$

and, for all three loci,

$$\text{overall } EP = 1 - (1 - 0.5791)(1 - 0.7056)(1 - 0.6806) = 0.9604.$$

This quantity can be interpreted as: given the genotypes of the mother and child at three loci (i.e. D3S1358: $M = 15/16, C = 15/17$; vWA: $M = 18/19, C = 18/18$; and FGA: $M = 20/21, C = 20/21$), there is a 0.9604 probability that a random unrelated man of the male population is excluded from paternity, i.e. his genotype is not consistent with the genotype of the child. In other words, there is about a 4% chance that a random unrelated man (who is in fact not the father of the child) in the male population will not be excluded from paternity using the DNA test at three loci of the mother and child. Now the genotype of the alleged father matches with the genotype of the child and so the alleged father is not excluded from paternity. It is then the duty of the jury and the judge to decide whether or not the alleged father is the father of the child. (Note: in practice, about 10 or more loci will usually be used, often resulting in an overall exclusion probability greater than 0.999.)

As can be observed from the above derivation, the exclusion probability evaluates

$$P(\text{a random man is excluded from paternity} \mid M, C).$$

This is rather different from the likelihood ratio (= paternity index) and the Bayesian posterior probability/odds approaches. One crucial difference is that the exclusion probability approach does not explicitly take the DNA profile of the alleged father into account in the probability calculation; the genotype of the alleged father AF is not needed in Table 4.8 at all. What it requires is only whether or not that DNA profile is consistent with the genotype of the child. For example, in the illustrative example, the exclusion probability remains the same no matter whether $AF = 17/18, 17/17$ or $17/20$ at D3S1358. As long as the genotype of the alleged father is consistent with that of the child, the exclusion probability, which depends on the genotypes of the mother and child, remains unchanged. This is, however, not true for the other two approaches.

The exclusion probability measure has been advocated by Li and Chakravarti (1988). However, some researchers such as Kaye (1989) pointed out the drawback that we have illustrated; the explicit genotype of the alleged father is irrelevant for the exclusion probability calculation provided that there is a match in the genotypes of the alleged father and child. Nevertheless, the exclusion probability provides a useful measure on the strength of the genotypes for a particular mother–child pair in excluding a random man from paternity of the child. Further discussion of the exclusion probability approach can be found in Balding (2005).

The idea of exclusion probability can also be used in the motherless case. The EP_l's at any particular locus l are referred to Table 4.9. The overall exclusion probability is evaluated in the same way as Equation (4.18).

Table 4.9   Probability (EP_l) that a random man is excluded from paternity of the child, given the child's genotype C at a particular locus l.

C	EP_l
$A_i A_i$	$(1 - p_i)^2$
$A_i A_j$	$(1 - p_i - p_j)^2$

4.9   Power of exclusion

4.9.1   A random man case

The effectiveness of a genetic marker as a tool for resolving paternity disputes can be characterized by its ability to exclude false fathers. One general measure that is commonly used for this purpose is the power or probability of exclusion (PE). The notation EP used in the last section refers to the probability of exclusion corresponding to a particular paternity case, whereas the notation PE used here corresponds to all possible paternity combinations and is *not* restricted to any particular case. The power of exclusion was first discussed by Wiener *et al.* (1930) on two allele systems. Ohno *et al.* (1982) and Garber and Morris (1983) developed general formulas for systems with any numbers of codominant alleles.

Consider a locus with n alleles $A_1, A_2, \ldots, A_n$ having corresponding allele frequencies $p_1, p_2, \ldots, p_n$. Given the genotypes of a child and the mother, C and M, respectively, we assess the probability of exclusion for a particular mother–child genotype combination, i.e. the individual probability or power of exclusion (IPE), which is the proportion of random men that can be excluded from being the father of the child, based on C and M.

Suppose that the genotypes of the mother and child are $M = A_i A_j$ and $C = A_i A_k$, respectively. Any man without the A_k allele will be excluded as the father of the child, and so the individual power of exclusion is

$$IPE = P(\text{a random man is excluded from paternity} \,|\, M = A_i A_j, C = A_i A_k) = (1 - p_k)^2.$$

The probability of that particular genotype combination for the mother and child is

$$P(M = A_i A_j, C = A_i A_k) = 2 p_i p_j (p_k / 2) = p_i p_j p_k.$$

The other genotype combinations for the mother and child are listed in Table 4.8, and the associated probabilities can be derived similarly (Evett and Weir 1998; Ohno *et al.* 1982). The power of exclusion PE is then obtained by summing the IPE's for all mother–child combinations, weighted by the corresponding genotype probabilities

$$PE_{WM} = \sum_{M,C} P(\text{a random man is excluded from paternity} \,|\, M, C) \times P(M, C)$$

$$= \sum_{i=1}^{n} p_i (1 - p_i + p_i^2)(1 - p_i)^2 + \sum_{i=1}^{n-1} \sum_{j=i+1}^{n} p_i p_j (p_i + p_j)(1 - p_i - p_j)^2.$$

The subscript '*WM*' stands for 'with mother' case, in contrast to the 'no mother' case to be discussed below. An equivalent but simpler expression is taken as

$$PE_{WM} = \sum_{i=1}^{n} p_i(1 - p_i)^2 - \sum_{i=1}^{n-1} \sum_{j=i+1}^{n} p_i^2 p_j^2 (4 - 3p_i - 3p_j). \tag{4.19}$$

Sometimes, the genotype of the mother may not be available. The formula for the power of exclusion in the no-mother case is

$$PE_{NM} = \sum_{i=1}^{n} p_i^2(1 - p_i)^2 + \sum_{i=1}^{n-1} \sum_{j=i+1}^{n} 2p_i p_j(1 - p_i - p_j)^2. \tag{4.20}$$

Since it is easier to exclude a man from being the child's father if the mother's genotype is available, we have $PE_{WM} \geq PE_{NM}$; the analytical proof is referred to in Fung *et al.* (2002). The power of exclusion in the no-mother case was also discussed in Garber and Morris (1983), Lee *et al.* (1980) and Jamieson and Taylor (1997).

When the power of exclusion P_i is calculated at locus i, $1 \leq i \leq K$, then the overall power of exclusion at all these K loci based on at least one or more loci exclusions is

$$PE = 1 - \prod_{i=1}^{K}(1 - P_i). \tag{4.21}$$

4.9.2   A relative case

When documentary proof is lacking or deemed inadequate, genetic testing is often required to verify parent–child claims in relation to immigration applications around the world (Fung *et al.* 2003b). Gorlin and Polesky (2000) reported a case in which the US embassy rejected an immigration application that involved a claim for the reunion of a boy with his parents. On the basis that the alleged father was suspected of being the boy's brother, the case was rejected, though no exclusions of paternity were found in the genetic tests. The boy and alleged father shared both alleles at three of the five RFLP loci tested, however.

In parentage testing for immigration purposes, one of the aims is to help deny those applications in which the claimed parent–child relationships are not substantiated. The above overall power of exclusion *PE* in Equation (4.21) is a way to express the ability of a panel of DNA markers for such a purpose. The ability is reasonably high when the number of typing loci is appropriately large whether the mother is available or not (Chakraborty *et al.* 1999). However, the powers of exclusion computed from Equations (4.19) and (4.20) can only reveal the power of a system to exclude a random man as the biological father. Unlike illegitimacy cases, the false father in immigration or inheritance disputes would be less likely to be an unrelated man, but rather a relative of the true father, e.g. his brother (see, for example, the above US immigration application). It is harder to exclude this man from paternity than an unrelated man, since the relative has a high chance of sharing genes with the true father. Knowing the power of a battery of tests to exclude a relative of the true father from paternity can help a parentage testing laboratory to interpret results more properly so as not to make undue claims to establishing the paternity of a particular child (Fung *et al.* 2002; Melvin *et al.* 1998).

To assess the power of a test from another perspective, the scope of computation can be limited to relatives of the true father. The calculation of power of exclusion under such consideration can be done by using the relatedness coefficients $(k_0, 2k_1, k_2)$. Fung *et al.* (2002) provided the following formulation of the power of excluding relatives of the true father from paternity based on autosomal markers. The power of excluding relatives of the true father for X-linked markers is referred to in Hu and Fung (2005c).

Suppose R is a relative of the true father (TF) and this relationship can be expressed in terms of their relatedness coefficients $(k_0, 2k_1, k_2)$. On the assumption that the mother (M) of the child (C) is unrelated to both TF and R, the child and TF will share exactly one ibd allele and the relationship between C and R can be described by the following probabilities:

$$P(\text{both alleles of } C \text{ and } R \text{ are ibd}) = 0,$$

$$P(\text{exactly one allele of } C \text{ and one allele of } R \text{ are ibd}) = k_1 + k_2,$$

$$P(\text{none of the alleles of } C \text{ and } R \text{ is ibd}) = k_0 + k_1.$$

If C and R share no ibd allele, R can be treated as a random man unrelated to C concerning the alleles in question. According to the law of total probability, since R can be excluded only when he shares no ibd allele with C, the probability of excluding a relative R as the father can be computed by

$$PER_{WM} = P(R \text{ and } C \text{ share no ibd allele})$$

$$\times P(R \text{ can be excluded} | R \text{ and } C \text{ share no ibd allele})$$

$$= (k_0 + k_1) PE_{WM}. \tag{4.22}$$

The following simple relationship between the PER_{WM} and the common PE_{WM} is found to be held: when we are concerned with the probability of the exclusion of a relative of the true father instead of a random man, the power of exclusion is reduced by a proportion equal to

$$\frac{PE_{WM} - PER_{WM}}{PE_{WM}} = 1 - k_0 - k_1$$

$$= k_1 + k_2$$

$$= \frac{1}{2}(\text{mean number of ibd alleles of } R \text{ and } TF).$$

It is obvious from this result that the closer the relationship between R and TF, the smaller the power of exclusion. This is consistent with the foregoing that it will be harder to exclude R from paternity, as R has a higher chance to inherit and share the same genotypes with TF. For the no-mother case, the corresponding PER can also be expressed as

$$PER_{NM} = (k_0 + k_1) PE_{NM}. \tag{4.23}$$

The above simple relationship between the PER and the common PE holds for situations as long as the mother can be assumed to be unrelated to both R and TF. It must be stressed that a change in the calculations would result if the mother bears a biological relationship with the relative R and true father TF. Thus, Equations (4.22) and (4.23) cannot be employed to answer the question 'what proportion of full sibling pairs disguising as parent/child can be discriminated by a test battery?' (Fung *et al.* 2004), since the sibling and the mother of the child are biologically related. This question is to be answered below.

In the following, we study the no-mother case first. We consider generally the probability that one relative of the child, whether or not he is related to the mother, is excluded from paternity. Let ϕ_0 denote the probability that the relative and the child share no ibd alleles (note, in the above discussion, the k-coefficients between the relative and the true father are used). For a child with homozygous $C = A_iA_i$, the relative is excluded from paternity if and only if $R = A_mA_n$ $(m, n \neq i)$. For a child with heterozygous $C = A_iA_j$ $(i < j)$, the relative is excluded from paternity if and only if $R = A_mA_n$ $(m, n \neq i, j)$. As the relative is excluded from paternity of the child, it can be concluded that the relative shares no ibd alleles with the child at that particular locus; so the joint genotype probability $P(C = A_iA_i, R = A_mA_n) = \phi_0 P(C = A_iA_i)P(R = A_mA_n)$ for $m, n \neq i$ and $P(C = A_iA_j, R = A_mA_n) = \phi_0 P(C = A_iA_j) \times P(R = A_mA_n)$ for $m, n \neq i, j$. Hence, the probability of excluding a relative of the child from paternity is obtained by summing over all possible exclusion configurations of R and C; that is

$$PER_{NM} = \phi_0 \left[\sum_{i;m,n\neq i} P(C = A_iA_i)P(R = A_mA_n) \right.$$

$$\left. + \sum_{i<j;m,n\neq i,j} P(C = A_iA_j)P(R = A_mA_n) \right]$$

$$= \phi_0 PE_{NM}. \tag{4.24}$$

The term inside the square bracket is just Equation (4.20). Thus, the second equality follows immediately.

Note that in Equation (4.24), the involved relative of the child can be paternal or maternal, but the involved relative in Equation (4.23) is confined to the paternal relative of the child, and so cannot be the elder brother of the child. It is shown that $\phi_0 = k_0 + k_1$ when the relative is paternal (Fung et al. 2004), so Equation (4.24) covers Equation (4.23).

4.9.3   An elder brother case: mother available

When the mother of a child is not available for typing, Fung et al. (2004) have shown that full brothers impersonating a father/child situation is very difficult to discredit with DNA profiling alone. When the mother is available, the relationship in Equation (4.22), however, does not hold for relatives who are biologically related to the mother (e.g. an elder brother of the child). In the following, we are going to derive the power of exclusion for an elder brother case when the mother is available (Hu and Fung 2005b).

Let M, C and EB denote the genotypes of the mother, child and elder brother, respectively. The power of excluding the elder brother of the child from paternity, termed as $PEEB$, is given by

$$PEEB_{WM} = \sum_{M, C, EB} P(M, C, EB), \tag{4.25}$$

where $P(M, C, EB)$ corresponds to the joint genotype probability for a particular paternity exclusion configuration of the mother–child–elder brother trio, and the summation sums over all possible configurations. Table 4.10 presents a summary of all the paternity exclusion configurations together with the associated probabilities. Summing over all possible configurations with the associated probabilities given in the last column of Table 4.10 yields the power of

Table 4.10   Paternity exclusion configurations and their joint genotype probabilities for the mother–child–elder brother trios having genotypes M, C and EB.

M	C	EB	Joint probability
A_iA_i	A_iA_j	A_iA_i	$p_i^3 p_j/2$
		A_iA_k	$p_i^2 p_j p_k/2$
A_iA_j	A_iA_i	A_jA_j	$p_i^2 p_j^3/4$
		A_jA_k	$p_i^2 p_j p_k/4$
	A_jA_j	A_iA_i	$p_i^2 p_j^2/4$
		A_iA_k	$p_i p_j^2 p_k/4$
	A_iA_k	A_iA_i	$p_i^2 p_j p_k/4$
		A_iA_l	$p_i p_j p_k p_l/4$
		A_iA_j	$p_i^2 p_j p_k/4 + p_i p_j^2 p_k/4$
		A_jA_j	$p_i p_j^2 p_k/4$
		A_jA_l	$p_i p_j p_k p_l/4$
	A_jA_k	A_iA_i	$p_i^2 p_j p_k/4$
		A_iA_l	$p_i p_j p_k p_l/4$
		A_iA_j	$p_i^2 p_j p_k/4 + p_i p_j^2 p_k/4$
		A_jA_j	$p_i p_j^2 p_k/4$
		A_jA_l	$p_i p_j p_k p_l/4$

exclusion in the with-mother case (Hu and Fung 2005b):

$$PEEB_{\text{WM}} = \frac{1}{4} \sum_i p_i(2 - p_i)(1 - p_i)^2$$

$$= \frac{1}{2} - \frac{5}{4} \sum_i p_i^2 + \sum_i p_i^3 - \frac{1}{4} \sum_i p_i^4. \tag{4.26}$$

When the population is subdivided with a degree of subdivision θ, Hu and Fung (2005b) provided an analogous formula for the power of exclusion in the with-mother case [see also Hu et al. (2004)].

The different measures of the power of exclusion are illustrated using the Hong Kong Chinese population data at 12 STR loci (Wong et al. 2001). The powers of excluding a random man, and a paternal uncle and an elder brother of the child from paternity, for the with-mother and no-mother cases, are listed in Table 4.11. The powers of excluding a random man as the true father range from 33 to 73% across loci when the genotype of the mother is available. Nevertheless, when the paternal uncle of a child claims to be the true father *in the absence of the mother* for testing, as in an immigration application for reunion, the powers of exclusion across loci become much smaller, ranging from 9 to 29%. The overall power at all loci is only 93.7%, implying the insufficiency of this system in resolving paternity disputes for such cases. In other words, the panel of 12 STR loci system cannot exclude 6.3% of the alleged fathers in nephew/niece–uncle cases for paternity determinations when the mother of the child

Table 4.11   Powers of excluding a random man (PE), and a paternal uncle (PER_1) and an elder brother (PER_2) of the child from paternity based on Hong Kong Chinese population data, for the with-mother and no-mother cases, from Hu and Fung (2005b). (Reproduced by permission of Elsevier.)

Locus	With-mother			No-mother		
	PE	PER_1	PER_2	PE	PER_1	PER_2
D3S1358	0.4745	0.2372	0.2314	0.3037	0.1519	0.0759
vWA	0.6099	0.3049	0.2944	0.4325	0.2162	0.1081
FGA	0.7317	0.3658	0.3531	0.5748	0.2874	0.1437
THO1	0.4496	0.2248	0.2177	0.2798	0.1399	0.0699
TPOX	0.3303	0.1651	0.1616	0.1862	0.0931	0.0466
CSF1PO	0.4992	0.2496	0.2425	0.3244	0.1622	0.0811
D5S818	0.5919	0.2960	0.2861	0.4139	0.2069	0.1035
D13S317	0.5694	0.2847	0.2751	0.3905	0.1953	0.0976
D7S820	0.5481	0.2740	0.2646	0.3680	0.1840	0.0920
D8S1179	0.7023	0.3512	0.3387	0.5368	0.2684	0.1342
D21S11	0.6622	0.3311	0.3191	0.4913	0.2456	0.1228
D18S51	0.7315	0.3658	0.3530	0.5748	0.2874	0.1437
Overall[a]	0.99998	0.98357	0.98068	0.99849	0.93659	0.72528
Overall[b]	0.99957	0.90213	0.88943	0.98487	0.73738	0.34857
Overall[c]	0.99622	0.71846	0.69326	0.92950	0.45378	0.11400

[a]Overall power of exclusion on the basis of at least one or more loci exclusions
[b]Overall power of exclusion on the basis of at least two or more loci exclusions
[c]Overall power of exclusion on the basis of at least three or more loci exclusions

is not available, although it performs well in the child–random man case ($PE = 0.99849$). It is also noted that when the mother is not available, the power of excluding an elder brother of the child from paternity using the said STR battery is only about 73%, indicating that about 27% of pairs of two full siblings impersonating father and child would not be discounted correctly. As the traditional PE may overstate the exclusion power in some situations, it is recommended to also compute the PER for a better assessment of the effectiveness of the test battery.

Considering the high mutation rates (Brinkmann *et al.* 2001; Chakraborty and Stivers 1996; Gunn *et al.* 1997) of STR loci, the American Association of Blood Banks recommends declaring non-paternity based on exclusions at two or more loci tested. To address this, we let P_i be the power of exclusion based upon the ith locus, $i = 1, \ldots, K$. The overall power of exclusion for a panel of tests on the basis of at least two or more loci exclusions is

$$PE' = 1 - \prod_{i=1}^{K}(1 - P_i) - \sum_{i=1}^{K} P_i \prod_{\substack{j=1 \\ j \neq i}}^{K}(1 - P_j)$$

$$= PE - \prod_{i=1}^{K}(1 - P_i) \sum_{i=1}^{K} \frac{P_i}{1 - P_i}, \tag{4.27}$$

and, on the basis of three or more loci exclusions, is

$$PE'' = PE' - \sum_{i<j} P_i P_j \prod_{\substack{k=1 \\ k\neq i, k\neq j}}^{K} (1 - P_k)$$

$$= PE' - \prod_{i=1}^{K}(1 - P_i) \sum_{i<j} \frac{P_i P_j}{(1 - P_i)(1 - P_j)}, \tag{4.28}$$

where the form of PE is provided in Equation (4.21).

Taking the possibility of mutation in STR loci into consideration and on the basis of at least two or more loci exclusions, the powers of excluding relatives from paternity are: in the with-mother case, 90% for a paternal uncle and 89% for an elder brother of the child; in the no-mother case, 74% for a paternal uncle and 35% for an elder brother of the child. All these values are 90% or below. On the basis of at least three or more loci exclusions, the powers of excluding the said relatives from paternity are all below 72% and can be as low as 11%. These results illustrate well the difficulty of excluding relatives of the child from paternity when the possibility of mutation in STR is taken into consideration. This may have serious consequences for parentage testing laboratories and immigration authorities in verifying parent/child claims. New sets of tests with much higher PER's are needed to serve the purpose of determining parentage and kinship (Fung *et al.* 2004; Wenk *et al.* 2003).

4.10   Other issues

4.10.1   Reverse parentage

Consider the following murder case about reverse parentage. A blood stain is found and the evidence is believed to be that of a murdered (missing) child of two known parents. The hypotheses of interest are

H_p : the blood stain came from the missing child of two known parents;
H_d : the blood stain did not come from the missing child.

The genotypes of the blood stain (BS) and the couple (AM and AF) are listed in Table 4.12. It is obvious that this problem is equivalent to the situation of determination of both parents as given in Section 4.7. The likelihood ratios can be obtained based on the formulas of Table 4.6 in which the genotype C is replaced by BS. The ratios are evaluated as

D3S1358 : $LR = 1/(8 p_{15} p_{17}) = 1/(8 \times 0.331 \times 0.239) = 1.58$,
   vWA : $LR = 1/(4 p_{16}^2) = 1/(4 \times 0.156^2) = 10.27$,
   FGA : $LR = 1/(2 p_{24} p_{25}) = 1/(2 \times 0.166 \times 0.110) = 27.38$.

The overall likelihood ratio is $1.58 \times 10.27 \times 27.38 = 444.28$. The software EasyDNA_BothParents can also be used to evaluate the likelihood ratios in this situation.

In situations in which only one parent is available, the formulas and software given in Section 4.5 for the motherless case would then be relevant. Other complex missing person problems are referred to in Section 5.8.

Table 4.12   A reverse parentage case with genotype data of the blood stain (BS) which is hypothesized to be that of a missing child of two known parents (AM and AF).

Locus	BS	AM	AF
D3S1358	15/17	15/16	14/17
vWA	16/16	16/17	16/19
FGA	24/25	24/24	25/25

4.10.2   Mutation

The high mutation rates of STR loci (Brinkmann *et al.* 2001; Chakraborty and Stivers 1996) cannot be neglected. It may happen in parentage testing that the genotype of the alleged father matches with the child at all except one or two loci. This situation might be explained by mutation. Brinkmann *et al.* (1998) investigated the estimation of mutation rates for various STR loci used in forensic and paternity testing. Thomson *et al.* (1999) concluded that a single paternal mutation event might occur about 1% of the time. Ayres (2000) reported the paternity index in the with-mother case and in the no-mother case, incorporating the mutation rate, in a subdivided population. Ayres (2002) reported the paternal exclusion in the presence of substructure, which extends the results listed in Dawid *et al.* (2001) to the subdivided population, where the stepwise stationary mutation model was employed.

According to the recommendations of the American Association of Blood Banks, non-paternity may be declared when there are mismatches at two or more loci tested. The average mutation paternity index (AMPI) is then used for the mismatch locus found between the alleged father and the child. This index can be derived in the following way.

Consider a standard trio case in which the genotypes of the child, mother and alleged father are typed. The hypotheses of interest are

H_p : the alleged father is true father of the child;

H_d : the true father of the child is a random unrelated man. $\qquad$ (4.29)

Suppose that there is a mismatch in one particular locus of the test battery, and let the genotypes of the child and mother be C and M at this locus, respectively. As a general index, the AMPI considers only the information that the genotype of the alleged father does not match, but not this person's particular genotype. The likelihood ratio at the mismatch locus is evaluated as

$$
\begin{aligned}
LR &= \frac{P(C, M, \text{the child's and alleged father's genotypes not match} \mid H_p)}{P(C, M, \text{the child's and alleged father's genotypes not match} \mid H_d)} \\
&= \frac{P(\text{the child's and alleged father's genotypes not match} \mid H_p, C, M)\ P(C, M \mid H_p)}{P(\text{the child's and alleged father's genotypes not match} \mid H_d, C, M)\ P(C, M \mid H_d)} \\
&= \frac{P(\text{the child's and alleged father's genotypes not match} \mid H_p, C, M)}{P(\text{the child's and alleged father's genotypes not match} \mid H_d, C, M)}.
\end{aligned}
$$

As for the numerator, the genotype of the alleged father (who is the true father of the child under H_p) does not match the genotype of the child due to mutation, and so this probability is equal to the (average) mutation rate μ. The denominator, under H_d that the man is not the

Table 4.13   Genotype data of the mother, child and alleged father at 12 loci, in which a mismatch is found at locus D18S51.

Locus	Child	Mother	Alleged father	*LR*
D3S1358	16/17	17/18	15/16	1.54
vWA	14/18	14/19	14/18	3.13
FGA	20/24	20/22	22/24	3.01
THO1	6/7	6/8	7/9	1.58
TPOX	8/11	8/9	11/11	3.2
CSF1PO	12/12	12/12	10/12	1.38
D5S818	11/12	12/13	10/11	1.96
D13S317	10/10	10/10	9/10	3.23
D7S820	8/8	8/10	8/11	4.15
D8S1179	14/16	16/18	11/14	3.29
D21S11	30/32.2	30/31	29/32.2	2.62
D18S51*	13/14	14/14	12/17	0.00414*

*A mismatch of the genotypes of the alleged father and child; the *LR* is evaluated using the average mutation paternity index (AMPI)

true father, is just the power or probability of excluding a random man from paternity *PE*. Thus, the likelihood at this locus (Fimmer *et al.* 1992) is evaluated as

$$LR = \frac{\mu}{PE}, \tag{4.30}$$

which is termed the average mutation paternity index (AMPI). There are other mutation models suggested in the literature (Dawid *et al.* 2002; Rolf *et al.* 2001; Valdes *et al.* 1993) which may also be employed for evaluating the likelihood ratio.

Consider a standard trio case example (Table 4.13) for the Hong Kong Chinese population. The genotype of the alleged father matches with that of the child at all 12 except the last locus. Using the software, we can obtain individual likelihood ratios and they are shown in the last column of Table 4.13. The last ratio 0.00414 at D18S31 is evaluated using Equation (4.30) with $\mu = 0.00303$ and $PE = 0.732$. The paternity index based on the match loci is called the residual paternity index, which is equal to $1.54 \times 3.13 \times \cdots \times 2.62 = 22926$. The overall paternity index is evaluated as $22926 \times 0.00414 = 94.9$, which is reduced substantially.

4.11   Problems

1. Obtain the paternity index (*PI*) for a standard trio where $C = A_1 A_2$, $M = A_1 A_2$ and $AF = A_2 A_3$, and the population is in Hardy–Weinberg equilibrium. Moreover, use the computer software EasyDNA_Trio to evaluate the *PI* for this case with $A_1 = 15$, $A_2 = 16$ and $A_3 = 17$ at locus D3S1358 and the corresponding allele frequencies specified in Table 4.3.

2. In a paternity testing where $C = A_1 A_2$, $M = A_1 A_3$ and $AF = A_2 A_3$, we are interested in the hypotheses:

H_p: the alleged father (AF) is the true father of the child (C);
H_d: a full sibling of AF is the true father of C.

Find the likelihood ratio.

3. Suppose in a paternity testing $C = A_1 A_2$, $M = A_1 A_2$ and a full sibling R of the alleged father is typed with genotype $R = A_2 A_3$. Find the likelihood ratio about the following two competing hypotheses:

H_p: the alleged father, a relative R, is the true father of the child;
H_d: the true father is a random unrelated man.

4. Derive the following relationship between the paternity index (PI) and the avuncular index (AI) for paternity testing in trio cases:

$$AI = (1 - 2F) + 2F \times PI,$$

where F is the kinship coefficient between the alleged father and the typed relative R (see details in Section 4.4).

5. In a paternity testing in which the mother is not available, we are interested in

H_p: the alleged father is the true father of the child;
H_d: the true father is a random unrelated man.

Evaluate the paternity indices for (i) $AF = A_1 A_2$ and $C = A_1 A_3$, (ii) $AF = A_1 A_2$, $C = A_1 A_1$; (iii) $AF = A_1 A_1$, $C = A_1 A_1$.

6. In a paternity testing without the mother's information, the genotypes of the child and the alleged father are $A_1 A_2$ and $A_2 A_3$, respectively. Find the paternity index for following two competing hypotheses:

H_p: the alleged father (AF) is the true father of the child (C);
H_d: a full sibling of AF is the true father of C.

7. Consider a paternity testing in the no-mother case, where the child is typed as $A_1 A_2$ and a full sibling R of the alleged father is typed as $A_1 A_2$. Find the paternity index about the following two competing propositions:

H_p: the alleged father, a relative of R, is the true father of the child;
H_d: a random unrelated man is the true father of the child.

8. In the motherless case, verify the relationship between the paternity index (PI) and avuncular index (AI):

$$AI = (1 - 2F) + 2F \times PI,$$

where F is the kinship coefficient between the alleged father and the typed relative R (see details in Section 4.6.2).

9. Suppose the genotypes of the alleged father, the alleged mother and the child are A_1A_2, A_3A_3 and A_2A_3, respectively. Find the likelihood ratio about the following two competing propositions:

   H_p: the alleged parents are true parents of the child;
   H_d: a random unrelated couple are true parents of the child.

10. Consider a paternity testing in the no-mother case where the genotypes of the child C and the alleged father AF are: $C = 16/17$, $AF = 17/17$ at locus D3S1358; $C = 17/18$, $AF = 17/18$ at locus vWA; $C = 24/25$, $AF = 25/26$ at locus FGA. The following hypotheses are of interest:

   H_p: the alleged father is the true father of the child;
   H_{d1}: a random unrelated man is the true father of the child;
   H_{d2}: a half sibling of the alleged father is the true father of the child.

   Obtain the likelihood ratios for H_p versus H_{d1} and H_p versus H_{d2} using (i) the formulas given in Table 4.5, and (ii) the software EasyDNA_Motherless, by having the allele frequencies specified in Table 4.3. Check whether the corresponding results in (i) and (ii) are the same.

5

Testing for kinship

In Chapter 4, we discussed a number of paternity problems such as paternity testing for the with-mother and without-mother cases, incest cases and determinations of both parents, etc. We have also considered situations in which relatives of the alleged father are involved, for example the defense proposition that a relative of the alleged father is the true father of the child, and when the alleged father is not available but his relative is. All of the above analyses are concerned about the determination of the 'father and child' relationship. In this particular chapter, we are going to investigate more general relationships between two persons (Fung et al. 2003a; Li and Sacks 1954) and those among three persons (Fung et al. 2005, 2006). Besides, unlike in Chapter 4, in which Hardy–Weinberg equilibrium (HWE) is assumed, the relationships of the persons involved here are determined under the situation that they belong to a subdivided or structured population. More complex paternity and kinship problems (Fung 2003b) with Hardy–Weinberg equilibrium are also investigated.

5.1 Kinship testing of any two persons: HWE

In addition to the parent–child determination in traditional parentage testing (Fung et al. 2002; Lee et al. 2000, 1999; Thomson et al. 1999), other kinds of relationships between individuals also need to be tested in practice. For example, Thomson et al. (2001) analyzed sibling relationships using STR loci; Gaytmenn et al. (2002) studied the sensitivity and specificity of sibship calculations. The use and abuse of the full sibling and half sibling indices in immigration cases were discussed by Gorlin and Polesky (2000).

We would like to determine a specific relationship between two typed persons. The following propositions are of interest:

H_p: the two persons are biologically related;
H_d: the two persons are biologically unrelated. $\hspace{2em}$ (5.1)

The relationship between the two persons can be of various sorts, for example parent–offspring, uncle–nephew, half siblings, etc. In this particular section, Hardy–Weinberg equilibrium is assumed. Let the genotypes of the two persons be denoted by Y and Z, respectively. For

Statistical DNA Forensics: Theory, Methods and Computation   Wing Kam Fung and Yue-Qing Hu
© 2008 John Wiley & Sons, Ltd

Table 5.1   The joint genotype probabilities $P(Y, Z)$ for all Y and Z combinations when the population is in Hardy–Weinberg equilibrium.

Y	Z	$P(Y, Z)$
$A_i A_i$	$A_i A_i$	$k_0 p_i^4 + 2k_1 p_i^3 + k_2 p_i^2$
$A_i A_i$	$A_i A_j$	$2k_0 p_i^3 p_j + 2k_1 p_i^2 p_j$
$A_i A_i$	$A_j A_j$	$k_0 p_i^2 p_j^2$
$A_i A_i$	$A_j A_k$	$2k_0 p_i^2 p_j p_k$
$A_i A_j$	$A_i A_j$	$4k_0 p_i^2 p_j^2 + 2k_1 p_i^2 p_j + 2k_1 p_i p_j^2 + 2k_2 p_i p_j$
$A_i A_j$	$A_i A_k$	$4k_0 p_i^2 p_j p_k + 2k_1 p_i p_j p_k$
$A_i A_j$	$A_k A_l$	$4k_0 p_i p_j p_k p_l$

simplicity, we use the following notation to describe the relationship between the two persons in the hypotheses. The pair of hypotheses in (5.1) is then formulated as

$$H_p : (Y, Z) \sim (k_0, 2k_1, k_2);$$
$$H_d : (Y, Z) \sim (1, 0, 0),$$

(5.2)

where $(k_0, 2k_1, k_2)$ are the relatedness coefficients [see Equation (3.18)] of the two persons with common values such as $(0, 1, 0)$ for parent–offspring, $(0.5, 0.5, 0)$ for half siblings and $(1, 0, 0)$ for unrelated persons, etc. The joint genotype probabilities $P(Y, Z)$ for all possible genotype combinations of Y and Z are listed in Table 5.1 when the population is in Hardy–Weinberg equilibrium. The results in Table 5.1 can be derived using a general formula given in Equation (7.21).

The likelihood ratio about the hypothesis pair in (5.1) is

$$\begin{aligned} LR &= \frac{P(\text{evidence}|H_p)}{P(\text{evidence}|H_d)} \\ &= \frac{P(Y, Z|H_p)}{P(Y, Z|H_d)} \\ &= \frac{P(Z|Y, H_p)}{P(Z|Y, H_d)} \frac{P(Y|H_p)}{P(Y|H_d)} \\ &= \frac{P(Z|Y, H_p)}{P(Z|Y, H_d)}. \end{aligned}$$

(5.3)

Suppose that the two persons have genotypes $Y = A_i A_j$ and $Z = A_i A_k$ at a particular locus. The numerator of the likelihood ratio in Equation (5.3), based on the law of total probability in Equation (2.19), can be evaluated as

$$P(Z = A_i A_k | Y = A_i A_j, H_p)$$

$$= \sum_{t=0}^{2} P(Z = A_i A_k | Y = A_i A_j, H_p, \text{ the two persons have } t \text{ ibd alleles})$$

$$\times P(\text{the two persons have } t \text{ ibd alleles} | Y = A_i A_j, H_p)$$

$$= (2p_i p_k)k_0 + (p_k \times 1/2)2k_1 + 0 \times k_2.$$

The second term ($p_k \times 1/2$) is explained as follows: given $Y = A_i A_j$ and the two persons have one ibd allele, the probability of the ibd allele being A_i is $1/2$ and the probability of the remaining allele being A_k is p_k. Hence,

$$P(Z = A_i A_k | Y = A_i A_j, H_p) = 2 p_i p_k k_0 + p_k k_1.$$

The denominator of the likelihood ratio is simply

$$P(Z = A_i A_k | Y = A_i A_j, H_d) = 2 p_i p_k,$$

since, under H_d that the two persons are unrelated, the probability that the genotype $Z = A_i A_k$ is independent of the genotype $Y = A_i A_j$. Thus, the likelihood ratio corresponding to the set of hypotheses (5.1) or (5.2) on kinship determination is

$$LR = (2 p_i p_k k_0 + p_k k_1) / (2 p_i p_k)$$

$$= k_0 + k_1 / (2 p_i).$$

The likelihood ratios for other combinations of genotypes Y and Z can be derived in similar ways. These ratios are all listed in Table 5.2, which can also be derived based on Table 5.1 [see also Li and Sacks (1954)].

The likelihood ratios in Table 5.2 correspond to the hypothesis pair (5.1) in which the relatedness coefficients $(k_0, 2k_1, k_2)$ are used to describe the relationship between the two persons under H_p. When the coefficients take values (0, 1, 0) for father–child, the likelihood ratios given in Table 5.2 reduce to the paternity indices (PI's), as reported in Table 4.5 for paternity testing in a motherless case.

Sometimes, the defense proposition H_d is that the two persons are not unrelated: consider the pedigree diagram in Figure 5.1 in which persons 5 and 6 are couple, and it is also known that person 5 is the biological mother of person 8. Suppose that there is a query if in fact person 4 instead of person 6 is the biological father of person 8. Suppose persons 4, 5 and 6 are unavailable, and only persons 7 and 8 (see diagram) are available for typing; in this case, we have the following propositions which describe whether persons 7 and 8 are related as half siblings or first cousins, i.e.

H_p: $(Y, Z) \sim (0.5, 0.5, 0)$;
H_d^*: $(Y, Z) \sim (0.75, 0.25, 0)$. $\hspace{2cm}$ (5.4)

Table 5.2   The likelihood ratios about two competing hypotheses $H_p : (Y, Z) \sim (k_0, 2k_1, k_2)$ versus $H_d : (Y, Z) \sim (1, 0, 0)$.

Y	Z	Likelihood ratio
$A_i A_i$	$A_i A_i$	$k_0 + 2k_1/p_i + k_2/p_i^2$
$A_i A_i$	$A_i A_j$	$k_0 + k_1/p_i$
$A_i A_i$	$A_j A_j$	k_0
$A_i A_i$	$A_j A_k$	k_0
$A_i A_j$	$A_i A_j$	$k_0 + k_1(p_i + p_j)/(2 p_i p_j) + k_2/(2 p_i p_j)$
$A_i A_j$	$A_i A_k$	$k_0 + k_1/(2 p_i)$
$A_i A_j$	$A_k A_l$	k_0

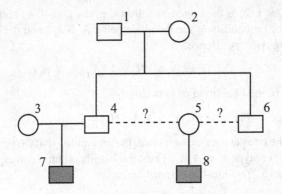

Figure 5.1   A pedigree diagram with only persons 7 and 8 available for typing. Interested in testing whether persons 7 and 8 are related as half siblings or first cousins.

The associated likelihood ratios can be obtained in the following way.

We consider the hypotheses with relationship half siblings versus unrelated:

$$H_p: (Y, Z) \sim (0.5, 0.5, 0); \\ H_d: (Y, Z) \sim (0, 0, 1), \tag{5.5}$$

and relationship first cousins versus unrelated:

$$H_d^*: (Y, Z) \sim (0.75, 0.25, 0); \\ H_d: (Y, Z) \sim (0, 0, 1). \tag{5.6}$$

Suppose that the associated likelihood ratios are, respectively, LR_1 and LR_2, which can be evaluated from Table 5.2. It is obvious that the likelihood ratio for hypotheses set (5.4) can be obtained as

$$LR = LR_1/LR_2. \tag{5.7}$$

We consider the genotypes of the two persons (Table 5.3) and are interested in testing whether they are half siblings or first cousins; the pair of hypotheses is as given in (5.4). We first evaluate the likelihood ratios for the hypothesis pair (5.5):

$$D3S1358 : LR_1 = k_0 + k_1(p_{15} + p_{17})/(2p_{15}p_{17}) + 0$$

$$= 0.5 + 0.25 \times (0.331 + 0.239)/(2 \times 0.331 \times 0.239) = 1.401,$$

$$vWA : LR_1 = k_0 + k_1/(2p_{15}) = 0.5 + 0.25/(2 \times 0.035) = 4.071,$$

$$FGA : LR_1 = k_0 + k_1/p_{22} = 0.5 + 0.25/0.178 = 1.904.$$

Table 5.3   Genotype data of two persons Y and Z at loci D3S1358, wWA and FGA.

Locus	Y	Z
D3S1358	15/17	15/17
vWA	14/15	15/19
FGA	22/22	22/23

Then, we assess the likelihood ratios for the hypothesis pair (5.6) in a similar way. They are

$$D3S1358 : LR_2 = 0.75 + 0.125 \times (0.331 + 0.239)/(2 \times 0.331 \times 0.239) = 1.2,$$

$$vWA : LR_2 = 0.75 + 0.125/(2 \times 0.035) = 2.536,$$

$$FGA : LR_2 = 0.75 + 0.125/0.178 = 1.452.$$

Thus, the likelihood ratios for the pair of hypotheses (5.4) at the three loci, based on Equation (5.7), are, respectively, $1.401/1.2 = 1.17$, $4.071/2.536 = 1.61$, and $1.904/1.452 = 1.31$. The overall likelihood ratio is then $1.17 \times 1.61 \times 1.31 = 2.47$, which seems to provide a larger support to the hypothesis that the two persons are half siblings related.

5.2   Computer software

A computer software has been developed to deal with various two-person kinship problems. The software is named EasyDNA_2Persons which consists of the following steps:

Steps in running the EasyDNA 2Persons software

1 Click the *Load frequency file* button after loading the EasyDNA program, then select the appropriate file

2 Choose the allele pairs at the locus for Y and Z

3a Choose the appropriate relation between Y and Z under H_p (which is, for the above example, *Half siblings*)

3b Choose the appropriate relation between Y and Z under H_d (which is, for the above example, *First cousins*)

4 Click the *Calculate* button

5 Repeat steps 2 and 4 for each of the remaining loci; step 3 (3a–3b) is blocked, since it is no longer needed for the remaining loci.

The procedure steps are straightforward and readers can easily get familiar with the running of the software. It is noted that the theory provided in Section 5.1 and the associated computer software can be used to determine the relationship between any two persons. For illustration, we analyze the example given in Table 5.3 using the EasyDNA_2Persons software. Figure 5.2 presents the captured screen in the running of the software. The likelihood ratios for individual loci are obtained as 1.17, 1.61 and 1.31, with an overall likelihood ratio of 2.47. These values are the same as those obtained above by formulas.

5.3   Kinship testing of two persons: subdivided populations

5.3.1   Joint genotype probability

The issue of population subdivision for paternity and kinship determination has been addressed. Balding and Nichols (1995) considered paternity testing for the case in which the mother, alleged father and 'alternative father' all belong to the same subpopulation. Ayres (2000) proposed tests for kinships in subdivided/structured populations. Clayton *et al.* (2002)

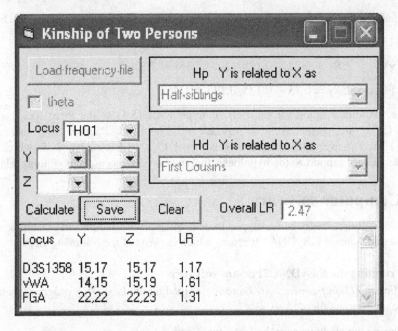

Figure 5.2   Captured screen for running the EasyDNA_2Persons software for determination of kinship for two persons Y and Z whose genotypes are provided in Table 5.3.

discussed that it might make more sense to take account of population subdivision in paternity testing and they referred to the results of Ayres (2000).

In this section, we are using the conditional probability formula for a subdivided population as given in Equation (3.17), where θ there measures the degree of subdivision. We shall derive expressions of the joint genotype probabilities for kinship of any two persons in a subdivided population and likelihood ratios for testing kinship of the two individuals (Fung et al. 2003a).

In order to test whether two given persons have the specific relationship claimed, we first need to find the joint genotype probability $P(Y, Z)$, where Y and Z are respectively genotypes of the two persons who belong to the same subdivided population. Denote respectively the paternal and maternal alleles of Y and Z as Y_P, Z_P, Y_M and Z_M, then the relatedness coefficients $(k_0, 2k_1, k_2)$ can be expressed as

$$k_2 = P(Y_P \equiv Z_P, Y_M \equiv Z_M) + P(Y_P \equiv Z_M, Y_M \equiv Z_P),$$

$$2k_1 = P(Y_P \equiv Z_P) + P(Y_P \equiv Z_M) + P(Y_M \equiv Z_P) + P(Y_M \equiv Z_M),$$

and
$$k_0 = P(\text{no ibd alleles}) = 1 - 2k_1 - k_2,$$

where the symbol '$\equiv$' denotes the ibd relationship of alleles (Evett and Weir 1998).

It is obvious that the relatedness coefficients will play an important role in the evaluation of joint genotype probability $P(Y, Z)$. For two related individuals described with relatedness coefficients $(k_0, 2k_1, k_2)$, there are seven possible combinations of the alleles of Y and Z (irrespective of order). In the following, we consider the simple case in which $Y = Z = A_i A_i$

and demonstrate the principle for the evaluation of their joint genotype probability $P(Y, Z)$. In this case, we have $Y_P = Y_M = Z_P = Z_M = A_i$, so

$P(Y = A_i A_i, Z = A_i A_i)$

$= P(Y_P = Y_M = Z_P = Z_M = A_i)$

$= \sum_{t=0}^{2} P(Y_P = Y_M = Z_P = Z_M = A_i, t \text{ ibd alleles})$

$= P(Y_P = Y_M = Z_P = Z_M = A_i, \text{ no ibd alleles})$

$\quad + P(Y_P = Y_M = Z_P = Z_M = A_i, Y_P \equiv Z_P)$

$\quad + P(Y_P = Y_M = Z_P = Z_M = A_i, Y_P \equiv Z_M)$

$\quad + P(Y_P = Y_M = Z_P = Z_M = A_i, Y_M \equiv Z_P)$

$\quad + P(Y_P = Y_M = Z_P = Z_M = A_i, Y_M \equiv Z_M)$

$\quad + P(Y_P = Y_M = Z_P = Z_M = A_i, Y_P \equiv Z_P, Y_M \equiv Z_M)$

$\quad + P(Y_P = Y_M = Z_P = Z_M = A_i, Y_P \equiv Z_M, Y_M \equiv Z_P)$

$= P(\text{no ibd alleles}) P(A_i, A_i, A_i, A_i)$

$\quad + [P(Y_P \equiv Z_P) + P(Y_P \equiv Z_M) + P(Y_M \equiv Z_P) + P(Y_M \equiv Z_M)] P(A_i, A_i, A_i)$

$\quad + [P(Y_P \equiv Z_P, Y_M \equiv Z_M) + P(Y_P \equiv Z_M, Y_M \equiv Z_P)] P(A_i, A_i).$

This gives immediately the corresponding result reported in the first genotype combination in Table 5.4. The joint genotype probabilities for the other six possible genotype combinations can be derived similarly and we omit the details.

Note that the results in Table 5.4 are general results that can be applied in various ways for the evaluation of joint genotype probabilities. For example, in the penultimate row, under Hardy–Weinberg equilibrium, the probabilities $P(A_i, A_i, A_j, A_k)$ and $P(A_i, A_j, A_k)$ are evaluated as $p_i p_i p_j p_k$ and $p_i p_j p_k$, respectively. Thus, the joint genotype probability $P(Y = A_i A_j, Z = A_i A_k)$ is obtained as $4k_0 p_i^2 p_j p_k + 2k_1 p_i p_j p_k$ under Hardy–Weinberg equilibrium.

In a subdivided population in which Hardy–Weinberg equilibrium does not hold, the evaluation of probabilities is implemented by employing the recursive formula in Equation (3.17). For example, in row 4 of Table 5.4,

$P(A_i, A_i, A_j, A_k) = P(A_i) P(A_i | A_i) P(A_j | A_i, A_i) P(A_k | A_i, A_i, A_j)$

$$= \left[\frac{(1-\theta) p_i}{1 + (0-1)\theta}\right] \left[\frac{\theta + (1-\theta) p_i}{1 + (1-1)\theta}\right] \left[\frac{(1-\theta) p_j}{1 + (2-1)\theta}\right] \left[\frac{(1-\theta) p_k}{1 + (3-1)\theta}\right]$$

$$= \frac{(1-\theta)^2 p_i p_j p_k [\theta + (1-\theta) p_i]}{(1+\theta)(1+2\theta)}$$

and the genotype probability $P(Y, Z)$ can be obtained accordingly.

Table 5.4   The joint genotype probabilities $P(Y, Z)$ for all Y and Z combinations where Y and Z come from the same subdivided population, from Fung *et al.* (2003a). (Reproduced by permission of Elsevier.)

Y	Z	$P(Y, Z)$
$A_i A_i$	$A_i A_i$	$k_0 P(A_i, A_i, A_i, A_i) + 2k_1 P(A_i, A_i, A_i) + k_2 P(A_i, A_i)$
$A_i A_i$	$A_i A_j$	$2k_0 P(A_i, A_i, A_i, A_j) + 2k_1 P(A_i, A_i, A_j)$
$A_i A_i$	$A_j A_j$	$k_0 P(A_i, A_i, A_j, A_j)$
$A_i A_i$	$A_j A_k$	$2k_0 P(A_i, A_i, A_j, A_k)$
$A_i A_j$	$A_i A_j$	$4k_0 P(A_i, A_i, A_j, A_j) + 2k_1 P(A_i, A_i, A_j) + 2k_1 P(A_i, A_j, A_j)$ $+ 2k_2 P(A_i, A_j)$
$A_i A_j$	$A_i A_k$	$4k_0 P(A_i, A_i, A_j, A_k) + 2k_1 P(A_i, A_j, A_k)$
$A_i A_j$	$A_k A_l$	$4k_0 P(A_i, A_j, A_k, A_l)$

One nice feature of the probabilities presented in Table 5.4 is that they can be applied for testing for kinship of any two persons in a subdivided population. Consider the same set of hypotheses as given in (5.2):

$$H_p : (Y, Z) \sim (k_0, 2k_1, k_2);$$

$$H_d : (Y, Z) \sim (1, 0, 0).$$

The genotype probabilities $P(Y, Z|H_p)$ and $P(Y, Z|H_d)$ are straightforward from Table 5.4 and their ratios, i.e. the likelihood ratios for all seven genotype combinations of Y and Z, are listed in Table 5.5. For example in the second row, where $Y = A_i A_i$ and $Z = A_i A_j$, we have from Table 5.4 that

$$LR = \frac{2k_0 P(A_i, A_i, A_i, A_j) + 2k_1 P(A_i, A_i, A_j)}{2P(A_i, A_i, A_i, A_j)}$$

$$= k_0 + \frac{k_1}{P(A_i|A_i, A_i, A_j)}$$

$$= k_0 + \frac{k_1(1 + 2\theta)}{2\theta + (1 - \theta)p_i}.$$

The likelihood ratios for the other six cases can be obtained similarly.

For the usual paternity testing in the no-mother case, the two competing hypotheses are

$$H_p: (C, AF) \sim (0, 1, 0);$$

$$H_d: (C, AF) \sim (1, 0, 0).$$

The paternity indices (PI's) can be obtained from Table 5.5, with specific values of $k_0 = 0$ and $2k_1 = 1$. These indices are reported in Table 5.6. They can be used when the alleged father and the child belong to a subdivided population with the degree of subdivision θ. When the population is in Hardy–Weinberg equilibrium, i.e. $\theta = 0$, the PI's in Table 5.6 reduce to those reported in Table 4.5.

Table 5.5   The likelihood ratios about two competing hypotheses $H_p : (Y, Z) \sim (k_0, 2k_1, k_2)$ versus $H_d : (Y, Z) \sim (1, 0, 0)$ in a subdivided population, from Fung *et al.* (2003a). (Reproduced by permission of Elsevier.)

Y	Z	Likelihood ratio
A_iA_i	A_iA_i	$k_0 + \dfrac{2k_1(1+2\theta)}{3\theta + (1-\theta)p_i} + \dfrac{k_2(1+\theta)(1+2\theta)}{[2\theta + (1-\theta)p_i][3\theta + (1-\theta)p_i]}$
A_iA_i	A_iA_j	$k_0 + \dfrac{k_1(1+2\theta)}{2\theta + (1-\theta)p_i}$
A_iA_i	A_jA_j	k_0
A_iA_i	A_jA_k	k_0
A_iA_j	A_iA_j	$k_0 + \dfrac{k_1(1+2\theta)[2\theta + (1-\theta)(p_i + p_j)] + k_2(1+\theta)(1+2\theta)}{2[\theta + (1-\theta)p_i][\theta + (1-\theta)p_j]}$
A_iA_j	A_iA_k	$k_0 + \dfrac{k_1(1+2\theta)}{2[\theta + (1-\theta)p_i]}$
A_iA_j	A_kA_l	k_0

5.3.2   Relatives involved

In fact, Table 5.5 also provides the likelihood ratio for any two propositions H_p and H_d, which is simply the ratio of the likelihood ratio about H_p versus unrelated and the likelihood ratio about H_d versus unrelated. Particularly, we consider the paternity testing in the no-mother

Table 5.6   Paternity index (*PI*) for the competing hypotheses H_p: AF is true father of the child versus H_d: the father is a random unrelated mean, i.e. $H_p : (C, AF) \sim (0, 1, 0)$ versus $H_d : (C, AF) \sim (1, 0, 0)$, in a subdivided population.

C	AF	PI
A_iA_i	A_iA_i	$\dfrac{1+2\theta}{3\theta + (1-\theta)p_i}$
A_iA_i	A_iA_j	$\dfrac{1+2\theta}{2[2\theta + (1-\theta)p_i]}$
A_iA_j	A_iA_i	$\dfrac{1+2\theta}{2[2\theta + (1-\theta)p_i]}$
A_iA_j	A_iA_j	$\dfrac{(1+2\theta)[2\theta + (1-\theta)(p_i + p_j)]}{4[\theta + (1-\theta)p_i][\theta + (1-\theta)p_j]}$
A_iA_j	A_iA_k	$\dfrac{1+2\theta}{4[\theta + (1-\theta)p_i]}$

Table 5.7 The likelihood ratios about two competing hypotheses $H_p : AF$ is the true father of the child versus $H_d : AF$ is a paternal relative of the child, i.e. $H_p : (C, AF) \sim (0, 1, 0)$ versus $H_d : (C, AF) \sim (k_0, 2k_1, 0)$, in a subdivided population, from Fung *et al.* (2003a). (Reproduced by permission of Elsevier.)

C	AF	Likelihood ratio
$A_i A_i$	$A_i A_i$	$\dfrac{1 + 2\theta}{k_0[3\theta + (1 - \theta)p_i] + 2k_1(1 + 2\theta)}$
$A_i A_i$	$A_i A_j$	$\dfrac{1 + 2\theta}{2k_0[2\theta + (1 - \theta)p_i] + 2k_1(1 + 2\theta)}$
$A_i A_j$	$A_i A_i$	$\dfrac{1 + 2\theta}{2k_0[2\theta + (1 - \theta)p_i] + 2k_1(1 + 2\theta)}$
$A_i A_j$	$A_i A_j$	$\dfrac{(1 + 2\theta)[2\theta + (1 - \theta)(p_i + p_j)]}{4k_0[\theta + (1 - \theta)p_i][\theta + (1 - \theta)p_j] + 2k_1(1 + 2\theta)[2\theta + (1 - \theta)(p_i + p_j)]}$
$A_i A_j$	$A_i A_k$	$\dfrac{1 + 2\theta}{4k_0[\theta + (1 - \theta)p_i] + 2k_1(1 + 2\theta)}$

case, where the two competing hypotheses are described by

H_p: $(C, AF) \sim (0, 1, 0)$;

H_d: $(C, AF) \sim (k_0, 2k_1, 0)$.

Under H_p, AF is the true father of the child, while under the alternative proposition H_d, the defendant argued that AF is only a paternal relative (such as uncle, say) of the child. The likelihood ratios for all possible genotype combinations of C and AF are listed in Table 5.7, which are derived directly from Table 5.5.

When the alleged father is not available but his relative Z is, we can type the relative instead. The hypotheses of interest are

H_p: a relative of Z is the true father of the child Y;

H_d: the true father is a random unrelated man.

That is,

H_p: $(Y, Z) \sim (k_0, 2k_1, 0)$;

H_d: $(Y, Z) \sim (1, 0, 0)$.

If the likelihood ratio for the hypotheses is denoted by LR, then the following simple relationship can be obtained:

$$LR = k_0 + (1 - k_0)PI = (1 - 2k_1) + 2k_1 PI, \tag{5.8}$$

which can be verified throughout all of the seven cases listed in Table 5.5. The PI's are listed in Table 5.6.

Using the notation δ_0 introduced in Evett and Weir (1998), Equation (5.8) can be expressed equivalently as

$$LR = \delta_0 + (1 - \delta_0)PI. \tag{5.9}$$

In fact, δ_0 is defined as the probability that no alleles in the two individuals Y and Z are ibd, which is obviously k_0. Ayres (2000) reported Equation (5.9) when δ_0 takes the specific values of half siblings and first cousin relationships.

A measure of relatedness θ_{AT} (Evett and Weir 1998) for individuals AF and the true father TF of the child is defined as the probability that two alleles, one taken at random from each of AF and TF, are ibd, which is just the kinship coefficient F between AF and TF defined in Equation (3.21). Since each of the two alleles of TF is equally likely of being transmitted to the child, θ_{AT} and k_1 are equivalent. So, Equation (5.8) can also be expressed as

$$LR = (1 - 2\theta_{AT}) + 2\theta_{AT} PI. \tag{5.10}$$

Equation (5.10) was reported in the special case that θ is taken as zero (Evett and Weir 1998), which is applicable in the population when the Hardy–Weinberg law holds.

5.4   Examples with software

The computer software EasyDNA_2Persons discussed earlier in Section 5.2 can also be used for kinship testing of any two persons in a subdivided population. The steps in running the software are exactly the same as those listed in Section 5.2 except for the addition of a step 1a after step 1:

1a Click the *theta* button and input the appropriate θ.

The program gives the likelihood ratios under Hardy–Weinberg equilibrium ($\theta = 0$) and under a subdivided population having the chosen θ value. Two real case examples reported in Fung *et al.* (2003a) are considered.

The first case of disputed paternity testing was provided by the Hong Kong Government Laboratory, where 12 STR loci (D3S1358, vWA, FGA, D5S818, D13S317, D7S820, D8S1179, D21S11, D18S51, THO1, TPOX, CSF1PO) were typed for a child and an alleged father [see Table 5.8 for information on the genotypes and, for the allele frequencies, one can refer to Wong *et al.* (2001)]. The following four hypotheses are proposed to describe the relationship between the alleged father and the child:

H_p: the alleged father is the true father of the child;

H_{d1}: the alleged father is unrelated to the child;

H_{d2}: the alleged father is the uncle of the child;

H_{d3}: the alleged father and the child are full siblings.

The example is analyzed using the EasyDNA_2Persons software. The overall likelihood ratios about H_p versus H_{di}, $i = 1, 2, 3$ for various values of θ are also obtained and they are shown in Table 5.9. In testing H_p versus H_{d1}, the *PI* when $\theta = 0$ is equal to 428, which is not too large. The *PI* decreases when the population structure is taken into account. When $\theta = 0.03$, the *PI* drops by about 70% to 136 and the genetic evidence may not be strong enough for paternity.

If we are testing H_p against other relationships such as uncle and nephew (H_{d2}), the genetic evidence would become much weaker. The *PI* is only 9.7 when $\theta = 0$, and is even smaller

Table 5.8   The genotypes of the alleged father and the child of the two disputed paternity testing cases in Hong Kong and Spain, from Fung *et al.* (2003a). (Reproduced by permission of Elsevier.)

Locus	Hong Kong		Spain	
	Alleged father	Child	Alleged father	Child
D3S1358	15/16	16/17	16/18	16/18
vWA	14/18	14/18	16/18	18/18
FGA	22/24	20/24	22/24	21/22
THO1	7/9	6/7	9/9.3	7/9.3
TPOX	11/11	8/11	8/9	9/11
CSF1PO	10/12	12/12	9/12	9/11
D5S818	10/11	11/12	11/11	11/13
D13S317	9/10	10/10	12/13	8/12
D7S820	8/11	8/8	11/11	11/11
D8S1179	11/14	14/16	10/13	10/13
D21S11	29/32.2	30/32.2	30/30	30/31
D18S51	13/14	13/14	14/14	14/18
D16S539	—	—	9/11	9/12

when the population subdivision is taken into account. Similar findings are observed when we are testing H_p versus H_{d3}.

The second case of disputed paternity testing comes from a Spanish population. The same set of 12 STR loci with an additional locus D16S539 were typed for a child and an alleged father [also see Table 5.8 for the genotypes and, for the allele frequencies, one can refer to Gusmão *et al.* (2000)]. The same sets of hypotheses are chosen.

In testing H_p versus H_{d_1}, unlike the case in Hong Kong, the overall *PI* when $\theta = 0$ is equal to 135 689 (see Table 5.9) which is very large, giving very strong evidence for paternity. When we increase the value of θ from 0.01, 0.02 to 0.03, the *PI* becomes 30, 12 and 5.9% of the *PI* when $\theta = 0$. The value drops substantially with the increase in θ. If we investigate the individual *PI* value (not shown) at each locus, we notice that for all loci, except CSF1PO,

Table 5.9   Likelihood ratios with different θ values for the two disputed paternity testing cases in Hong Kong and Spain.

Hypotheses[a]	$\theta = 0$	0.01	0.02	0.03
(Hong Kong)				
H_p versus H_{d1}	428	280	192	136
H_p versus H_{d2}	9.7	8.6	7.6	6.8
H_p versus H_{d3}	12.2	11.9	11.6	11.4
(Spain)				
H_p versus H_{d1}	135 689	41 148	16 766	7 989
H_p versus H_{d2}	45.5	37.5	31.2	26.2
H_p versus H_{d3}	12.4	12.4	12.4	12.4

[a] H_p: father and son; H_{d1}: unrelated persons; H_{d2}: uncle and nephew; H_{d3}: full siblings

the *PI* drops by a few percent to about 30% when θ is increased from 0 to 0.03. The *PI* value at CSF1PO, however, has a large drop from 20.8 to 11.7, 8.2 and 6.4 for $\theta = 0.01, 0.02$ and 0.03, respectively. If we look at the genotypes of the alleged father and the child, we find that they share one common allele (9) at CSF1PO, which is a very rare allele in the Spanish population (with frequency 0.012). The value of θ has a crucial effect on *PI* for the case with a rare allele.

Table 5.9 also shows the *PI's* for the other two sets of hypotheses. From both paternity cases in Hong Kong and Spain, we notice that the paternity indices for testing H_p (father and son) versus H_{d3} (full siblings) have values of about 10. This phenomenon is not unusual, and it may have implications for some paternity cases such as those found in immigration (Fung *et al.* 2002, see also Section 4.9.2).

In the majority of paternity cases, *PI* values are so high that even if there is strong population structure, the final consequences will generally be of little importance. But, in deficiency paternity testing and many immigration cases, the effect of population subdivision may be of importance and mistakes could be made if this effect is not properly taken into account in the calculations.

5.5   Three persons situation: HWE

The testing for a biological relationship between two persons in a population with Hardy–Weinberg equilibrium was studied in detail by Li and Sacks (1954). Ayres (2000) and Fung *et al.* (2003a) have successfully generalized Li and Sack's results to a subdivided population. In the following, we consider an extension of the results to a three persons situation.

Let X, Z denote the maternal and paternal relatives of Y, respectively, and suppose that X and Z are unrelated. The relatedness coefficients between X and Y, and between Y and Z are denoted as $(k_0^{XY}, 2k_1^{XY}, 0)$ and $(k_0^{YZ}, 2k_1^{YZ}, 0)$, respectively. The population is assumed to be in Hardy–Weinberg equilibrium. In order to determine the biological relationship among the three individuals X, Y, and Z, we list in Table 5.10 all the possible joint genotype probabilities $P(X, Y, Z)$.

To see the derivation of the joint genotype probabilities given in Table 5.10, we consider $Y = A_i A_i$, $X = A_i A_j$ and $Z = A_k A_l$, $j \neq i, k \neq i, l \neq i$. It is concluded from the genotypes of X, Y and Z that X and Y may share ibd allele A_i, and Y and Z share no ibd alleles. The joint genotype probability can then be evaluated as

$$P(X = A_i A_j, Y = A_i A_i, Z = A_{kl})$$

$$= P(X = A_i A_j, Y = A_i A_i)P(Z = A_{kl}) \times k_0^{YZ}$$

$$= \sum_{t=0}^{2} P(X = A_i A_j, Y = A_i A_i | X \text{ and } Y \text{ share } t \text{ ibd alleles})$$

$$\times P(X \text{ and } Y \text{ share } t \text{ ibd alleles}) \times P(Z = A_{kl}) \times k_0^{YZ}$$

$$= [P(X = A_i A_j)P(Y = A_i A_i)k_0^{XY} + P(A_i, A_i, A_j) \times 2k_1^{XY}] \times P(Z = A_k A_l) \times k_0^{YZ}$$

$$= k_0^{XY} k_0^{YZ} p_i^2 P(X = A_i A_j)P(Z = A_k A_l) + 2k_1^{XY} k_0^{YZ} p_i^2 p_j P(Z = A_k A_l)$$

$$= k_0^{XY} k_0^{YZ} p_i^2 P(X)P(Z) + 2k_1^{XY} k_0^{YZ} p_i^2 p_j P(Z), \tag{5.11}$$

where $P(X)$ and $P(Z)$ are abbreviated forms of $P(X = A_i A_j)$ and $P(Z = A_k A_l)$, respectively.

Table 5.10   The joint genotype probabilities $P(X, Y, Z)$, for all possible combinations of X, Y and Z (regardless of order X and Z), where X and Z are the maternal and paternal relatives of Y, respectively; X and Z are unrelated; $(k_0^{XY}, 2k_1^{XY}, 0)$ are the relatedness coefficients of X and Y; and $(k_0^{YZ}, 2k_1^{YZ}, 0)$ are the relatedness coefficients of Y and Z, from Fung *et al.* (2006). (Reproduced by permission of Elsevier.)

Y	X	Z	$P(X, Y, Z)$
A_iA_i	A_iA_j	A_iA_k	$k_0^{XY}k_0^{YZ}p_i^2 P(X)P(Z) + 2k_0^{XY}k_1^{YZ}p_i^2 p_k P(X)$
			$\quad + 2k_1^{XY}k_0^{YZ}p_i^2 p_j P(Z) + 4k_1^{XY}k_1^{YZ}p_i^2 p_j p_k$
	A_iA_j	A_kA_l	$k_0^{XY}k_0^{YZ}p_i^2 P(X)P(Z) + 2k_1^{XY}k_0^{YZ}p_i^2 p_j P(Z)$
		$(k, l \neq i)$	
	A_jA_k	A_lA_m	$k_0^{XY}k_0^{YZ}p_i^2 P(X)P(Z)$
	$(j, k \neq i)$	$(l, m \neq i)$	
A_iA_j	A_iA_j	A_iA_j	$8k_0^{XY}k_0^{YZ}p_i^3 p_j^3 + 4k_0^{XY}k_1^{YZ}(p_i + p_j)p_i^2 p_j^2$
$(j \neq i)$	$(j \neq i)$	$(j \neq i)$	$\quad + 4k_1^{XY}k_0^{YZ}(p_i + p_j)p_i^2 p_j^2 + 8k_1^{XY}k_1^{YZ}p_i^2 p_j^2$
		A_iA_k	$4k_0^{XY}k_0^{YZ}p_i^2 p_j^2 P(Z) + 4k_0^{XY}k_1^{YZ}p_i^2 p_j^2 p_k$
		$(k \neq j)$	$\quad + 2k_1^{XY}k_0^{YZ}(p_i + p_j)p_i p_j P(Z) + 4k_1^{XY}k_1^{YZ}p_i^2 p_j p_k$
		A_kA_l	$4k_0^{XY}k_0^{YZ}p_i^2 p_j^2 P(Z)$
		$(k, l \neq i, j)$	$\quad + 2k_1^{XY}k_0^{YZ}(p_i + p_j)p_i p_j P(Z)$
	A_iA_k	A_iA_l	$2k_0^{XY}k_0^{YZ}p_i p_j P(X)P(Z) + 2k_0^{XY}k_1^{YZ}p_i p_j p_l P(X)$
	$(k \neq j)$	$(l \neq j)$	$\quad + 2k_1^{XY}k_0^{YZ}p_i p_j p_k P(Z)$
		A_jA_l	$2k_0^{XY}k_0^{YZ}p_i p_j P(X)P(Z) + 2k_0^{XY}k_1^{YZ}p_i p_j p_l P(X)$
		$(l \neq i)$	$\quad + 2k_1^{XY}k_0^{YZ}p_i p_j p_k P(Z) + 4k_1^{XY}k_1^{YZ}p_i p_j p_k p_l$
		A_lA_m	$2k_0^{XY}k_0^{YZ}p_i p_j P(X)P(Z) + 2k_1^{XY}k_0^{YZ}p_i p_j p_k P(Z)$
		$(l, m \neq i, j)$	
	A_kA_l	A_mA_n	$2k_0^{XY}k_0^{YZ}p_i p_j P(X)P(Z)$
	$(k, l \neq i, j)$	$(m, n \neq i, j)$	

The above derivation considers the situation that $j \neq i$. When $j = i$, i.e. $X = A_iA_i$ and $Y = A_iA_i$, it looks as though X and Y may share two ibd A_i alleles. This is, however, impossible, since X and Y are only maternally related and so they cannot share two ibd alleles, i.e. $k_2^{XY} = 0$. Hence, the same formula in Equation (5.11) results when $j = i$. Thus, we have obtained the joint genotype probability Equation (5.11) for $Y = A_iA_i$, $X = A_iA_j$ and $Z = A_kA_l$, $k, l \neq i$, which is shown in the second row of Table 5.10.

The other joint genotype probabilities in Table 5.10 can be shown in a similar way [see also Fung *et al.* (2006)]. The details are omitted for brevity. The expressions in Table 5.10 can be used to examine the biological relationship among any three persons X, Y, and Z where X and Z are unrelated. For example, we can use one maternal relative and one paternal relative to identify a missing person. We can also examine the biological relationship between Y and Z when the biological relationship between X and Y are known without error such as in the paternity testing case.

For two competing hypotheses H_p and H_d, the likelihood ratio is

$$LR = \frac{P(\text{evidence}|H_p)}{P(\text{evidence}|H_d)} = \frac{P(X, Y, Z|H_p)}{P(X, Y, Z|H_d)}. \tag{5.12}$$

It is a ratio of two like genotype probabilities, one evaluated under H_p and the other under H_d. These probabilities can be obtained from Table 5.10, with values of $(k_0^{XY}, 2k_1^{XY}, k_0^{YZ}, 2k_1^{YZ})$ determined under H_p and H_d. To illustrate this, we consider a paternity testing problem with genotypes of three persons provided in Table 5.11. Person Y is always regarded as the child in the following consideration:

(i) X is the mother of Y and Z is the alleged father with propositions

H_p : Z is the true father of the child Y;
H_d : the true father is a random unrelated man. $\tag{5.13}$

In this case, the relatedness coefficients for X and Y are $k_0^{XY} = 0$ and $2k_1^{XY} = 1$, and for Y and Z are $k_0^{YZ} = 0$ and $2k_1^{XY} = 1$. Plugging them into the appropriate formulas in Table 5.10 can provide the likelihood ratio we want. In fact, this is just a standard trio problem. The overall likelihood ratio for genotypes in Table 5.11 is obtained as 37.36. The details are omitted for brevity.

(ii) The mother is unavailable but her brother is. Then X is the uncle of the child Y and Z is the alleged father. The propositions are the same as those listed in (5.13). The relatedness coefficients are

$$k_0^{XY} = 2k_1^{XY} = 0.5, \quad k_0^{YZ} = 0 \quad \text{and} \quad 2k_1^{YZ} = 1, \quad \text{under } H_p;$$
$$k_0^{XY} = 2k_1^{XY} = 0.5, \quad k_0^{YZ} = 1 \quad \text{and} \quad 2k_1^{YZ} = 0, \quad \text{under } H_d.$$

Table 5.11   Genotype data of three persons Y, X and Z at loci D3S1358, wWA and FGA.

Locus	Y	X	Z
D3S1358	15/17	15/16	17/18
vWA	18/18	18/19	18/18
FGA	20/21	20/21	19/20

Suppose we write the likelihood ratio in Equation (5.12) as $LR = Num/Den$. Based on the formulas in Table 5.10 and the genotypes in Table 5.11, we have

$$D3S1358: \quad Num = 2k_0^{XY}k_0^{YZ}p_ip_jP(X)P(Z) + 2k_0^{XY}k_1^{YZ}p_ip_jp_lP(X)$$

$$+ 2k_1^{XY}k_0^{YZ}p_ip_jp_kP(Z) + 4k_1^{XY}k_1^{YZ}p_ip_jp_kp_l$$

$$= 2 \times 0.5 \times 0 + 2 \times 0.5 \times 0.5 \times p_{15}p_{17}p_{18} \times 2p_{15}p_{16}$$

$$+ 0.5 \times 0 + 0.5 \times p_{15}p_{17}p_{16}p_{18}$$

$$= 2 \times 0.5 \times 0.5 \times 0.331 \times 0.239 \times 0.056 \times 2 \times 0.331$$

$$\times 0.326 + 0.5 \times 0.331 \times 0.239 \times 0.326 \times 0.056$$

$$= 1.20 \times 10^{-3},$$

$$Den = 2 \times 0.5 \times 1 \times 0.331 \times 0.239 \times 2 \times 0.331 \times 0.326$$

$$\times 2 \times 0.239 \times 0.056 + 0.5 \times 0 + 0.5 \times 1 \times 0.331$$

$$\times 0.239 \times 0.326 \times 2 \times 0.239 \times 0.056 + 2 \times 0.5 \times 0$$

$$= 8.02 \times 10^{-4},$$

$$LR = 1.20 \times 10^{-3}/(8.02 \times 10^{-4}) = 1.50,$$

and the likelihood ratios for vWA and FGA can be obtained similarly. They are

$$vWA : LR = 6.25, \quad \text{and} \quad FGA : LR = 3.19,$$

giving an overall likelihood ratio $LR = 29.9$.

(iii) Both the mother and alleged father are unavailable, but the brother of the mother and the father of the alleged father are. Then X is the maternal uncle of the child Y, and Z is the paternal grandfather of the child under H_p. Thus, the propositions become

H_p : Z is the paternal grandfather of the child Y;
H_d : the true father is a random unrelated man. $\hspace{1cm}$ (5.14)

The relatedness coefficients are

$$k_0^{XY} = 2k_1^{XY} = 0.5, \quad k_0^{YZ} = 2k_1^{YZ} = 0.5, \quad \text{under} \quad H_p;$$

$$k_0^{XY} = 2k_1^{XY} = 0.5, \quad k_0^{YZ} = 1 \text{ and } 2k_1^{YZ} = 0, \quad \text{under} \quad H_d.$$

Based on the formulas in Table 5.10 and the genotypes in Table 5.11, we have

$$D3S1358: \quad Num = 2k_0^{XY}k_0^{YZ}p_ip_jP(X)P(Z) + 2k_0^{XY}k_1^{YZ}p_ip_jp_lP(X)$$

$$+ 2k_1^{XY}k_0^{YZ}p_ip_jp_kP(Z) + 4k_1^{XY}k_1^{YZ}p_ip_jp_kp_l$$

$$= 2 \times 0.5 \times 0.5 \times 0.331 \times 0.239 \times 2 \times 0.331$$

$$\times 0.326 \times 2 \times 0.239 \times 0.056 + 0.5 \times 0.5$$

$$\times 0.331 \times 0.239 \times 0.056 \times 2 \times 0.331 \times 0.326$$

$$+ 0.5 \times 0.5 \times 0.331 \times 0.239 \times 0.326$$

$$\times 2 \times 0{,}239 \times 0.056 + 0.5 \times 0.5 \times 0.331$$
$$\times 0.239 \times 0.326 \times 0.056$$

$$= \quad 1.001 \times 10^{-3},$$

$$Den \quad = \quad 8.02 \times 10^{-4}, \text{ as obtained previously in (ii)},$$

$$LR \quad = \quad 1.001 \times 10^{-3}/(8.02 \times 10^{-4}) = 1.25,$$

and the likelihood ratios at vWA and FGA can be obtained similarly. They are

$$\text{vWA}: LR = 3.62, \quad \text{and} \quad \text{FGA}: LR = 2.09,$$

giving an overall likelihood ratio $LR = 9.46$.

As we can see from previous discussions, the overall likelihood ratio is the highest in case (i) of the standard trio problem, becomes smaller in case (ii) in which the mother of the child is not available for typing but her brother is, and drops again in case (iii), in which, additionally, the alleged father is unavailable but his father is. In other words, the likelihood ratio becomes smaller and smaller when the biological relationship between the child and his/her maternal and paternal relatives who provide genotyping information becomes looser and looser. This phenomenon is generally true in kinship testing.

5.6 Computer software and example

Although we have extended Li and Sacks' (1954) joint genotype probability for two persons to the case of three persons X, Y and Z, where X and Z are biologically unrelated, the formulas given in Table 5.10 are, however, rather lengthy. We have developed a computer software named EasyDNA_3Persons to deal with the associated kinship problems.

Steps in running the EasyDNA 3Persons software

1 Click the *Load frequency file* button after loading the EasyDNA program, then select the appropriate file

2 Choose the allele pairs at the locus for Y, X and Z

3a Choose the appropriate maternal relation between Y and X under H_p [which is, for the example in case (iii) above, *Nephew–uncle*]

3b Choose the appropriate paternal relation between Y and Z under H_p [which is, for the example in case (iii) above, *Child–grandparent*]

3c Choose the appropriate maternal relation between Y and X under H_d [which is, for the example in case (iii) above, *Nephew–uncle*]

3d Choose the appropriate paternal relation between Y and Z under H_d [which is, for the example in case (iii) above, *unrelated*]

4 Click the *Calculate* button

5 Repeat steps 2 and 4 for each of the remaining loci; step 3 (3a–3d) is blocked, since it is no longer needed for the remaining loci.

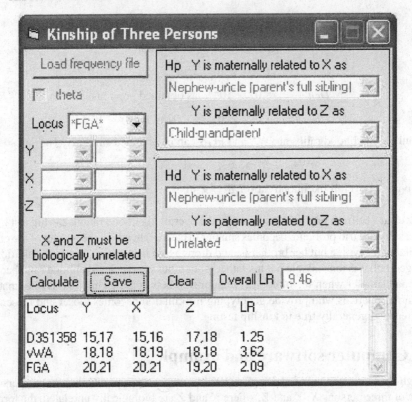

Figure 5.3   Captured screen for running the EasyDNA_3Persons software for analyzing the example given in case (iii) of Section 5.5.

The procedure steps are straightforward and easy to follow.

We use the software to deal with the example in case (iii) above. Figure 5.3 gives the screen capture in the running of the program. Although we have shown earlier that the numerical calculations are rather tedious, we can see from the figure that our EasyDNA_3Persons can handle the problem easily. The likelihood ratios are obtained as 1.25, 3.62 and 2.09 for individual loci, giving an overall ratio of 9.46.

5.7   Three persons situation: subdivided populations

5.7.1   Standard trio

Consider the trio problem in which the DNA profiles of the child, mother and alleged father are typed. Suppose that the mother, alleged father and biological father of the child are assumed to be unrelated to one another. The usual hypotheses are given as

H_p : the alleged father is the true father of the child;

H_d : the true father is a random unrelated man.

(5.15)

Let M, C and AF be the genotypes of the mother, her child and the alleged father, respectively. The paternity index can be expressed as (Section 4.1.1)

$$PI = \frac{P(C|M, AF, H_p)}{P(C|M, AF, H_d)}. \tag{5.16}$$

Consider a particular locus that $C = A_i A_j$, $M = A_i A_k$ and $AF = A_j A_l$. In this situation, the numerator of the paternity index is $(1/2) \times (1/2)$. However, the denominator is not $(1/2)p_j$ because the population is not in Hardy–Weinberg equilibrium. It is in fact equal to

$$P(C = A_i A_j | M = A_i A_k, AF = A_j A_l, H_d) = (1/2)P(A_j | A_i, A_k, A_j, A_l, H_d),$$

since the mother has $1/2$ chance of passing A_i to the child. The conditional probability of observing the other allele A_j for the child is obtained according to Equation (3.17). The denominator then becomes

$$(1/2)[\theta + (1 - \theta)p_j]/[1 + (4 - 1)\theta].$$

Thus, the paternity index is

$$PI = \frac{(1/4)}{(1/2)[\theta + (1 - \theta)p_j]/(1 + 3\theta)}$$

$$= \frac{(1 + 3\theta)}{2[\theta + (1 - \theta)p_j]}.$$

The paternity indices for other combinations of genotypes of C, M and AF can be derived similarly, and they are all shown in Table 5.12 [see also Evett and Weir (1998)].

5.7.2   A relative of the alleged father is the true father

In the situation in which the alleged father gives an alternative explanation that his relative is the true father of the child, the defense proposition becomes

H_d : a relative of the alleged father is the true father of the child.

The prosecution proposition H_p remains unchanged, as in (5.15). Suppose that the genotypes of the child, mother and alleged father are obtained as $C = A_i A_j$, $M = A_i A_k$ and $AF = A_j A_l$, respectively. The numerator of the likelihood ratio in Equation (5.16) is $(1/2) \times (1/2) = 1/4$. For the denominator, it is concluded from the genotypes of the child and the mother that $C_M = A_i$ and $C_P = A_j$. So

$$P(C = A_i A_j | M = A_i A_k, AF = A_j A_l, H_d)$$

$$= P(C_M = A_i, C_P = A_j | M = A_i A_k, AF = A_j A_l, H_d)$$

$$= (1/2)P(C_P = A_j | M = A_i A_k, AF = A_j A_l, H_d).$$

Let $(k_0, 2k_1, k_2)$ be the relatedness coefficients between C and AF. Consider the probability that $C_P = A_j$ is not ibd with the A_j allele of AF is k_0 and the probability that $C_P = A_j$ is ibd with the A_j allele of AF is k_1, so

$$P(C_P = A_j | M = A_i A_k, AF = A_j A_l, H_d)$$

$$= k_0 P(A_j | A_i, A_j, A_k, A_l) + k_1$$

$$= k_0 \frac{\theta + (1 - \theta)p_j}{1 + 3\theta} + k_1.$$

Table 5.12   Paternity index (*PI*) for a standard trio case in a subdivided population.

C	M	AF	PI
A_iA_i	A_iA_i	A_iA_i	$\dfrac{1+3\theta}{4\theta+(1-\theta)p_i}$
		A_iA_j	$\dfrac{1+3\theta}{2[3\theta+(1-\theta)p_i]}$
	A_iA_j	A_iA_i	$\dfrac{1+3\theta}{3\theta+(1-\theta)p_i}$
		A_iA_j	$\dfrac{1+3\theta}{2[2\theta+(1-\theta)p_i]}$
		A_iA_k	$\dfrac{1+3\theta}{2[2\theta+(1-\theta)p_i]}$
A_iA_j	A_iA_i	A_iA_j	$\dfrac{1+3\theta}{2[\theta+(1-\theta)p_j]}$
		A_jA_j	$\dfrac{1+3\theta}{2\theta+(1-\theta)p_j}$
		A_jA_k	$\dfrac{1+3\theta}{2[\theta+(1-\theta)p_j]}$
	A_iA_j	A_iA_i	$\dfrac{1+3\theta}{4\theta+(1-\theta)(p_i+p_j)}$
		A_iA_j	$\dfrac{1+3\theta}{4\theta+(1-\theta)(p_i+p_j)}$
		A_iA_k	$\dfrac{1+3\theta}{2[3\theta+(1-\theta)(p_i+p_j)]}$
	A_iA_k	A_iA_j	$\dfrac{1+3\theta}{2[\theta+(1-\theta)p_j]}$
		A_jA_j	$\dfrac{1+3\theta}{2\theta+(1-\theta)p_j}$
		A_jA_k	$\dfrac{1+3\theta}{2[\theta+(1-\theta)p_j]}$
		A_jA_l	$\dfrac{1+3\theta}{2[\theta+(1-\theta)p_j]}$

If follows that the likelihood ratio is

$$LR = \frac{1/4}{(1/2)\left[k_1+k_0\frac{\theta+(1-\theta)p_i}{1+3\theta}\right]}$$

$$= \frac{1+3\theta}{2k_1(1+3\theta)+2k_0[\theta+(1-\theta)p_j]}$$

$$= \frac{1 + 3\theta}{2F(1 + 3\theta) + 2(1 - 2F)[\theta + (1 - \theta)p_j]},$$

where F is the kinship coefficient between the alleged father and his relative who is the true father of the child under H_d (see Section 4.3). This likelihood ratio is reported in the last row of Table 5.13.

The likelihood ratios for all other genotype combinations of C, M and AF can be derived similarly. These ratios are all shown in Table 5.13. In particular, we also show the likelihood ratios for the defense proposition H_d^*: a brother of the alleged father is the true father of the child, in which the kinship coefficient between the alleged father and the true father is $F = 1/4$. The ratios for this particular H_d^* proposition are presented in the last column of Table 5.13, and have also been reported by Buckleton *et al.* (2005).

5.7.3   Alleged father unavailable but his relative is

When the alleged father is not available and his relative R is tested instead, then the hypotheses of interest are given as

H_p : a relative of R is the true father of the child;

H_d : the true father is a random unrelated man.

Based on a similar argument as presented in Section 4.4, in which Hardy–Weinberg equilibrium holds, we can derive the avuncular index for the above hypotheses as

$$AI = \frac{PI}{LR},$$

where PI and LR are provided in Tables 5.12 and 5.13, respectively, and the genotypes of R are listed as those shown in the AF columns.

Morris *et al.* (1988) noticed the following relationship under the standard trio case with Hardy–Weinberg equilibrium:

$$AI = (1 - 2F) + 2F \times PI.$$

After some simple derivations, this relationship can be shown to hold true in the current situation in which the mother, alleged father, R and true father belong to the same subdivided population. In addition to the findings we obtained earlier for the no-mother case, this relationship is found to hold true for populations with Hardy–Weinberg equilibrium or with subdivision, and in the with-mother or without-mother case.

5.7.4   Example

We consider the standard trio example given in Table 4.2 in which the mother, alleged father and true father come from a subdivided population. The value of θ is taken to be 0.01. The hypotheses of interest are

H_p : the alleged father is the true father of the child;
H_d : the true father is a random unrelated man.   (5.17)

Based on the formulas given in Table 5.12, the paternity indices are obtained as

$$\text{D3S1358} : \quad PI = \frac{1 + 3\theta}{2[\theta + (1 - \theta)p_{17}]} = \frac{1 + 3 \times 0.01}{2 \times [0.01 + (1 - 0.01) \times 0.239]} = 2.088,$$

Table 5.13   Likelihood ratio for a trio case in a subdivided population with H_p: the alleged father is the true father of the child versus H_d: a relative of the alleged father is the true father; F is the kinship coefficient for the alleged father and his relative who is the true father under H_d, with $F = 1/4$ being the coefficient for brothers.

C	M	AF	LR	LR($F = 1/4$)
A_iA_i	A_iA_i	A_iA_i	$\dfrac{1+3\theta}{2F(1+3\theta)+(1-2F)[4\theta+(1-\theta)p_i]}$	$\dfrac{2(1+3\theta)}{1+7\theta+(1-\theta)p_i}$
		A_iA_j	$\dfrac{1+3\theta}{2F(1+3\theta)+2(1-2F)[3\theta+(1-\theta)p_i]}$	$\dfrac{2(1+3\theta)}{1+9\theta+2(1-\theta)p_i}$
A_iA_j	A_iA_i	A_iA_i	$\dfrac{1+3\theta}{2F(1+3\theta)+(1-2F)[3\theta+(1-\theta)p_i]}$	$\dfrac{2(1+3\theta)}{1+6\theta+(1-\theta)p_i}$
		A_iA_j	$\dfrac{1+3\theta}{2F(1+3\theta)+2(1-2F)[2\theta+(1-\theta)p_i]}$	$\dfrac{2(1+3\theta)}{1+7\theta+2(1-\theta)p_i}$
		A_iA_k	$\dfrac{1+3\theta}{2F(1+3\theta)+2(1-2F)[2\theta+(1-\theta)p_i]}$	$\dfrac{2(1+3\theta)}{1+7\theta+2(1-\theta)p_i}$
A_iA_j	A_iA_i	A_iA_j	$\dfrac{1+3\theta}{2F(1+3\theta)+2(1-2F)[\theta+(1-\theta)p_j]}$	$\dfrac{2(1+3\theta)}{1+5\theta+2(1-\theta)p_j}$
		A_jA_j	$\dfrac{1+3\theta}{2F(1+3\theta)+(1-2F)[2\theta+(1-\theta)p_j]}$	$\dfrac{2(1+3\theta)}{1+5\theta+(1-\theta)p_j}$
		A_jA_k	$\dfrac{1+3\theta}{2F(1+3\theta)+2(1-2F)[\theta+(1-\theta)p_j]}$	$\dfrac{2(1+3\theta)}{1+5\theta+2(1-\theta)p_j}$
A_iA_j	A_iA_i	A_iA_i	$\dfrac{1+3\theta}{2F(1+3\theta)+(1-2F)[4\theta+(1-\theta)p_0^*]}$	$\dfrac{2(1+3\theta)}{1+7\theta+(1-\theta)p_0}$
		A_iA_j	$\dfrac{1+3\theta}{2F(1+3\theta)+(1-2F)[4\theta+(1-\theta)p_0]}$	$\dfrac{2(1+3\theta)}{1+7\theta+(1-\theta)p_0}$
		A_iA_k	$\dfrac{1+3\theta}{2F(1+3\theta)+2(1-2F)[3\theta+(1-\theta)p_0]}$	$\dfrac{2(1+3\theta)}{1+9\theta+2(1-\theta)p_0}$
A_iA_k	A_iA_j	A_iA_j	$\dfrac{1+3\theta}{2F(1+3\theta)+2(1-2F)[\theta+(1-\theta)p_j]}$	$\dfrac{2(1+3\theta)}{1+5\theta+2(1-\theta)p_j}$
		A_jA_j	$\dfrac{1+3\theta}{2F(1+3\theta)+(1-2F)[2\theta+(1-\theta)p_j]}$	$\dfrac{2(1+3\theta)}{1+5\theta+(1-\theta)p_j}$
		A_jA_k	$\dfrac{1+3\theta}{2F(1+3\theta)+2(1-2F)[\theta+(1-\theta)p_j]}$	$\dfrac{2(1+3\theta)}{1+5\theta+2(1-\theta)p_j}$
		A_jA_l	$\dfrac{1+3\theta}{2F(1+3\theta)+2(1-2F)[\theta+(1-\theta)p_j]}$	$\dfrac{2(1+3\theta)}{1+5\theta+2(1-\theta)p_j}$

$^*p_0 = p_i + p_j$

$$\text{FGA}: \quad PI = \frac{1+3\theta}{3\theta+(1-\theta)p_{18}} = \frac{1+3\times0.01}{3\times0.01+(1-0.01)\times0.160} = 5.467,$$

$$\text{vWA}: \quad PI = \frac{1+3\theta}{2[3\theta+(1-\theta)(p_{20}+p_{21})]}$$

$$= \frac{1+3\times0.01}{2\times[3\times0.01+(1-0.01)\times(0.044+0.131)]}$$

$$= 2.534.$$

The overall paternity index is 28.93.

Suppose that the defendant provides an alternative explanation that his brother is the true father of the child. Then, the defense proposition becomes

H_d^* : the brother of the alleged father is the true father of the child.   (5.18)

In this situation, the child and the alleged father are nephew–uncle related under H_d, i.e. $(k_0, 2k_1, k_2) = (0.5, 0.5, 0)$. Using the formulas given in Table 5.13, we obtain the likelihood ratios

$$D3S1358 : LR = 1.352,$$

$$FGA : LR = 1.691,$$

$$vWA : LR = 1.434.$$

The overall likelihood ratio is 3.278, which is (much) smaller than 28.93–the likelihood ratio under the alternative explanation H_d given in (5.17). In other words, to the defendant, the DNA evidence against him is weaker under the alternative explanation H_d^* that his brother is the true father of the child.

5.7.5   General method and computer software

The joint genotype probabilities for the special three person cases under Hardy–Weinberg equilibrium can be categorized into 10 different scenarios and they have been summarized in Table 5.10. However, when there is population subdivision, the situations become much more complicated. To illustrate the way of obtaining the joint genotype probability, we consider $Y = A_i A_i$, $X = A_i A_j$ and $Z = A_k A_k$, where i, j, k are all distinct. Recall that Y and X are taken to be maternally related, Y and Z paternally related, while Y and Z are unrelated. It is clear from the genotypes of X, Y and Z that X and Y may share an ibd allele A_i, and Y and Z share no ibd alleles. If X, Y and Z come from the same subdivided population, using the law of total probability, the joint genotype probability can be obtained as

$$P(X = A_i A_j, Y = A_i A_i, Z = A_k A_k)$$

$$= \sum_{t=0}^{2} P(X = A_i A_j, Y = A_i A_i, Z = A_k A_k | Y \text{ and } Z \text{ share } t \text{ ibd alleles})$$

$$\times P(Y \text{ and } Z \text{ share } t \text{ ibd alleles})$$

$$= P(X = A_i A_j, Y = A_i A_i, A_k, A_k) k_0^{YZ}.$$

Again, using the law of total probability, it becomes

$$[2k_0^{XY} P(A_i, A_j, A_i, A_i, A_k, A_k) + 2k_1^{XY} P(A_i, A_j, A_i, A_k, A_k)] k_0^{YZ}.$$

Apply the conditional probability formula in Equation (3.17) recursively to $P(A_i, A_j, A_i, A_i, A_k, A_k)$ and $P(A_i, A_j, A_i, A_k, A_k)$, and the joint genotype probability can be obtained as

$$P(X = A_i A_j, Y = A_i A_i, Z = A_k A_k) = 2k_0^{XY} k_0^{YZ}$$

$$\times \frac{(1 - \theta) p_i [\theta + (1 - \theta) p_i][2\theta + (1 - \theta) p_i](1 - \theta) p_j (1 - \theta) p_k [\theta + (1 - \theta) p_k]}{(1 - \theta) \times 1 \times (1 + \theta)(1 + 2\theta)(1 + 3\theta)(1 + 4\theta)}$$

$$+ 2k_1^{XY} k_0^{YZ} \times \frac{(1-\theta)p_i[\theta + (1-\theta)p_i](1-\theta)p_j(1-\theta)p_k[\theta + (1-\theta)p_k]}{(1-\theta) \times 1 \times (1+\theta)(1+2\theta)(1+3\theta)}.$$

The probabilities for other combinations of genotypes of X, Y and Z can be obtained in similar ways. In fact, there are more than 100 such combinations, and it is not feasible to list all these probabilities. Instead, we have developed a computer software which incorporates all these possibilities. The software can be used to test for kinship among three persons X, Y and Z who belong to the same subdivided population, and X and Z are taken to be unrelated.

In fact, the software EasyDNA_3Persons mentioned in Section 5.6 can deal with the problems in subdivided populations. The steps in running the software are exactly the same as those listed in Section 5.6, except for the addition of the following step:

1a Click the *theta* button and input the appropriate θ.

We illustrate using the data set given in Table 5.11, in which Y is regarded as the child and X is the half-brother of the mother of the child. The following hypotheses are of interest:

H_p : the alleged father Z is the true father of Y;

H_{d1} : the true father is a random man;   (5.19)

H_{d2} : the brother of the alleged father is the true father.

H_p versus H_{d1}, and H_p versus H_{d2} with $\theta = 0.01$ are considered respectively. The likelihood ratios are summarized in Table 5.14. We notice that, as usual, the likelihood ratio decreases when θ increases. This is true for all loci except D3S1358. The overall likelihood ratios for H_p versus H_{d1} are much larger than those for H_p versus H_{d2}. The captured screen for the competing hypotheses H_p versus H_{d2} is displayed in Figure 5.4.

5.8   Complex kinship determinations: method and software

All of the above discussions on paternity and kinship problems consider, at most, three persons. Analytical formulas are derived and computer programs have been developed. In practice, we also encounter complicated paternity problems which are difficult to handle analytically (e.g. a case in which the alleged father cannot be typed but several of his relatives can), complex and missing person problems in which relatives of the missing persons are typed.

Table 5.14   Likelihood ratios for paternity testing problems with hypotheses given in (5.19) and genotypes in Table 5.11, where Y is the child, X is the half-brother of the mother of the child and Z is the alleged father.

	H_p versus H_{d1}		H_p versus H_{d2}	
Locus	$\theta = 0$	0.01	0	0.01
D3S1358	1.26	1.27	1.11	1.11
vWA	6.25	5.35	1.72	1.68
FGA	3.66	3.06	1.57	1.51
Overall	28.82	20.79	3.00	2.84

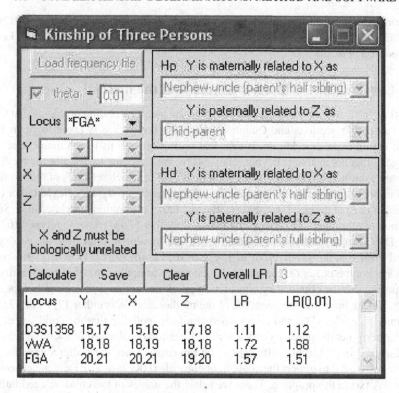

Figure 5.4   Captured screen with hypotheses H_p versus H_{d2} given in (5.19) and genotypes in Table 5.11, where Y is the child, X is the half-brother of the mother of the child and Z is the alleged father.

Dawid *et al.* (2002) and Egeland *et al.* (1997), respectively, used the probabilistic expert system and an algorithm resembling Elston–Stewart to handle complex pedigrees. There have also been discussions on the theory on general kinship determinations, with computer software developed accordingly (Brenner 1997; Egeland *et al.* 1997; Fung 2000, 2003b). The EasyDNA_In_1_Minute (Fung 2000, 2003b) is one such software that is easy to use.

The EasyDNA_In_1_Minute is a package consisting of four computer modules or programs developed for handling paternity and kinship determinations, including the statistical calculations for (a) alleged fathers, (b) alleged fathers where DNA typing is absent, (c) missing persons, and (d) incest cases. The programs can deal with both civil and criminal paternity cases. Computer enumeration is used in the calculations for complex paternity and kinship problems. The programs employ the pedigree tree design, and so are very easy to understand and use. The developed programs have wide applicability, for example the program EasyPA_In_1_Minute can handle the calculations both for the standard trio case and for the motherless paternity case, with or without DNA typing for the relatives of the mother. The program can deal with problems with more than one relative typed, and handle non-standard alternative hypotheses.

In the following sections, we describe the main features of the programs and explain the background theory and methods. We assume Hardy–Weinberg and linkage equilibrium, which is commonly taken in paternity testing and kinship determinations (Brenner 1997; Dawid *et al.* 2002; Egeland *et al.* 1997, 2000; Fung *et al.* 2002, 1996; Gaytmenn *et al.* 2002; Lee *et al.* 1999; Thomson *et al.* 2001).

5.8.1   EasyPA_In_1_Minute software and the method

The EasyPA_In_1_Minute software can deal with the paternity testing problems that we have discussed in earlier sections and Chapter 4 when the population is taken to be in Hardy–Weinberg equilibrium. In addition, it can deal with problems in which many relatives are typed, e.g. mother not available but her relatives are. We are going to describe the method that the software is built upon, based on the motherless case in which relatives of the mother (M) provide the genetic information. Consider the usual hypotheses H_p: the alleged father (AF) is the true father (TF) of the child (C), and H_d: the true father is a random unrelated man. Suppose that the mother of mother (MoM) and the father of mother (FoM) have genotypes 16/17 and 17/19 at D3S1358, respectively (see Table 5.15). We are able to infer from the genotypes of MoM and FoM that the genotype of M is either 16/17, 16/19, 17/17 or 17/19. Given that the child's genotype is 17/18, the mother's genotype cannot be 16/19. The paternity index in this case can then be obtained by considering all of the mother's possible genotypes. As in D3S1358, we can infer that the genotype of the mother at vWA is either 17/19 or 17/20. So, the paternity index for vWA can be obtained similarly, noticing that the child's genotype is 17/19. Furthermore, the paternity index for FGA can also be derived in a similar way.

The EasyPA_In_1_Minute software can be run easily, since the pedigree tree diagram is shown. First, we need to import the allele frequency file (HKChinese.af) and the genotype file (GenotypePA.txt) to the program. Then, we select the names of the child, alleged father and relatives of the mother in the genotype file (in the file, they are called Name-C, Name-AF, Name-FoM and Name-MoM, and the corresponding names are C, AF, FoM and MoM in this particular example) using the built-in combo box. The paternity index for each locus and the overall paternity index are calculated and displayed immediately after the *Calculate* button is clicked. In other words, the paternity indices at *all loci* can be obtained immediately by clicking a few buttons. The paternity and kinship problem can be solved *within one minute*, no matter how many loci one has in the battery of tests. The captured screen in Figure 5.5 shows the details of the results. Another useful feature of the program is that the input names and the output findings can be saved in a file, which can used for checking and/or reporting purposes. The findings for the above problem obtained by the program are summarized in the fourth column of Table 5.16.

In the above situation, genotypes of both parents of M are available, from which we can derive possible genotypes of M. This makes the calculations easy to handle. However, the situation becomes more complicated when the genotypes of neither parent, or only one parent,

Table 5.15   Genotype data of the child (C), alleged father (AF) and relatives (FoM, MoM, $S1oM$, $S2oM$) of the mother.

Locus	C	AF	FoM	MoM	$S1oM$	$S2oM$
D3S1358	17/18	18/20	16/17	17/19	17/17	17/17
vWA	17/19	19/19	17/17	19/20	17/19	17/19
FGA	20/22	22/23	20/21	22/23	20/22	21/23

are available. We consider below the situations in which only the siblings of M ($S1oM$) and/or the father of M are available for typing. Table 5.16 gives the paternity indices obtained by the EasyPA_In_1_Minute for various relatives combinations (see Table 5.15 for the genotypes). A method that the EasyPA_In_1_Minute or the general EasyDNA_In_1_Minute is based upon is to evaluate from the available genotype information of relatives the possible genotype(s) of the parent(s) of M by enumeration, which may possibly transmit on to M and then to C. The law of total probability, Bayes Theorem and conditional probability formulas are employed for assessing the probabilities of having those possible genotypes. For example, in the C-FoM-$S1oM$-AF case at D3S1358, we can use the genotypes of FoM, $S1oM$ and C (see Table 5.15) to infer the genotype of MoM, which must be $17/y$, where y can be any allele at D3S1358. As a result, the genotype of M can be either one of $16/17$, $17/17$, $16/y$ or $17/y$. From this information, and using the conditional probability of observing each of these possible genotypes, we can compute the paternity index based on all possible values of y. Figure 5.6 illustrates some of the ideas which can be generalized to deal with other situations.

Suppose that we have another sibling of M ($S2oM$) typed, and he/she has the same genotype $17/17$ at D3S1358 as the first sibling ($S1oM$). In this case, $S2oM$ does not provide extra genotype information that the possible genotype of M is still $16/17$, $17/17$, $16/y$ or $17/y$. This may give rise to the assumption that the paternity index will remain unchanged. In fact this assumption is incorrect, because the conditional probability of observing a possible

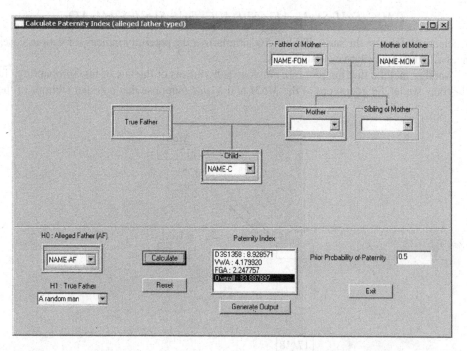

Figure 5.5   Captured screen for running the EasyPA_In_1_Minute software for paternity testing in a motherless case with relatives of mother typed. $H0$ and $H1$ are used in the software to represent H_p and H_d.

Table 5.16   Paternity indices for H_p: *TF* of *C* is *AF* versus (a) H_d: *TF* of *C* is a random man, or (b) H_d: *TF* of *C* is a brother of *AF*.

Locus	C-M-AF	C-AF	C-FoM-MoM-AF	C-FoM-AF	C-FoM-S1oM-AF	C-FoM-S1oM-S2oM-AF	C-S1oM-AF
(a) H_d: *TF* of *C* is a random man							
D3S1358	8.93	4.46	8.93	6.75	8.07	8.26	7.48
vWA	9.42	4.71	4.18	7.79	4.24	4.04	3.16
FGA	2.25	1.40	2.25	2.59	2.19	2.25	2.14
Overall	18.9	29.5	83.9	136	74.9	75.0	50.6
(b) H_d: *TF* of *C* is a brother of *AF*							
D3S1358	1.80	1.63	1.80	1.74	1.78	1.78	1.76
vWA	1.81	1.65	1.61	1.77	1.62	1.61	1.52
FGA	1.38	1.17	1.38	1.44	1.37	1.38	1.36
Overall	4.50	3.15	4.02	4.46	3.95	3.96	3.65

genotype is no longer the same as before. The conditional probabilities in the two situations are

$$P(M|C, FoM, S1oM, AF) \text{ and } P(M|C, FoM, S1oM, S2oM, AF),$$

which are clearly not the same. Table 5.16 summarizes the paternity indices for various cases involving different relative combinations.

Another method that the program employs is by means of the law of total probability. To illustrate, we let the genotypes of the *MoM* and *S1oM* (suppose that no other siblings of the

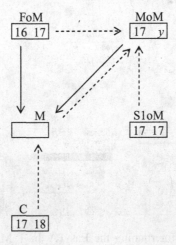

Figure 5.6   A diagram to illustrate some of the ideas used in the calculations in the EasyDNA_In_1_Minute software.

mother are available) be (x, y) and (u, v), where x, y, u and v may take any possible allelic values. By the law of total probability in Equation (2.19), we obtain $P(x, y) = \sum_{u,v} P(x, y, u, v)$. The genotype probability of MoM can be obtained from the joint genotype probabilities $P(x, y, u, v)$'s, of which many are zeros, since MoM and $S1oM$ have at least one common allele.

5.8.2   EasyPAnt_In_1_Minute

When the alleged father (AF) is not available, his relatives may have to be typed. This is by no means a rare occurrence, and frequently arises in inheritance disputes, where the AF is deceased. Although there are methods provided in Chapter 4 and earlier sections of Chapter 5, they can only handle the situation with only one relative of AF typed. A computer program EasyPAnt_In_1_Minute with a more complicated pedigree diagram has been developed for this purpose. Previous ideas in Section 5.8.1 can be generalized, though the theory here would be more involved. For example, consider the case in which the AF is not available and siblings 1 and 2 of the AF are typed with genotypes 19/20 and 16/19 at D3S1358, respectively. Suppose that the M is not available but the FoM and MoM are. In this case, neither the M nor the AF can be typed, and, instead, two relatives for each of them are typed. A total of five persons (including the C) are involved. Relatively little attention has been paid so far in the literature to complex paternity cases of this kind, except Brenner (1997), Egeland et $al.$ (2000) and Fung (2003b). Based on the software, we find that the paternity index of this C-FoM-MoM-$S1oAF$-$S2oAF$ case is 0.404, which is much smaller than the paternity index, 8.93, of the C-FoM-MoM-AF case that the AF is typed (Table 5.16). At this particular locus D3S1358, the new paternity index is smaller than 1 and so it does not seem to support the null hypothesis that the AF (who is not typed) is the TF of the C. Such a low value is, however, not surprising, since the two siblings of the AF do not even have allele 18, which the C has inherited from his TF.

5.8.3   EasyIN_In_1_Minute

Some researchers find it hard to deal with incest cases because the AF and the M are biologically related, but, in fact, these cases are usually not difficult to handle (see Section 4.2.1). Consider a criminal paternity incest case with the genotype information given in Table 5.17. A child ('child 1 of F and M', called Name-$C1$ in the genotype file) and his mother are accused of having an incestuous relationship, from which the mother has given birth to another child (C). The hypotheses of interest are

H_p : the TF of C is 'child 1 of F and M';

H_d : the TF of C is a random unrelated man.

(Notice that $H0$ and $H1$, instead of H_p and H_d, are used in the software.) This is not a difficult problem and our program finds the overall paternity index at all three loci equal to 13.4 (details omitted). Suppose that the accused puts up an alternative explanation H_{d1}: the TF of C is F, and there is no incestuous relationship. How should we compute the paternity index?

If the genotype of F is available, the problem can be easily solved. If it is not, the problem is non-trivial and not many discussions are observed. Consider the case in which the genotype of F is unavailable, but the genotype of his two siblings and the M are. (They are called Name-$S1oF$, Name-$S2oF$ and Name-M in the genotype file, for genotypes; see Table 5.17.)

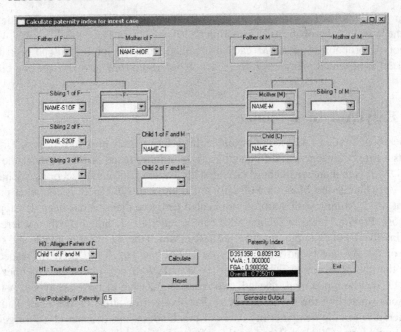

Figure 5.7   Captured screen for running the EasyIN_In_1_Minute software for an incest case with a special alternative explanation $H1$ (i.e. H_d).

Based on the ideas of pedigree analysis, the law of total probability and the Bayes formula, the EasyIN_In_1_Minute can solve this problem by just clicking in the available genotypes information. By choosing the appropriate option in the combo box $H1$ in the software (meaning H_d here), the paternity index can be obtained immediately. The paternity index in this case is reduced from 13.4 to 0.735 (see Figure 5.7). The index, which is even smaller than 1 may suggest that the genetic evidence is more in favor of the accused. Of course, the genetic evidence at other loci as well as the non-genetic evidence have to be considered in order to come up with a more definite answer.

5.8.4   EasyMISS_In_1_Minute

Suppose that a person (X) went missing and his family members reported his disappearance to local police. A dead body (Alleged X, abbreviated as AX) was found a few months later. In order to determine if the dead body is X or not, we type a total of eight family members

Table 5.17   An incest case in which 'Child 1 of F and M' and his mother (M) are accused of having an incestuous relationship with genotype data of C, M, Child 1 and relatives (MoF, $S1oF$ and $S2oF$) of F.

Locus	C	M	Child 1	MoF	$S1oF$	$S2oF$
D3S1358	16/18	17/18	16/18	15/16	15/18	16/18
vWA	17/18	17/17	17/18	15/19	15/19	18/19
FGA	21/22	22/23	21/22	21/23	23/24	21/24

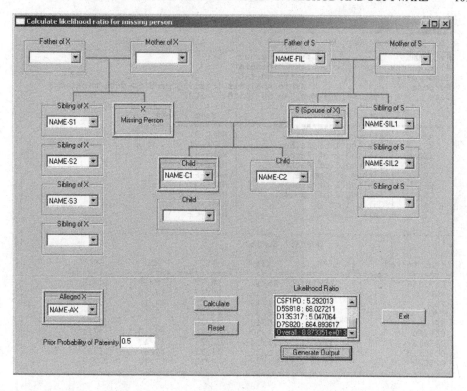

Figure 5.8   Captured screen for running the EasyMISS_In_1_Minute software for a missing person problem with genotypes of eight family members provided in Table 5.18.

of X, i.e., his three sibs (genotype data labeled as $S1$, $S2$, $S3$), his two children ($C1$, $C2$), his father-in-law (FIL) and two sisters-in-law ($SIL1$, $SIL2$). These genotype data at nine loci obtained from the AmpFℓSTR Profiler kit are put in a file (Missing.txt) as shown in Table 5.18. We are interested in the following hypotheses:

H_p : the dead body (Alleged X) is the missing person X;

H_d : the dead body is an unrelated random man.

Although the problem looks complicated, the computer program EasyMISS_In_1_Minute can deal with it easily. We first import the allele frequency file (HKChinese.af) and the genotype file (Missing.txt). Then we select the names of Alleged X and the eight family members in the genotype file using the built-in combo boxes. The likelihood ratio at each locus and the overall likelihood ratio are calculated and displayed almost instantly when we click the *Calculate* button (see the captured screen shown in Figure 5.8 for details).

Figure 5.9 shows the captured screen for the output file, in which we can check whether we have input correctly. Notice that in the EasyDNA_In_1_Minute software, there would be little manual handling error, since only very minimal information is needed for the input. Moreover, the findings can be obtained quickly, *within one minute*.

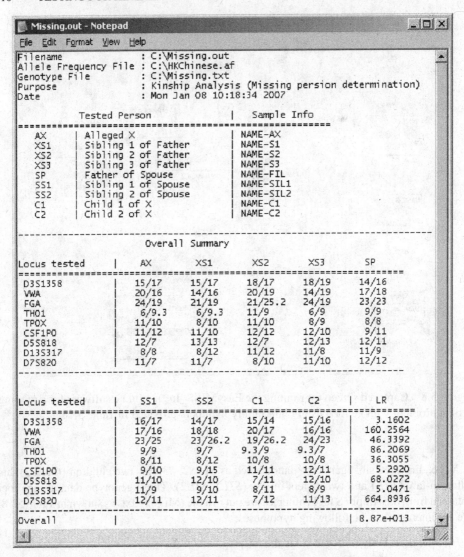

Figure 5.9 Captured screen for the output file of the missing person example.

5.8.5 Other considerations: probability of paternity and mutation

Another feature found in the EasyDNA_In_1_Minute software is that prior probabilities that the prosecution proposition H_p holds true have been built in. Besides, there is an option to choose your own prior; see, for example, the lower left boxes in Figures 5.7 and 5.8. The posterior probabilities or probabilities of paternity are automatically evaluated after obtaining the likelihood ratio/paternity index for the problem of kinship determination.

In the case of paternity testing, there is a possibility that the genotypes of all except one or two loci of the AF and C are found to match one another. This phenomenon may be explained

Table 5.18   Names and genotype data of nine persons for a missing person example, from Fung *et al.* (2006). (Reproduced by permission of Elsevier.)

Sample	D3S1358	vWA	FGA	THO1	TPOX	CSF1PO	D5S818	D13S317	D7S820
AX	15/17	20/16	24/19	6/9.3	11/10	11/12	12/7	8/8	11/7
S1	15/17	14/16	21/19	6/9.3	8/10	11/10	13/13	8/12	11/7
S2	18/17	20/19	21/25.2	11/9	11/10	12/12	12/7	11/12	8/10
S3	18/19	14/19	24/19	6/9	8/9	12/10	12/13	11/8	11/10
C1	15/14	20/17	19/26.2	9.3/9	10/8	11/11	7/11	8/11	7/12
C2	15/16	16/16	24/23	9.3/7	10/8	12/11	12/10	8/9	11/13
FIL	14/16	17/18	23/23	9/9	8/8	9/11	12/11	11/9	12/12
SIL1	16/17	17/16	23/25	9/9	8/11	9/10	11/10	11/9	12/11
SIL2	14/17	18/18	23/26.2	9/7	8/12	9/15	12/10	9/10	12/11

by mutation. The EasyPA_In_1_Minute program also allows the possibility of mutation and the simple average mutation paternity index (Section 4.10.2) is adopted:

$$AMPI = \frac{\text{average mutation rate } (AMR)}{\text{power of exclusion } (PE)}$$

for the mismatch locus. A standard trio case example with one mismatch locus is given in Section 4.10.

5.9   Problems

1. Let $X = A_1 A_2$ and $Y = A_2 A_2$, with $p_1 = 0.12$ and $p_2 = 0.37$. Test whether X and Y are first cousins versus whether they are unrelated, and obtain its likelihood ratio. The population is in Hardy–Weinberg equilibrium.

2. In order to test whether Y is the nephew or unrelated to X, we type Y and a son of X. The DNA profiles of Y and Z (the son of X) are $A_1 A_2$ and $A_1 A_3$, respectively. Obtain the likelihood ratio for the kinship determination. Hardy–Weinberg law is assumed.

3. In a subdivided population with the degree of subdivision θ, test whether $X = A_1 A_2$ and $Y = A_1 A_2$ are parent–child versus whether they are full siblings, and obtain its likelihood ratio. (Note: this situation may happen in immigration applications.) Evaluate the likelihood ratio when $p_1 = 0.18$, $p_2 = 0.43$ and $\theta = 0.03$.

4. In a subdivided population with the degree of subdivision θ, find the paternity index for a standard trio case in which the genotypes of the child, mother and alleged father are $C = A_1 A_2$, $M = A_1 A_1$ and $AF = A_2 A_3$, respectively, and the two competing hypotheses are

H_p : the alleged father is the true father of the child;
H_d : the alleged father and the child are biologically unrelated.

Evaluate the paternity index when $p_1 = 0.18$, $p_2 = 0.23$, $p_3 = 0.31$ and $\theta = 0.03$.

5. In a paternity testincase, the genotypes of the child, mother and alleged father are $A_1 A_1$, $A_1 A_2$ and $A_1 A_3$, respectively. Find the paternity index about the following two competing

hypotheses:

H_p : the alleged father is the true father of the child;
H_d : a full sibling of the alleged father is the true father of the child.

The population is subdivided with the degree of subdivision θ. Evaluate the paternity index when $p_1 = 0.12$, $p_2 = 0.23$, $p_3 = 0.38$ and $\theta = 0.03$.

6. In a paternity testing case, the alleged father is not available and a full sibling R of the alleged father is typed instead. Suppose the genotypes of the child, mother and R are A_1A_1, A_1A_1 and A_1A_2, respectively. All involved people come from the same subdivided population with the degree of subdivision θ. Find the likelihood ratio about the following two competing hypotheses:

H_p : the alleged father, a brother of R, is the true father of the child;
H_d : a random unrelated man is the true father of the child.

7. Suppose $X = A_1A_1$, $Y = A_1A_2$ and $Z = A_2A_3$. Test whether X is the maternal uncle of Y and Z is the paternal grandfather of Y versus X, Y and Z are biologically unrelated. The population is in Hardy–Weinberg equilibrium.

8. Let $X_1 = A_1A_2$, $X_2 = A_3A_3$, $X_3 = A_1A_4$, $X_4 = A_2A_3$ and $X_5 = A_1A_3$. The family relationship among X_1, X_2, X_3, X_4 and X_5 is shown in the figure on the right. Find $P(X_1, X_2, X_3, X_4, X_5)$ and $P(X_1, X_2, X_3, X_5)$ if X_4 is unavailable. The population to which the family belongs is in Hardy–Weinberg equilibrium.

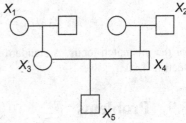

9. In order to determine the relationship between two individuals Y and Z, their genotypes at three loci are provided as follows: at locus D3S1358, $Y = 13/13$, $Z = 13/14$; at locus vWA, $Y = 16/18$, $Z = 16/18$; at locus FGA, $Y = 19/19$, $Z = 20/21$. The following three hypotheses are of interest:

H_{p1} : Y and Z are full siblings;
H_{p2} : Y and Z are half siblings;
H_d : Y and Z are biologically unrelated.

The allele frequencies are listed in Table 4.3. For $\theta = 0$ and 0.03, test H_{p1} versus H_d, and H_{p2} versus H_d.

(a) Use the computer program EasyDNA_2Persons to obtain the likelihood ratios at these three loci.

(b) Use Table 5.5 to evaluate the likelihood ratios at these three loci.

(c) Check whether the corresponding results in (a) and (b) are the same.

6

Interpreting mixtures

It is not uncommon in practice for the stain discovered in the scene to be contributed by more than one person. This kind of mixture renders complexity for evaluating the weight of the DNA evidence. The likelihood ratio is a useful tool to measure the weight of the evidence. In this chapter, we first give an illustrative example and then some common cases to show the steps in deriving the likelihood ratio, where a detailed description of the method for evaluating the DNA evidence is described. Three kinds of populations are considered, namely a population in Hardy–Weinberg equilibrium, a subdivided population, as well as a population with multiple ethnic groups. The associated formulas under each situation are reported, while the more technical derivations are deferred to the last section of this chapter. Thus, the reader can focus on the application of the calculating formulas in practical problems. Meanwhile, computer software is provided to demonstrate how to process the statistical evaluation of DNA mixtures.

In this and the next chapters, the peak height and peak area information is not incorporated into the calculation. The issue of taking account of peak information in the evaluation of DNA evidence is left to Chapter 8. We also assume in Chapters 6 and 7 that the number of unknown contributors is known and the profiles of mixture and the involved persons are typed without errors. A likelihood approach was proposed in Egeland *et al.* (2003) to estimate the number of contributors and determine whether a stain was a mixture or not. The approach in Mortera *et al.* (2003) can readily handle cases in which the number of contributors to the mixture cannot be regarded as known in advance. When the number of unknown contributors is not known for sure, we can also try different choices of the number and report their likelihood ratios, or give an overall likelihood ratio by weighting the individual ones.

6.1 An illustrative example

Simpson case This is the well known case of People v. Simpson (Los Angeles County Case BA097211), in which a three-band profile $A_1 A_2 A_3$ at the RFLP locus D2S44 was obtained for DNA recovered from the center console of an automobile owned by the defendant (Weir *et al.* 1997). The profiles of the defendant, Mr Simpson, and a victim, Mr Goldman, were found

Statistical DNA Forensics: Theory, Methods and Computation   Wing Kam Fung and Yue-Qing Hu
© 2008 John Wiley & Sons, Ltd

to be A_1A_2 and A_1A_3, respectively. The population frequencies of alleles A_1, A_2 and A_3 are, respectively, $p_1 = 0.0316$, $p_2 = 0.0842$ and $p_3 = 0.0926$, and they are rather small, which is typical for RFLP loci.

Based on some facts of this crime, it is postulated that the mixture was contributed by the victim and the perpetrator. To judge whether the suspect was the perpetrator, two alternative propositions (hypotheses or explanations) are proposed, as follows:

H_p : the victim and the suspect were contributors to the mixed stain;

H_d : the victim and one unknown were the contributors

(6.1)

The likelihood ratio

$$LR = \frac{P(\text{evidence}|H_p)}{P(\text{evidence}|H_d)}$$

defined in Equation (2.27) is now used to evaluate the weight of the DNA evidence. Specifically, the DNA evidence is composed of the mixture M, the victim's genotype V and the suspect's genotype S. For convenience, let K generally denote the collection of all the typed genotypes involved in a case. So, the evidence can be expressed simply as (M, K). From the third law of probability, as described in Equation (2.4), the likelihood ratio can be transformed further as

$$LR = \frac{P(M, K|H_p)}{P(M, K|H_d)}$$

$$= \frac{P(M|K, H_p)}{P(M|K, H_d)} \frac{P(K|H_p)}{P(K|H_d)}$$

$$= \frac{P(M|K, H_p)}{P(M|K, H_d)}.$$

The last equality holds because the probability of observing the known genotype K does not depend on whether H_p or H_d holds or not, and so $P(K|H_p) = P(K|H_d)$. Thus, the evaluation of the likelihood ratio is induced to the calculation of the conditional probability $P(M|K, H)$ for some proposition H about the contributors of the mixture M. Hence, the calculation of $P(M|K, H)$ is the focus in the statistical evaluation of the DNA mixture.

Suppose that the population is under Hardy–Weinberg equilibrium. For the Simpson case described above, under the prosecution proposition, based on the victim's genotype $V = A_1A_2$ and the suspect's genotype $S = A_1A_3$, all the alleles in the mixture M can be explained by the genotypes of the victim and the suspect. So, we have $P(M|K, H_p) = 1$. However, under the defense proposition H_d, the alleles A_1 and A_2 in the mixture M are explained by the victim's genotype V and the allele A_3 remains to be explained by the unknown contributor. That is to say, the perpetrator involved in this case must carry the allele A_3. Of course, the perpetrator cannot carry alleles which are not elements in the mixture set M, so the genotype of the perpetrator, G, must be one of the following three types: A_1A_3, A_2A_3 and A_3A_3. It implies that

$$P(M|K, H_d) = P(G = A_1A_3) + P(G = A_2A_3) + P(G = A_3A_3)$$

$$= 2p_1p_3 + 2p_2p_3 + p_3^2,$$

where p_1, p_2 and p_3 are, respectively, the population frequencies of alleles A_1, A_2 and A_3. It follows immediately that

$$LR = \frac{1}{2p_1p_3 + 2p_2p_3 + p_3^2}.$$

Table 6.1 All 12 possible combinations of the genotypes G_1 and G_2 comprising A_1, A_2 and A_3, and the corresponding joint genotype probabilities $P(G_1, G_2)$.

G_1	G_2	$P(G_1, G_2)$	G_1	G_2	$P(G_1, G_2)$
A_1A_1	A_2A_3	$2p_1^2 p_2 p_3$	A_1A_3	A_2A_2	$2p_1 p_2^2 p_3$
A_2A_2	A_1A_3	$2p_1 p_2^2 p_3$	A_1A_3	A_1A_2	$4p_1^2 p_2 p_3$
A_3A_3	A_1A_2	$2p_1 p_2 p_3^2$	A_1A_3	A_2A_3	$4p_1 p_2 p_3^2$
A_1A_2	A_3A_3	$2p_1 p_2 p_3^2$	A_2A_3	A_1A_1	$2p_1^2 p_2 p_3$
A_1A_2	A_1A_3	$4p_1^2 p_2 p_3$	A_2A_3	A_1A_2	$4p_1 p_2^2 p_3$
A_1A_2	A_2A_3	$4p_1 p_2^2 p_3$	A_2A_3	A_1A_3	$4p_1 p_2 p_3^2$

If the defense proposition H_d is altered as

H_d^* : two unknowns were contributors of the mixture,

then the calculation of the denominator of the likelihood ratio becomes a little more complicated. With the constraint that the two contributors must carry and only carry the three alleles A_1, A_2, and A_3 in the mixture M, all the possible combinations of the genotypes G_1 and G_2 of these two unknown contributors are listed in Table 6.1. Also listed in Table 6.1 are the joint genotype probabilities $P(G_1, G_2)$. For example, when $G_1 = A_1A_1$ and $G_2 = A_2A_3$, we have $P(G_1, G_2) = P(A_1A_1)P(A_2A_3) = 2p_1^2 p_2 p_3$. The summation over all those 12 probabilities in the last column of Table 6.1 leads to $12p_1 p_2 p_3(p_1 + p_2 + p_3)$ and so

$$LR = \frac{1}{12p_1 p_2 p_3(p_1 + p_2 + p_3)}. \tag{6.2}$$

In the following section, we are going to derive the likelihood ratios for some commonly encountered cases.

6.2 Some common cases and a case example

Let A_1, A_2, ... be the alleles at an autosomal locus, and the corresponding allele frequencies are denoted as p_1, p_2, ..., respectively. Generally, A_i, A_j, A_k, A_l, ... are used to denote distinct alleles, unless otherwise stated. In the following, we are going to show the derivation of the likelihood ratios when the DNA profile of the mixed stain ranges from two alleles to four alleles under different scenarios of the prosecution and defense propositions. Hardy–Weinberg equilibrium is taken to be held in this section. A case example is provided in detail for the calculation of the likelihood ratio at three loci.

6.2.1 One victim, one suspect and one unknown

Suppose that a mixed stain M was recovered, and the victim and a suspect were typed. The two competing propositions are

H_p : the contributors of M were the victim and the suspect;
H_d : the contributors of M were the victim and one unknown person. $\qquad$ (6.3)

Consider the case in which $M = \{A_i, A_j, A_k\}$, $V = A_iA_j$ and $S = A_kA_k$. Under the prosecution proposition H_p, the three alleles A_i, A_j, A_k are explained by the victim's genotype

Table 6.2 Likelihood ratio for the case of one victim, one suspect and one unknown with H_p: the contributors were the victim and the suspect, and H_d: the contributors were the victim and one unknown person.

Mixture	Victim	Suspect	LR
$\{A_i, A_j\}$	$A_i A_i$	$A_i A_j$	$1/[p_j(2p_i + p_j)]$
		$A_j A_j$	$1/[p_j(2p_i + p_j)]$
	$A_i A_j$	$A_i A_i$	$1/(p_i + p_j)^2$
		$A_i A_j$	$1/(p_i + p_j)^2$
$\{A_i, A_j, A_k\}$	$A_i A_i$	$A_j A_k$	$1/(2p_j p_k)$
	$A_i A_j$	$A_i A_k$	$1/[p_k(2p_i + 2p_j + p_k)]$
		$A_k A_k$	$1/[p_k(2p_i + 2p_j + p_k)]$
$\{A_i, A_j, A_k, A_l\}$	$A_i A_j$	$A_k A_l$	$1/(2p_k p_l)$

and the suspect's genotype, so $P(M|K, H_p) = 1$. Under the defense proposition H_d, alleles A_i and A_j in the mixture are explained by the victim's genotype, and so the remaining allele A_k in the mixture is to be explained by the unknown contributor. Thus, the unknown's genotype G is one of $A_i A_k$, $A_j A_k$ and $A_k A_k$. Therefore,

$$P(M|K, H_d) = P(G = A_i A_k) + P(G = A_j A_k) + P(G = A_k A_k)$$
$$= 2p_i p_k + 2p_j p_k + p_k^2$$
$$= p_k(2p_i + 2p_j + p_k).$$

Finally, we have

$$LR = 1/[p_k(2p_i + 2p_j + p_k)].$$

Based on a similar approach, we can derive the likelihood ratios for the cases (i) $M = \{A_i, A_j\}$, $V = A_i A_i$, $S = A_i A_j$; (ii) $M = \{A_i, A_j\}$, $V = A_i A_i$, $S = A_j A_j$; (iii) $M = \{A_i, A_j\}$, $V = A_i A_j$, $S = A_i A_i$; (iv) $M = \{A_i, A_j\}$, $V = A_i A_j$, $S = A_i A_j$; (v) $M = \{A_i, A_j, A_k\}$, $V = A_i A_i$, $S = A_j A_k$; (vi) $M = \{A_i, A_j, A_k\}$, $V = A_i A_j$, $S = A_i A_k$; (vii) $M = \{A_i, A_j, A_k\}$, $V = A_i A_j$, $S = A_k A_k$; (viii) $M = \{A_i, A_j, A_k, A_l\}$, $V = A_i A_j$, $S = A_k A_l$. All these likelihood ratios are listed in Table 6.2.

6.2.2 One suspect and two unknowns

In cases in which the mixed stain did not originate from the victim and one suspect was identified, the two competing propositions could be

H_p : the contributors were the suspect and one unknown;
H_d : the contributors were two unknowns.

Consider the situation in which $M = \{A_i, A_j, A_k\}$, $S = A_i A_j$. Observe that the prosecution proposition H_p here is equivalent to the defense proposition in Section 6.2.1, so $P(M|K, H_p) = p_k(2p_i + 2p_j + p_k)$. Under H_d, the alleles A_i, A_j, A_k are to be explained by the two unknowns. From Table 6.1, we have $P(M|K, H_d) = 12p_i p_j p_k(p_i + p_j + p_k)$.

Table 6.3   Likelihood ratio for a one suspect and two unknowns case with H_p: the contributors were the suspect and one unknown, and H_d: the contributors were two unknowns.

Mixture	Suspect	LR
$\{A_i, A_j\}$	A_iA_i	$(2p_i + p_j)/[2p_i(2p_i^2 + 3p_ip_j + 2p_j^2)]$
	A_iA_j	$(p_i + p_j)^2/[2p_ip_j(2p_i^2 + 3p_ip_j + 2p_j^2)]$
$\{A_i, A_j, A_k\}$	A_iA_i	$1/[6p_i(p_i + p_j + p_k)]$
	A_iA_j	$(2p_i + 2p_j + p_k)/[12p_ip_j(p_i + p_j + p_k)]$
$\{A_i, A_j, A_k, A_l\}$	A_iA_j	$1/(12p_ip_j)$

Therefore, the likelihood ratio becomes

$$LR = \frac{p_k(2p_i + 2p_j + p_k)}{12p_ip_jp_k(p_i + p_j + p_k)}$$

$$= \frac{2p_i + 2p_j + p_k}{12p_ip_j(p_i + p_j + p_k)}.$$

Based on a similar derivation, the likelihood ratios can be obtained for other combinations of the DNA mixture and the suspect's genotype. All the derived results are shown in Table 6.3.

6.2.3   Two suspects and two unknowns

When two suspects were identified, we may consider the two competing propositions as

H_p : the contributors were the two suspects;
H_d : the contributors were two unknown persons.

Suppose that the mixed stain is $M = \{A_i, A_j, A_k\}$, suspect 1 has genotype $S_1 = A_iA_j$, and suspect 2 has genotype $S_2 = A_iA_k$ (or $S_1 = A_iA_i$, $S_2 = A_jA_k$). Under H_p, there is no unknown contributor and so $P(M|K, H_p) = 1$. Under H_d, we have from the previous subsection that $P(M|K, H_d) = 12p_ip_jp_k(p_i + p_j + p_k)$. So, the likelihood ratio is

$$LR = 1/[12p_ip_jp_k(p_i + p_j + p_k)].$$

The other scenarios relating to this two suspects–two unknowns case were also considered. All the likelihood ratios are reported in Table 6.4. Note that the genotypes of the two tested suspects are not listed in Table 6.4. In fact, the results therein are irrelevant to the genotypes of the two suspects. The only requirement is that the genotypes of these two suspects explain all the alleles in the mixture.

Table 6.4   Likelihood ratio for a two suspects and two unknowns case with H_p: the contributors were two suspects, and H_d: the contributors were two unknowns.

Mixture	LR
$\{A_i, A_j\}$	$1/[2p_ip_j(2p_i^2 + 3p_ip_j + 2p_j^2)]$
$\{A_i, A_j, A_k\}$	$1/[12p_ip_jp_k(p_i + p_j + p_k)]$
$\{A_i, A_j, A_k, A_l\}$	$1/(24p_ip_jp_kp_l)$

6.2.4   Case example

Hong Kong case   Consider one rape case that occurred in Hong Kong (Fung and Hu 2000a), from which three loci–D3S1358, vWA and FGA–were selected. The DNA profiles for the crime stain, victim and suspect at these three loci are shown in Figure 6.1. The information of the alleles found in the mixture, victim and suspect are listed in Table 6.5. The population frequencies of alleles of these three loci can be referred to in Table 4.3.

It happened that the mixture had four, two and three alleles at loci D3S1358, vWA and FGA, respectively, thereby giving a range of examples. We offer the following propositions:

H_p : the victim and the suspect were contributors to the mixed stain;

H_d : the victim and one unknown were the contributors.   (6.4)

Let us first consider the locus D3S1358 with mixture $M = \{14, 15, 17, 18\}$, victim $V = 15/18$ and suspect $S = 14/17$. From Table 6.2, we have the likelihood ratio

$$LR = 1/(2p_{14}p_{17}) = 1/(2 \times 0.033 \times 0.239) = 63.40.$$

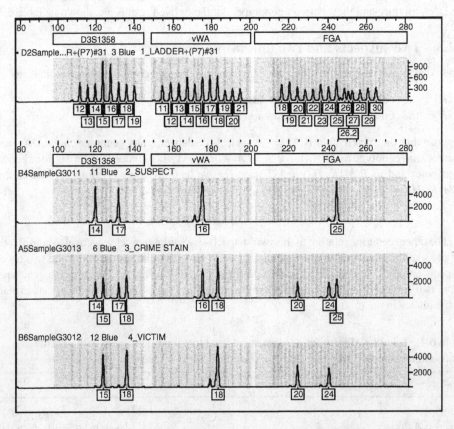

Figure 6.1   The DNA profiles for the crime stain, victim and suspect at loci D3S1358, vWA and FGA in a rape case.

Table 6.5   Alleles detected in a rape case in Hong Kong, from Hu and Fung (2003b). (Reproduced by permission of Springer-Verlag.)

Locus	Mixture (M)	Victim (V)	Suspect (S)	Frequency
D3S1358	14		14	0.033
	15	15		0.331
	17		17	0.239
	18	18		0.056
vWA	16		16	0.156
	18	18		0.160
FGA	20	20		0.044
	24	24		0.166
	25		25	0.110

Secondly, we consider locus vWA with $M = \{16, 18\}$, $V = 18/18$, $S = 16/16$. We have from Table 6.2 that

$$LR = 1/[p_{16}(p_{16} + 2p_{18})] = 1/[0.156 \times (0.156 + 2 \times 0.16)] = 13.47.$$

Thirdly, we consider the locus FGA with $M = \{20, 24, 25\}$, $V = 20/24$, and $S = 25/25$, having the likelihood ratio

$$LR = 1/[p_{25}(2p_{20} + 2p_{24} + p_{25})] = 1/[0.11 \times (2 \times 0.044 + 2 \times 0.166 + 0.11)] = 17.15.$$

Finally, the overall likelihood ratio can be obtained by multiplication, assuming linkage equilibrium, which is equal to $63.04 \times 13.47 \times 17.15 = 15\,695$.

Note that Tables 6.2–6.4 list the likelihood ratios only for the simple common cases, having, at most, four alleles found in the mixed stain. It is not possible to enumerate all the cases here. A general approach is therefore needed to calculate the likelihood ratio in the interpretation of DNA mixtures (see Section 6.3).

6.2.5   Exclusion probability

As in paternity testing (Section 4.8), besides the likelihood ratio, the exclusion probability is another measure that is used by some scientists or forensic laboratories in the interpretation of DNA mixture. Given the alleles found in the mixed stain, the exclusion probability (EP) is evaluated as the probability that a random man is excluded as a contributor to the mixture.

Suppose that the mixed stain has four alleles A_1, A_2, A_3 and A_4 at a particular locus l with corresponding allele frequencies p_1, p_2, p_3 and p_4. Denote $p = p_1 + p_2 + p_3 + p_4$. A person is excluded as a possible contributor to the mixture if at least one of his/her alleles does not belong to the DNA profile of the mixed stain. Thus, the exclusion probability at this locus is evaluated as

$$EP_l = 1 - p^2, \tag{6.5}$$

and the inclusion probability is $IP_l = 1 - EP_l = p^2$. When we consider a total of K loci, the overall exclusion probability is evaluated as

$$\text{overall } EP = 1 - \prod_{l=1}^{k}(1 - EP_l).$$

Using the Hong Kong case given in Table 6.5 as an example, the EP_l at those three loci are evaluated as

$$\text{D3S1358} : EP_1 = 1 - (0.033 + 0.331 + 0.239 + 0.056)^2 = 0.566,$$

$$\text{vWA} : EP_2 = 1 - (0.156 + 0.160)^2 = 0.900,$$

$$\text{FGA} : EP_3 = 1 - (0.044 + 0.166 + 0.110)^2 = 0.898,$$

and the overall exclusion probability is

$$\text{overall } EP = 1 - (1 - 0.566)(1 - 0.9)(1 - 0.898) = 0.9956.$$

This quantity may be interpreted as follows: given the DNA profile found in the mixture (i.e. D3S1358: $M = \{14, 15, 17, 18\}$; vWA: $M = \{16, 18\}$; FGA: $M = \{20, 24, 25\}$), there is a 0.9956 probability that a random person is excluded as a contributor to the mixture. In other words, there is 0.44% probability that a random person who is, however, not a contributor is not excluded. Since the suspect in the Hong Kong case example cannot be excluded as a possible contributor, it is often the duty of the jury and the judge to decide whether or not the suspect is a contributor to the observed DNA mixture.

In the likelihood ratio approach that we mentioned earlier, we find that the likelihood ratios in Sections 6.2.1–6.2.3 depend on how the prosecution and defense propositions and the numbers of contributors are postulated. The exclusion probability approach that we discussed here, however, does not take into account or assume the number of contributors. Moreover, the exclusion probability is only based on the alleles in the mixture; the exact profiles of the potential contributors are not needed in evaluating the probability. In other words, the exclusion probability remains the same, no matter whether the suspect $S = 14/15$, $15/18$ or $17/17, \ldots$ at locus D3S1358, i.e. provided that both alleles of the suspect belong to $\{14, 15, 17, 18\}$. This is regarded as a limitation of the exclusion probability approach by some researchers.

The exclusion probability approach also has a potential limitation when the DNA mixture contains many alleles. For example, if we have a mixture of six alleles $M = \{14, 15, 16, 17, 18, 19\}$ at D3S1358, the exclusion probability is then evaluated as

$$1 - (0.033 + 0.331 + 0.326 + 0.239 + 0.056 + 0.011)^2 = 0.007984,$$

which is very small. In other words, a very high majority of random persons who are not contributors to the mixture will not be excluded at this particular locus. It is also to be noted that the exclusion probability in Equation (6.5) always decreases when p increases, and approaches 0 when p is close to 1. The overall exclusion probability can be small if the observed number of alleles at each locus in the DNA mixture is high. This special phenomenon does not normally happen in the likelihood ratio approach. In this book, we employ the likelihood ratio approach which is commonly used in the interpretation of DNA mixtures.

6.3   A general approach

As demonstrated in Section 6.1, the likelihood ratio is a ratio of two conditional probabilities $P(M|K, H_p)$ and $P(M|K, H_d)$. So, it is sufficient to find a formula to calculate the probability $P(M|K, H)$, where H is a proposition specifying the contributors to the mixed stain. Let x be the number of unknown contributors to the mixed stain stated in the proposition H and X be the genetic profile (distinct alleles) of these x unknown contributors. Also stated in the proposition H is who the known contributors were. Note that the genotypes of the known contributors are listed in K. Considering that the mixture is contributed by the known as well as the unknown contributors, let U be the set of alleles present in the mixture but not present in the known contributors stated in H, and it implies $U \subset X \subset M$. So, we have $P(M|K, H) = P(U \subset X \subset M|K, H)$. The set-notation symbols, such as $\subset, \setminus, \cup, \cap, \in$ and $|\cdot|$, carry the meanings in the standard convention. Note that the set U is allowed to be empty in some situations in which all the alleles in the mixture are present in the genotypes of the known contributors. All the notations used in the evaluation of the DNA mixture are summarized in Table 6.6 for easy reference. Based on the principle of inclusion and exclusion as given in Equation (2.7), we have

$$P(M|K, H) = \sum_{M \setminus U \subset C \subset M} (-1)^{|M \setminus C|} W(C)$$

$$= W(M) - \sum_{A_i \in U} W(M \setminus \{A_i\})$$

$$+ \sum_{A_i, A_j \in U} W(M \setminus \{A_i, A_j\}) - \sum_{A_i, A_j, A_k \in U} W(M \setminus \{A_i, A_j, A_k\})$$

$$+ \cdots + (-1)^{|U|} W(M \setminus U), \tag{6.6}$$

where

$$W(C) = P(X \subset C|K) \tag{6.7}$$

Table 6.6   Notations for interpreting DNA mixtures, from Fung and Hu (2004). (Reproduced by permission of Blackwell Publishing.)

M	The DNA profile of a mixed stain
H	A proposition which specifies the known and unknown contributors to the mixed stain
K	The collection of genotypes of the typed persons
x	The number of unknown contributors stated in H
X	The genetic profile of the x unknown contributors stated in H
U	The set of distinct alleles present in the mixture M but not in the genotypes of the known contributors stated in H
$(k_0, 2k_1, k_2)$	The relatedness coefficient for two biologically related persons
θ	The degree of population subdivision
$A_1, A_2, \ldots$	The alleles at an autosomal chromosome
$p_1, p_2, \ldots$	The allele population frequencies of $A_1, A_2, \ldots$
c_l	The number of allele A_l present in $K, l = 1, 2, \ldots$
c	$\sum_l c_l$, the two times of the number of tested persons

is the conditional probability that every allele of the x unknown contributors is in set C given the genotypes K of the typed persons, C is an arbitrary subset of M, $W(\phi) = 0$, $|U|$ represents the cardinality of set U. It is noted that when $x = 0$ and $U = \phi$, we have $P(M|K, H) = 1$, and $|U|$ cannot exceed $2x$, otherwise $P(M|K, H) = 0$. The details of the derivation of Equation (6.6) are given in Section 6.9.1. It is seen from Equation (6.6) that the evaluation of the DNA mixture is now converted to the calculation of $W(C)$ defined in Equation (6.7) for any $C \subset M$. As we shall see in the later discussion, we are going to use this general formula in Equation (6.6) and evaluate the particular $W(C)$ in Equation (6.7) for the interpretation of DNA mixtures in different scenarios.

6.4   Population in Hardy–Weinberg equilibrium

When the people involved in a case come from the same population in Hardy–Weinberg equilibrium and these people are biologically unrelated, we have

$$W(C) = \left(\sum_{A_l \in C} p_l \right)^{2x},$$ (6.8)

for arbitrary subset C of M. Combining Equations (6.6) and (6.8) thus provides a general approach to calculate the likelihood ratio. The proof of Equation (6.8) is given in Section 6.9.2. Note that one equivalent formula was reported in Weir *et al.* (1997) and Fukshansky and Bär (1998) when the population under study is in Hardy–Weinberg equilibrium. Now let us go back to the Simpson case, introduced in Section 6.1, with $M = \{A_1, A_2, A_3\}$, to see the application of Equation (6.8) in real cases. The hypothesis pair in (6.1) is considered. Under the prosecution proposition H_p, there is no unknown contributor, i.e. $x = 0$, and all the alleles in the mixture are present in the genotypes of the stated contributors, the victim and the suspect, so $P(M|K, H_p) = 1$. Under the defense proposition H_d, $x = 1$, and $V = A_1 A_2$ is the only known contributor to the mixture M. It follows that $U = M \setminus \{A_1\} \cup \{A_2\} = \{A_3\}$. From Equations (6.6) and (6.8), we have

$$P(M|K, H_d) = W(M) - W(M \setminus \{A_3\})$$
$$= W(\{A_1, A_2, A_3\}) - W(\{A_1, A_2\})$$
$$= (p_1 + p_2 + p_3)^2 - (p_1 + p_2)^2$$
$$= 2p_1 p_3 + 2p_2 p_3 + p_3^2.$$

If we instead consider the defense proposition H_d^* that two unknowns were contributors of the mixture, we have $x = 2$ and $U = \{A_1, A_2, A_3\}$. From Equations (6.6) and (6.8), we have

$$P(M|K, H_d^*) = W(M) - W(M \setminus \{A_1\}) - W(M \setminus \{A_2\}) - W(M \setminus \{A_3\})$$
$$+ W(M \setminus \{A_1, A_2\}) + W(M \setminus \{A_1, A_3\}) + W(M \setminus \{A_2, A_3\})$$
$$= (p_1 + p_2 + p_3)^4 - (p_1 + p_2)^4 - (p_1 + p_3)^4 - (p_2 + p_3)^4$$
$$+ p_1^4 + p_2^4 + p_3^4$$
$$= 12 p_1 p_2 p_3 (p_1 + p_2 + p_3).$$

Both $P(M|K, H_d)$ and $P(M|K, H_d^*)$ are the same as those derived in Section 6.1.

In the following, the Hong Kong case described in Section 6.2.4 is used to illustrate the application of Equations (6.6) and (6.8) in the derivation of the likelihood ratio. The pair of hypotheses in (6.4) is considered. For the locus D3S1358 with mixture $M = \{14, 15, 17, 18\}$ and typed genotypes $K = 14/17, 15/18$, under H_p, there is no unknown contributor, i.e. $x = 0$; all the alleles in the mixture are present in the known contributors, thus $U = \phi$ and $P(M|K, H_p) = 1$. Under H_d, there is, however, one unknown contributor, i.e. $x = 1$. The alleles 15 and 18 in M are present in the known victim contributor; thus $U = \{14, 17\}$. Equivalently, the unknown contributor's genotype is definitely 14/17. So, from Equations (6.6) and (6.8), we have

$$P(M|K, H_d) = W(M) - W(M \setminus \{14\}) - W(M \setminus \{17\}) + W(M \setminus \{14, 17\})$$
$$= (p_{14} + p_{15} + p_{17} + p_{18})^2 - (p_{15} + p_{17} + p_{18})^2$$
$$- (p_{14} + p_{15} + p_{18})^2 + (p_{15} + p_{18})^2$$
$$= 2p_{14}p_{17}.$$

Secondly, we consider locus vWA. It is seen from Table 6.5 that the mixture $M = \{16, 18\}$ and the typed genotypes $K = 16/16, 18/18$. Under $H_p, x = 0$ and $U = \phi$, so $P(M|K, H_p) = 1$. Under $H_d, x = 1$ and $U = \{16\}$, so, from Equations (6.6) and (6.8), we have

$$P(M|K, H_d) = W(M) - W(M \setminus \{16\})$$
$$= (p_{16} + p_{18})^2 - p_{18}^2$$
$$= p_{16}^2 + 2p_{16}p_{18}.$$

Thirdly, we consider the locus FGA with $M = \{20, 24, 25\}$ and $K = 20/24, 25/25$. Under $H_p, x = 0$ and $U = \phi$, so $P(M|K, H_p) = 1$. Under $H_d, x = 1$ and $U = \{25\}$, so, from Equations (6.6) and (6.8), we have

$$P(M|K, H_d) = W(M) - W(M \setminus \{25\})$$
$$= (p_{20} + p_{24} + p_{25})^2 - (p_{20} + p_{24})^2$$
$$= p_{25}(2p_{20} + 2p_{24} + p_{25}).$$

Note that all three expressions of $P(M|K, H_d)$ derived above are the same as those given in Section 6.2.4. For practitioners' convenience, the corresponding formulas of calculating $P(M|K, H)$ for the commonly encountered situations are listed in Table 6.7, which covers the results reported in Tables 6.2–6.4. It is observed from Table 6.7 that in some situations, e.g. $x > 2$, the implementation of $P(M|K, H)$ is not simple. See also the detailed expressions of $P(M|K, H)$ reported in Weir et al. (1997).

Comparing the current general approach based on Equations (6.6) and (6.8) with the specific approach described in Sections 6.1 and 6.2, it is a matter for one to choose the approach according to one's experience and knowledge in deriving the likelihood ratio for simple DNA mixture problems such as the Simpson and the Hong Kong cases. However, the implementation of $P(M|K, H)$ by a computer program based on Equations (6.6) and (6.8) is not only easy to work on, but also good to deal with complex DNA mixture problems having more than two contributors.

Table 6.7 The calculating formulas of $P(M|K, H)$ for different combinations of M and U with x unknown contributors.

M	U	$P(M|K, H)$
$\{A_i\}$	ϕ	p_i^{2x}
	$\{A_i\}$	p_i^{2x}
$\{A_i, A_j\}$	ϕ	$(p_i + p_j)^{2x}$
	$\{A_i\}$	$(p_i + p_j)^{2x} - p_j^{2x}$
	$\{A_i, A_j\}$	$(p_i + p_j)^{2x} - p_i^{2x} - p_j^{2x}$
$\{A_i, A_j, A_k\}$	ϕ	$(p_i + p_j + p_k)^{2x}$
	$\{A_i\}$	$(p_i + p_j + p_k)^{2x} - (p_j + p_k)^{2x}$
	$\{A_i, A_j\}$	$(p_i + p_j + p_k)^{2x} - (p_j + p_k)^{2x}$ $- (p_i + p_k)^{2x} + p_k^{2x}$
	$\{A_i, A_j, A_k\}$	$(p_i + p_j + p_k)^{2x} - (p_j + p_k)^{2x} - (p_i + p_k)^{2x}$ $- (p_i + p_j)^{2x} + p_i^{2x} + p_j^{2x} + p_k^{2x}$
$\{A_i, A_j, A_k, A_l\}$	ϕ	$(p_i + p_j + p_k + p_l)^{2x}$
	$\{A_i\}$	$(p_i + p_j + p_k + p_l)^{2x} - (p_j + p_k + p_l)^{2x}$
	$\{A_i, A_j\}$	$(p_i + p_j + p_k + p_l)^{2x} - (p_j + p_k + p_l)^{2x}$ $- (p_i + p_k + p_l)^{2x} + (p_k + p_l)^{2x}$
	$\{A_i, A_j, A_k\}$	$(p_i + p_j + p_k + p_l)^{2x} - (p_j + p_k + p_l)^{2x}$ $- (p_i + p_k + p_l)^{2x} - (p_i + p_j + p_l)^{2x}$ $+ (p_k + p_l)^{2x} + (p_j + p_l)^{2x} + (p_i + p_l)^{2x}$ $- p_l^{2x}$
	$\{A_i, A_j, A_k, A_l\}$	$(p_i + p_j + p_k + p_l)^{2x} - (p_j + p_k + p_l)^{2x}$ $- (p_i + p_k + p_l)^{2x} - (p_i + p_j + p_l)^{2x}$ $- (p_i + p_j + p_k)^{2x} + (p_k + p_l)^{2x} + (p_j + p_l)^{2x}$ $+ (p_j + p_k)^{2x} + (p_i + p_l)^{2x} + (p_i + p_k)^{2x}$ $+ (p_i + p_j)^{2x} - p_i^{2x} - p_j^{2x} - p_k^{2x} - p_l^{2x}$

6.5 Population with multiple ethnic groups

All the people involved are assumed to be of the same ethnic group in the previous section. One fact that we have to face in the interpretation of DNA mixtures is contributors coming from different ethnic/racial groups. For example, the mixed stain collected from the crime scene contains material from the victim and the offender, who may belong to the Caucasian and African American ethnic groups, respectively. Extensive studies from a wide variety of databases show that there are indeed substantial differences between allele frequencies among the major racial and linguistic groups (National Research Council 1996). The ignorance of this phenomenon may not be allowed and may be misleading in the presentation of evidence in the court. Harbison and Buckleton (1998), following the sampling formula developed by Balding and Nichols (1994), discussed the interpretation of DNA mixtures when the two contributors come from two different races. Fukshansky and Bär (1999) obtained a formula for the calculation of the likelihood ratio for the situation in which the contributors belonged to different ethnic origins. Each ethnic group is in Hardy–Weinberg equilibrium. The independence of alleles between ethnic groups was employed.

Let us first investigate an example in which the mixture $M = \{A_1, A_2, A_3, A_4\}$, and two suspects are identified as $S_1 = A_1 A_4$ and $S_2 = A_2 A_3$, respectively. The two competing propositions about the source of the DNA mixture are as follows:

H_p : the contributors were the two suspects;
H_d : the contributors were two unknown persons: X_1 (ethnic group a) and
$\qquad X_2$ (ethnic group b).

Under H_p, all the four alleles in the mixture are present in the genotypes of the two typed suspects, so $P(M|K, H_p) = 1$. Under H_d, the two unknown contributors' genotypes can take one of the following six genotype combinations: $(A_1 A_2, A_3 A_4)$, $(A_1 A_3, A_2 A_4)$, $(A_1 A_4, A_2 A_3)$, $(A_2 A_3, A_1 A_4)$, $(A_2 A_4, A_1 A_3)$ and $(A_3 A_4, A_1 A_2)$. Noting the independence between two ethnic groups a and b, we have

$$P(X_1 = A_i A_j, X_2 = A_k A_l) = 2 p_{ai} p_{aj} \times 2 p_{bk} p_{bl} = 4 p_{ai} p_{aj} p_{bk} p_{bl},$$

where p_{ai} and p_{bi} are the population frequencies of allele A_i in ethnic groups a and b, respectively. So,

$$P(M|K, H_d) = 4 p_{a1} p_{a2} p_{b3} p_{b4} + 4 p_{a1} p_{a3} p_{b2} p_{b4} + 4 p_{a1} p_{a4} p_{b2} p_{b3}$$
$$+ 4 p_{a2} p_{a3} p_{b1} p_{b4} + 4 p_{a2} p_{a4} p_{b1} p_{b3} + 4 p_{a3} p_{a4} p_{b1} p_{b2}.$$

The ratio of $P(M|K, H_p)$ and $P(M|K, H_d)$ leads to the likelihood ratio. However, it is not easy to enumerate all the possible combinations when the situation becomes a little more complicated. So it is desired to develop a general method to handle the evaluation of DNA mixtures when the persons involved come from different ethnic groups.

As we did before, let A_1, A_2, ... denote the alleles at an autosomal locus, and $G = \{a, b, \ldots\}$ denote the ethnic group indices. The population frequencies of alleles A_1, A_2, ... in ethnic group g ($g = a, b, \ldots$) are denoted as p_{g1}, p_{g2}, ..., respectively. The number of unknown contributors is $x = \sum_g x_g$, where x_g is the number of unknown contributors belonging to ethnic group g, $g = a, b, \ldots$. Then, the formula for calculating the probability $W(C)$ defined in Equation (6.7) could be expressed as

$$W(C) = \prod_{g \in G} \left(\sum_{A_l \in C} p_{gl} \right)^{2 x_g}. \tag{6.9}$$

The proof of this formula is given in Section 6.9.3. The derivation of the general formula of $W(C)$ for problems with contributors from different ethnic groups can also be referred to in Fukshansky and Bär (1999) and Fung and Hu (2001). For the convenience of practitioners, the explicit expressions of the likelihood ratios for 14 common cases were presented in Fung and Hu (2001).

To illustrate the application of Equation (6.9), we consider the Simpson case, as described in Section 6.1, for the evaluation of the likelihood ratio. The court ordered that the number of contributors to the mixed sample be at least two, three and four. Here, we only take it equal to two for illustration. The following two competing propositions are of interest:

H_p : contributors were the victim and the suspect;
H_d : contributors were two unknown persons.

The defendant is an African American and the victim is a Caucasian. The two unknowns could be from different ethnic groups and we regard them as being African Americans (AA),

Caucasians (CA) and/or Chinese (CH). The following allele frequencies are taken: AA (ethnic group a): $p_{a1} = 0.0316$, $p_{a2} = 0.0842$, $p_{a3} = 0.0926$; CA (ethnic group b): $p_{b1} = 0.0859$, $p_{b2} = 0.0827$, $p_{b3} = 0.1073$; and CH (ethnic group c): $p_{c1} = 0.0169$, $p_{c2} = 0.0749$, $p_{c3} = 0.1522$ (Budowle et al. 1991b; Fung 1996; Tsui and Wong 1996). Taking the single-banded alleles as true homozygotes, the effect of different ethnic groups to the likelihood ratio is investigated and the results are shown in Table 6.8. In fact, when the two unknown persons come from the same ethnic group, for example Caucasian (ethnic group b), then it is easy to calculate the likelihood ratio by Equation (6.2) or Table 6.4 as follows:

$$LR = \frac{1}{12 \times 0.0859 \times 0.0827 \times 0.1073 \times (0.0859 + 0.0827 + 0.1073)} = 396.$$

When the two unknown contributors come from ethnic group a (African American), we have, similarly, $LR = 1623$. See the same result in Weir et al. (1997). But when the two unknown contributors are one African American and one Caucasian, the calculation becomes complicated. In this situation, under H_d, $M = \{A_1, A_2, A_3\}$, $U = \{A_1, A_2, A_3\}$, $x_a = x_b = 1$, so, from Equations (6.6) and (6.9), we have

$$\begin{aligned}
P(M|K, H_d) &= W(M) - W(M \setminus \{A_1\}) - W(M \setminus \{A_2\}) - W(M \setminus \{A_3\}) \\
&\quad + W(M \setminus \{A_1, A_2\}) + W(M \setminus \{A_1, A_3\}) + W(M \setminus \{A_2, A_3\}) \\
&= (p_{a1} + p_{a2} + p_{a3})^2 (p_{b1} + p_{b2} + p_{b3})^2 - (p_{a2} + p_{a3})^2 (p_{b2} + p_{b3})^2 \\
&\quad - (p_{a1} + p_{a3})^2 (p_{b1} + p_{b3})^2 - (p_{a1} + p_{a2})^2 (p_{b1} + p_{b2})^2 \\
&\quad + p_{a3}^2 p_{b3}^2 + p_{a2}^2 p_{b2}^2 + p_{a1}^2 p_{b1}^2 \\
&= (0.0316 + 0.0842 + 0.0926)^2 \times (0.0859 + 0.0827 + 0.1073)^2 \\
&\quad - (0.0842 + 0.0926)^2 \times (0.0827 + 0.1073)^2 \\
&\quad - (0.0316 + 0.0926)^2 \times (0.0859 + 0.1073)^2 \\
&\quad - (0.0316 + 0.0842)^2 \times (0.0859 + 0.0827)^2 \\
&\quad + 0.0926^2 \times 0.1073^2 + 0.0842^2 \times 0.0827^2 + 0.0316^2 \times 0.0859^2 \\
&= 0.001375.
\end{aligned}$$

So, the likelihood ratio is $LR = 1/0.001375 = 727$. In this situation, we can use the developed DOS-based computer program to tackle it. Table 6.8 shows the likelihood ratios for all possible combinations of the two unknowns' origins. It is observed from Table 6.8 that, compared with the likelihood ratio 1623 with two African Americans, when the two unknown persons were one African American and one Caucasian, the likelihood ratio drops to 727 (less than half) and drops further to 396 (less than a quarter) if the two unknowns were Caucasians. Thus, the effect of different ethnic groups could be large. It is to be noticed that the ethnic group of the defendant does not matter to the likelihood ratio when the ethnic groups are in Hardy–Weinberg equilibrium. Only the ethnic groups of the unknowns matter in the evaluation of DNA mixtures.

From Table 6.8, in which the Hardy–Weinberg law holds, we observe that the likelihood ratio gives the highest or the lowest value for the situation in which both unknown contributors come from the same ethnic group, the two unknowns are African Americans

Table 6.8   Likelihood ratios with two unknowns belonging to ethnic groups of African American (AA), Caucasian (CA) and Chinese (CH).

AA	CA	CH	LR
2	0	0	1623
0	2	0	396
0	0	2	1773
1	1	0	727
1	0	1	1519
0	1	1	599

and/or Caucasians (i.e. 727 lies between 396 and 1623), or the two unknowns are Caucasians and/or Chinese (i.e. 599 lies between 396 and 1773). This will in effect bracket the range of likelihood ratio values – the two ethnic group value will invariably fall between the one group values. So the one ethnic group scenarios can be conveyed as bounds, and this approach is used by some practitioners. However, such constructed bounds are not always valid. For example, in the case in which the two unknowns are African Americans and/or Chinese, the likelihood ratio 1519 for the one African American and one Chinese unknowns situation is smaller than the likelihood ratio 1623 with two African American unknowns or the likelihood ratio 1773 with two Chinese. So it is necessary to calculate the exact value of the likelihood ratio when the contributors to the mixture come from different ethnic groups.

For practitioners' convenience, Table 6.9 lists the conditional probability formulas $P(M|K, H)$ with two unknown contributors, respectively, from ethnic groups a and b and up to three alleles in DNA mixtures (Fung and Hu 2001), and it can meet the practical needs when the situation is not complicated.

Table 6.9   The calculating formula of $P(M|K, H)$ for different M and U with two unknown contributors respectively from ethnic groups a and b.

M	U	$P(M|K, H)$
$\{A_i\}$	ϕ	$p_{ai}^2 p_{bi}^2$
	$\{A_i\}$	$p_{ai}^2 p_{bi}^2$
$\{A_i, A_j\}$	ϕ	$(p_{ai} + p_{aj})^2(p_{bi} + p_{bj})^2$
	$\{A_i\}$	$(p_{ai} + p_{aj})^2(p_{bi} + p_{bj})^2 - p_{aj}^2 p_{bj}^2$
	$\{A_i, A_j\}$	$(p_{ai} + p_{aj})^2(p_{bi} + p_{bj})^2 - p_{ai}^2 p_{bi}^2 - p_{aj}^2 p_{bj}^2$
$\{A_i, A_j, A_k\}$	ϕ	$(p_{ai} + p_{aj} + p_{ak})^2(p_{bi} + p_{bj} + p_{bk})^2$
	$\{A_i\}$	$(p_{ai} + p_{aj} + p_{ak})^2(p_{bi} + p_{bj} + p_{bk})^2$ $- (p_{aj} + p_{ak})^2(p_{bj} + p_{bk})^2$
	$\{A_i, A_j\}$	$(p_{ai} + p_{aj} + p_{ak})^2(p_{bi} + p_{bj} + p_{bk})^2$ $- (p_{aj} + p_{ak})^2(p_{bj} + p_{bk})^2 - (p_{ai} + p_{ak})^2(p_{bi} + p_{bk})^2$
	$\{A_i, A_j, A_k\}$	$(p_{ai} + p_{aj} + p_{ak})^2(p_{bi} + p_{bj} + p_{bk})^2$ $- (p_{aj} + p_{ak})^2(p_{bj} + p_{bk})^2 - (p_{ai} + p_{ak})^2(p_{bi} + p_{bk})^2$ $- (p_{ai} + p_{aj})^2(p_{bi} + p_{bj})^2 + p_{ai}^2 p_{bi}^2 + p_{aj}^2 p_{bj}^2 + p_{ak}^2 p_{bk}^2$

6.6   Subdivided population

6.6.1   Single ethnic group: simple cases

Hardy–Weinberg equilibrium is assumed in the derivation of the formula for evaluating the DNA evidence in Equations (6.8) and (6.9). Clearly, Hardy–Weinberg equilibrium is seldom exactly certain or correct. As noted by Balding and Nichols (1994), the uncertainty in DNA profile analysis may be due to various factors such as population subdivision. Equation (3.17) was proposed by Balding and Nichols (1994) to evaluate the probability of a set of alleles.

Firstly, let us consider the case with $M = \{A_i, A_j, A_k\}$, $V = A_i A_j$ and $S = A_k A_k$, as reported in Section 6.2.1, to investigate the effect of population subdivision on the evaluation of the DNA mixture. The same proposition pair in (6.3) is taken. Under H_p that the victim and the suspect were the contributors of M, the three alleles A_i, A_j, A_k are present in the victim's genotype and the suspect's genotype, so $P(M|K, H_p) = 1$. Under H_d that the victim and one unknown were the contributors of M, however, the allele A_k in the mixture is to be explained by the unknown contributor. So the unknown's genotype G is one of $A_i A_k$, $A_j A_k$ and $A_k A_k$. Therefore,

$$
\begin{aligned}
& P(M|K, H_d) \\
&= P(G = A_i A_k | V = A_i A_j, S = A_k A_k) \\
&\quad + P(G = A_j A_k | V = A_i A_j, S = A_k A_k) \\
&\quad + P(G = A_k A_k | V = A_i A_j, S = A_k A_k) \\
&= 2P(A_i, A_k | A_i, A_j, A_k, A_k) + 2P(A_j, A_k | A_i, A_j, A_k, A_k) \\
&\quad + P(A_k, A_k | A_i, A_j, A_k, A_k) \\
&= 2P(A_i | A_i, A_j, A_k, A_k)P(A_k | A_i, A_i, A_j, A_k, A_k) \\
&\quad + 2P(A_j | A_i, A_j, A_k, A_k)P(A_k | A_j, A_i, A_j, A_k, A_k) \\
&\quad + P(A_k | A_i, A_j, A_k, A_k)P(A_k | A_k, A_i, A_j, A_k, A_k) \\
&= 2\left[\frac{\theta + (1 - \theta)p_i}{1 + 3\theta}\right]\left[\frac{2\theta + (1 - \theta)p_k}{1 + 4\theta}\right] + 2\left[\frac{\theta + (1 - \theta)p_j}{1 + 3\theta}\right]\left[\frac{2\theta + (1 - \theta)p_k}{1 + 4\theta}\right] \\
&\quad + \left[\frac{2\theta + (1 - \theta)p_k}{1 + 3\theta}\right]\left[\frac{3\theta + (1 - \theta)p_k}{1 + 4\theta}\right] \\
&= \frac{[2\theta + (1 - \theta)p_k][7\theta + (1 - \theta)(2p_i + 2p_j + p_k)]}{(1 + 3\theta)(1 + 4\theta)}.
\end{aligned}
$$

So we have the likelihood ratio as listed in Table 6.10. The other likelihood ratios listed in Table 6.10 can be derived in a similar way. Particularly when $\theta = 0$, the likelihood ratios listed in Table 6.10 are the same as those listed in Table 6.2.

6.6.2   Single ethnic group: general situations

In order to express the general formula for calculating $P(M|K, H)$ when the people involved come from the same subdivided population, we define for any given real r and non-negative

Table 6.10   Likelihood ratios for one victim, one suspect and one unknown case about H_p: the contributors were the victim and the suspect, and H_d: the contributors were the victim and one unknown person.

Mixture	Victim	Suspect	LR
$\{A_i, A_j\}$	$A_i A_i$	$A_i A_j$	$\dfrac{(1 + 3\theta)(1 + 4\theta)}{[\theta + (1 - \theta)p_j][8\theta + (1 - \theta)(2p_i + p_j)]}$
		$A_j A_j$	$\dfrac{(1 + 3\theta)(1 + 4\theta)}{[2\theta + (1 - \theta)p_j][7\theta + (1 - \theta)(2p_i + p_j)]}$
	$A_i A_j$	$A_i A_i$	$\dfrac{(1 + 3\theta)(1 + 4\theta)}{[4\theta + (1 - \theta)(p_i + p_j)][5\theta + (1 - \theta)(p_i + p_j)]}$
		$A_i A_j$	$\dfrac{(1 + 3\theta)(1 + 4\theta)}{[4\theta + (1 - \theta)(p_i + p_j)][5\theta + (1 - \theta)(p_i + p_j)]}$
$\{A_i, A_j, A_k\}$	$A_i A_i$	$A_j A_k$	$\dfrac{(1 + 3\theta)(1 + 4\theta)}{2[\theta + (1 - \theta)p_j][\theta + (1 - \theta)p_k]}$
	$A_i A_j$	$A_i A_k$	$\dfrac{(1 + 3\theta)(1 + 4\theta)}{[\theta + (1 - \theta)p_k)][8\theta + (1 - \theta)(2p_i + 2p_j + p_k)]}$
		$A_k A_k$	$\dfrac{(1 + 3\theta)(1 + 4\theta)}{[2\theta + (1 - \theta)p_k][7\theta + (1 - \theta)(2p_i + 2p_j + p_k)]}$
$\{A_i, A_j, A_k, A_l\}$	$A_i A_j$	$A_k A_l$	$\dfrac{(1 + 3\theta)(1 + 4\theta)}{2[\theta + (1 - \theta)p_k][\theta + (1 - \theta)p_l]}$

integers m and k that

$$r^{(m)}(k, \theta)$$

$$= \prod_{i=0}^{m-1}[(k + i)\theta + (1 - \theta)r]$$

$$= [k\theta + (1 - \theta)r][(k + 1)\theta + (1 - \theta)r] \cdots [(k + m - 1)\theta + (1 - \theta)r], \quad (6.10)$$

and $r^{(0)}(k, \theta) = 1$. Note that $r^{(m)}(k, \theta) = r^m$ when $\theta = 0$. For brevity, $r^{(m)}(k, \theta)$ is shortened to $r^{(m)}(k)$ when the parameter θ is specified and fixed. But, in some situations, for example, in the case of multiple ethnic groups, different θ values are taken for different groups, and so the parameter θ in $r^{(m)}(k, \theta)$ cannot be omitted.

Recall that there are x unknown contributors stated in the proposition H and K is the collection of all the typed genotypes. Let c_l denote the count of allele A_l present in K, $l = 1, 2, \ldots$. Then the formula for calculating $W(C)$ defined in Equation (6.7) for arbitrary subset C of the mixture M is provided as follows:

$$W(C) = \frac{\left(\sum_{A_l \in C} p_l\right)^{(2x)}\left(\sum_{A_l \in C} c_l\right)}{1^{(2x)}\left(\sum_l c_l\right)}, \quad (6.11)$$

where the parameter θ is omitted in the notation for brevity. The proof of Equation (6.11) is given in Section 6.9.4. The general formulas for calculating $P(M|K, H)$ can also be referred to in Curran *et al.* (1999) and Fung and Hu (2000b). Note that when the population is in Hardy–Weinberg equilibrium, we have $\theta = 0$ and $W(C) = (\sum_{A_l \in C} p_l)^{2x}$, which is reported in Equation (6.8).

For the Simpson case described in Section 6.1 with $M = \{A_1, A_2, A_3\}$, $V = A_1 A_3$ and $S = A_1 A_2$, now all the people involved are assumed to be coming from the same subdivided population with parameter θ. The measure θ of population subdivision is taken as 0, 0.01, and 0.03. The following two competing propositions are considered:

H_p : contributors were the victim and the suspect;
H_d : contributors were the victim and one unknown.

Then, from Table 6.10, we have

$$LR = \frac{(1 + 3\theta)(1 + 4\theta)}{[\theta + (1 - \theta)p_2][8\theta + (1 - \theta)(2p_1 + p_2 + 2p_3)]}.$$

On the other hand, we can also derive the same likelihood ratio from Equations (6.6) and (6.9). The details are provided as follows. Under H_p, $P(M|K, H_p) = 1$. Under H_d, $x = 1$ and $U = M \setminus \{A_1\} \cup \{A_3\} = \{A_2\}$, $c_1 = 2$, $c_2 = c_3 = 1$, so

$$P(M|K, H_d) = W(M) - W(M \setminus \{A_2\})$$

$$= W(\{A_1, A_2, A_3\}) - W(\{A_1, A_3\})$$

$$= \frac{(p_1 + p_2 + p_2)^{(2)}(c_1 + c_2 + c_3)}{1^{(2)}(c_1 + c_2 + c_3)} - \frac{(p_1 + p_3)^{(2)}(c_1 + c_3)}{1^{(2)}(c_1 + c_2 + c_3)}$$

$$= \frac{(p_1 + p_2 + p_2)^{(2)}(4)}{1^{(2)}(4)} - \frac{(p_1 + p_3)^{(2)}(3)}{1^{(2)}(4)}$$

$$= \frac{[4\theta + (1 - \theta)(p_1 + p_2 + p_3)][5\theta + (1 - \theta)(p_1 + p_2 + p_3)]}{(1 + 3\theta)(1 + 4\theta)}$$

$$- \frac{[3\theta + (1 - \theta)(p_1 + p_3)][4\theta + (1 - \theta)(p_1 + p_3)]}{(1 + 3\theta)(1 + 4\theta)}$$

$$= \frac{[\theta + (1 - \theta)p_2][8\theta + (1 - \theta)(2p_1 + p_2 + 2p_3)]}{(1 + 3\theta)(1 + 4\theta)}.$$

For example, when $\theta = 0.03$, we have further

$$LR$$

$$= \frac{(1 + 3 \times 0.03) \times (1 + 4 \times 0.03)}{[0.03 + 0.0842 \times (1 - 0.03)] \times [8 \times 0.03 + (1 - 0.03) \times (0.0632 + 0.0842 + 0.1852)]}$$

$$= 19.43.$$

Moreover, suppose that the prosecution and defense propositions are altered as

H_p : contributors were the victim, suspect and m unknowns;
H_d : contributors were n unknowns.

Under H_p, the known contributors have all three alleles A_1, A_2 and A_3 in the mixture M. Under H_d, all contributors are unknown and the alleles A_1, A_2, and A_3 should be explained by the n unknown contributors and $U = \{A_1, A_2, A_3\}$. Taking $m = 0$ and $n = 2$ for illustration, we have $P(M|K, H_p) = 1$ and, from Equation (6.6),

$$P(M|K, H_d) = W(\{A_1, A_2, A_3\}) - W(\{A_2, A_3\}) - W(\{A_1, A_3\})$$
$$- W(\{A_1, A_2\}) + W(\{A_1\}) + W(\{A_2\}) + W(\{A_3\}).$$

Note that the tested genotypes in this case are A_1A_3 and A_1A_2, so $c_1 = 2$, $c_2 = c_3 = 1$ (see notations listed in Table 6.6), which are used to calculate $W(C)$ based on Equation (6.11). For example,

$$W(\{A_1, A_2, A_3\}) = \frac{(p_1 + p_2 + p_3)^{(2n)}(c_1 + c_2 + c_3)}{1^{(2n)}(c_1 + c_2 + c_3)}$$
$$= \prod_{i=0}^{3} \frac{(4 + i)\theta + (1 - \theta)(p_1 + p_2 + p_3)}{(4 + i)\theta + (1 - \theta)},$$

$$W(\{A_2, A_3\}) = \frac{(p_2 + p_3)^{(2n)}(c_2 + c_3)}{1^{(2n)}(c_1 + c_2 + c_3)}$$
$$= \prod_{i=0}^{3} \frac{(2 + i)\theta + (1 - \theta)(p_2 + p_3)}{(4 + i)\theta + (1 - \theta)},$$

and the other values of $W(\{A_1, A_3\})$, $W(\{A_1, A_3\})$, $W(\{A_1\})$, $W(\{A_2\})$ and $W(\{A_3\})$ can be derived similarly. Based on all these values, we can obtain the likelihood ratio. Table 6.11 shows the effect of considering uncertainty and population subdivision with different θ values on the likelihood ratios under various combinations of m and n. In each of these combinations, the likelihood ratio at $\theta = 0$ is larger than that at $\theta \neq 0$. Thus, taking $\theta \neq 0$ would be more conservative and to the advantage of the defendant. Taking the extreme example of $n = 4$ and $m = 0$ for demonstration, the likelihood ratios are in the proportions of about $70 : 10 : 1$ for the three different values of $\theta = 0, 0.01$ and 0.03. The strength of the evidence is reduced dramatically if $\theta = 0.03$ is taken. When the 'more reasonable' scenario of $n = 2$ and $m = 0$ is

Table 6.11 Likelihood ratios for the Simpson case about two competing propositions H_p: contributors were the victim, suspect and m unknowns, and H_d: contributors were n unknowns, from Fung and Hu (2000b). (Reproduced by permission of Blackwell Publishing.)

		m		
n	θ	0	1	2
2	0.00	1 623	70	3.06
	0.01	739	44	2.88
	0.03	276	26	2.98
3	0.00	21 606	938	41
	0.01	5 853	345	23
	0.03	1 150	107	12
4	0.00	396 495	17 220	748
	0.01	58 264	3 434	227
	0.03	5 682	528	61

considered, the likelihood ratio drops from 1623 to 739 (half) when $\theta = 0.01$, and further to 276 (one-sixth) when $\theta = 0.03$. The value of θ can have a substantial effect on the likelihood ratio in this RFLP example with a high discriminating power where the allele frequencies p_1, p_2 and p_3 are small.

6.6.3   Multiple ethnic groups

When the persons involved come from different ethnic groups, the calculating formula of the likelihood ratio has to be adjusted accordingly. More parameters are needed to describe the model in this situation. Let p_{gl} be the allele proportion or frequency for type A_l in ethnic group g, $g \in G = \{a, b, \ldots\}$, $l = 1, 2, \ldots$, with measure θ_g for the degree of subdivision. In order to evaluate the conditional probability $P(M|K, H)$ for some proposition H using the formula in Equation (6.6), let x_g be the number of unknown contributors belonging to ethnic group g stated in H, and c_{gl} be the count of allele A_l ($l = 1, 2, \ldots$) present in the typed persons belonging to the ethnic group g, and $c_{g.} = \sum_l c_{gl}$, $g \in G$. The alleles between different ethnic groups are taken to be independent but, for within group, the alleles are not independent, since they belong to the same subdivided population [see Equation (3.17)]. Then, the corresponding formula for calculating $W(C)$ is given as follows:

$$W(C) = \prod_{g \in G} \left[1^{(2x_g)}(c_{g.}, \theta_g)\right]^{-1} \left(\sum_{A_l \in C} p_{gl}\right)^{(2x_g)} \left(\sum_{A_l \in C} c_{gl}, \theta_g\right). \tag{6.12}$$

Note that there could be different degrees of subdivision θ_g for different ethnic groups, so we keep parameter θ_g in Equation (6.12); see also Equation (6.10) for the definition of the expression $r^{(m)}(k, \theta)$. For easy reference, Table 6.12 lists the notations used in Equation (6.12). The proof of Equation (6.12) is given in Section 6.9.3. For practitioners' convenience, Table 6.13 lists the likelihood ratios with a typed victim, a suspect and one unknown contributor. The details of derivation are omitted for simplicity. The detailed expressions for six common mixture cases can be referred to in Fung and Hu (2002b). It is understood from Equation (6.12) and Table 6.13 that it is not easy to calculate the likelihood ratio when the people involved come from different subdivided populations.

In order to evaluate the weight of DNA evidence in this complex situation, a DOS-based computer program has been developed to tackle such problems. In the following, we consider again the Simpson case reported in Section 6.1 to see the effects of population subdivision measures in different ethnic groups. The following two competing propositions are considered (Hu and Fung 2003a):

Table 6.12   A list of notations used in Equation (6.12).

Group	Number of unknowns	Degree of subdivision	Allele frequency A_1	A_2	$\cdots$	A_n	Allele count A_1	A_2	$\cdots$	A_n
a	x_a	θ_a	p_{a1}	p_{a2}	$\cdots$	p_{an}	c_{a1}	c_{a2}	$\cdots$	c_{an}
b	x_b	θ_b	p_{b1}	p_{b2}	$\cdots$	p_{bn}	c_{b1}	c_{b2}	$\cdots$	c_{bn}
$\vdots$	$\vdots$	$\vdots$	$\vdots$	$\vdots$	$\vdots$	$\vdots$	$\vdots$	$\vdots$	$\vdots$	$\vdots$
	$\sum_{g \in G} x_g = x$					$\sum_{j=1}^{n} p_{gj} = 1, \sum_{j=1}^{n} c_{gj} = c_{g.}, g \in G$				

Table 6.13   Likelihood ratios for different mixture M, victim V and suspect S with H_p: the contributors were the victim V and the suspect S, and H_d: the contributors were the victim V and one unknown person X where the people involved come from different subdivided ethnic groups.

Ethnicity			
X	V	S	Likelihood ratio

$M = \{A_i, A_j, A_k\},\ S = A_iA_i,\ V = A_jA_k$

a	a	a	$\dfrac{(1+3\theta_a)(1+4\theta_a)}{[2\theta_a+(1-\theta_a)p_{ai}][7\theta_a+(1-\theta_a)(p_{ai}+2p_{aj}+2p_{ak})]}$
a	a	$\bar{a}$	$\dfrac{(1+\theta_a)(1+2\theta_a)}{(1-\theta_a)p_{ai}[5\theta_a+(1-\theta_a)(p_{ai}+2p_{aj}+2p_{ak})]}$
a	$\bar{a}$	a	$\dfrac{(1+\theta_a)(1+2\theta_a)}{[2\theta_a+(1-\theta_a)p_{ai}][3\theta_a+(1-\theta_a)(p_{ai}+2p_{aj}+2p_{ak})]}$
a	$\bar{a}$	$\bar{a}$	$\dfrac{1}{p_{ai}[\theta_a+(1-\theta_a)(p_{ai}+2p_{aj}+2p_{ak})]}$

$M = \{A_i, A_j, A_k\},\ S = A_iA_j,\ V = A_kA_k$

a	a	a	$\dfrac{(1+3\theta_a)(1+4\theta_a)}{2[\theta_a+(1-\theta_a)p_{ai}][\theta_a+(1-\theta_a)p_{aj}]}$
a	a	$\bar{a}$	$\dfrac{(1+\theta_a)(1+2\theta_a)}{2(1-\theta_a)^2 p_{ai}p_{aj}}$
a	$\bar{a}$	a	$\dfrac{(1+\theta_a)(1+2\theta_a)}{2[\theta_a+(1-\theta_a)p_{ai}][\theta_a+(1-\theta_a)p_{aj}]}$
a	$\bar{a}$	$\bar{a}$	$\dfrac{1}{2(1-\theta_a)p_{ai}p_{aj}}$

$M = \{A_i, A_j, A_k, A_l\},\ S = A_iA_j,\ V = A_kA_l$

a	a	a	$\dfrac{(1+3\theta_a)(1+4\theta_a)}{2[\theta_a+(1-\theta_a)p_{ai}][\theta_a+(1-\theta_a)p_{aj}]}$
a	a	$\bar{a}$	$\dfrac{(1+\theta_a)(1+2\theta_a)}{2(1-\theta_a)^2 p_{ai}p_{aj}}$
a	$\bar{a}$	a	$\dfrac{(1+\theta_a)(1+2\theta_a)}{2[\theta_a+(1-\theta_a)p_{ai}][\theta_a+(1-\theta_a)p_{aj}]}$
a	$\bar{a}$	$\bar{a}$	$\dfrac{1}{2(1-\theta_a)p_{ai}p_{aj}}$

$\bar{a}$ means not ethnic group a

H_p : the contributors were the victim, suspect and m unknowns;
H_d : the contributors were n unknowns

Note that the defendant and the victim were an African American and a Caucasian, respectively. The unknown persons could be from various ethnic groups and they are taken to be

Table 6.14   Likelihood ratios for the Simpson case example about H_p: the contributors were the victim, the suspect and m unknowns, versus H_d: the contributors were n unknowns. Scenario 1, $m = 0$; scenario 2, $m = 1$ unknown of African American; scenario 3, $m = 1$ unknown of Caucasian, from Hu and Fung (2003a). (Reproduced by permission of Springer-Verlag.)

	Under H_d, the number of unknowns belong to group[a]			Scenario					
				1		2		3	
n	AA	CA	CH	$\theta = 0$	0.03	0	0.03	0	0.03
2	2	0	0	1 623	518	70	36	124	56
	0	2	0	396	218	17	15	30	23
	0	0	2	1 773	1536	77	108	135	165
	1	1	0	727	329	32	23	55	35
	1	0	1	1 519	739	66	52	116	79
	0	1	1	599	420	26	29	46	45
3	3	0	0	21 606	2561	938	180	1645	275
	0	3	0	3 112	799	135	56	237	86
	0	0	3	16 007	7432	695	521	1218	798

[a]AA: African American; CA: Caucasian; CH: Chinese

African Americans (AA), Caucasians (CA) and/or Chinese (CH). The allele frequencies of A_1, A_2 and A_3 in ethnic groups AA, CA and CH refer to Section 6.5.

For brevity, Table 6.14 shows the results for $n = 2$ and 3, and $m = 0$ and 1. A few points are observed. First, the likelihood ratio is highly affected by the different sets of propositions, and this is not unusual. Second, ethnicities of the contributors could have a large effect on the size of the likelihood ratio. For example, in scenario 1 with $m = 0$ and $\theta = 0.03$, the likelihood ratio when the unknowns in H_d are Chinese is about seven times that when they are Caucasians. A similar phenomenon is also found for the other two scenarios with $m = 1$. Third, the effect of population subdivision on the value of the likelihood ratio can be substantial. In some cases, taking $\theta = 0.03$ can reduce the value of the likelihood ratio by a few times. However, in three cases, the likelihood ratio increases with θ, indicating that taking $\theta \neq 0$ is not always more conservative than the Hardy–Weinberg rule.

It is seen from the results that the effects of different ethnic groups on the weight of evidence are sometimes great. This example demonstrates the importance of taking ethnicities of contributors into account, and the flexibility of the developed computer program in dealing with various situations. Forensic scientists can choose one or some of the likelihood ratios in Table 6.14 that they find appropriate, or choose to average out different possibilities to obtain an overall likelihood ratio.

6.7   Computer software and example

The authors have developed Window-based user-friendly software and also some Dos-based computer programs for the evaluation of DNA mixtures. In the following, we first introduce the way to run the Window-based program. There are a total of 12 steps needed for the first locus and only three steps for subsequent loci.

Steps in running the EasyDNA_Mixture software

1 Input the population frequency file

2 Input θ values

3 Input the number of alleles in the mixture

4 Input the alleles in the mixture

5 Input the number of typed persons

6 Input the names of typed persons and their genotypes

7 Choose the known contributors for H_p

8 Input the number of unknown contributors for H_p

9 Choose the relationship of the involved persons for H_p (in the example given below, *All involved persons are unrelated*)

10-12 Execute steps 7–9 but for H_d, respectively.

Note that only steps 3, 4 and 6 are needed after processing the first locus.

Note that in step 4, the software will search automatically the frequency corresponding to the chosen allele. In step 6, it is recommended to call those involved persons with names such as victim, suspect, etc. for convenience. Potential contributors to the mixture and their names as well as the genotypes will appear on the screen for selection.

Take the Hong Kong case example introduced in Section 6.2.4 to illustrate the calculation of the likelihood ratio by the computer program. After inputing all the entries, e.g. allele names in the mixture, the two alleles of the typed victim and the typed suspect, for the first locus D3S1358, we can get the input screen (Figure 6.2), where multiple values of parameter θ are designed. We specify the victim and the suspect being the contributors to the mixed stain in the prosecution proposition H_p and the victim and one unknown person being the contributors to the mixed stain in the defense proposition H_d. We can then click the *Calculate* button and confirm the input entries to get the likelihood ratio for the first locus. As shown in Figure 6.2, the likelihood ratios when $\theta = 0$, 0.01 and 0.03 are, respectively, 63.4, 50.9 and 37.6. Afterwards, we can click the *Next Locus* button to start the processing of the second locus. Note that only steps 3, 4 and 6 are needed for this and the subsequent loci. After we complete steps 3, 4 and 6 for the remaining loci, we can get the likelihood ratio results for all loci and at various values of θ. The overall likelihood ratios will be displayed simultaneously. See Figure 6.3 for the captured screen of the computational results of the Hong Kong case example. Finally, we can also click the *Save* button to save the results in a text file for review and further investigation. Figure 6.4 shows the captured screen of the output file.

6.8 NRC II Recommendation 4.1

6.8.1 Single ethnic group

In Section 6.6.1, the subpopulation model of Balding and Nichols (1994) was selected to deal with the evaluation of the DNA mixture when Hardy–Weinberg equilibrium is violated. That model forms the basis of Recommendation 4.2 or Equations (4.9) and (4.10) of the NRC II

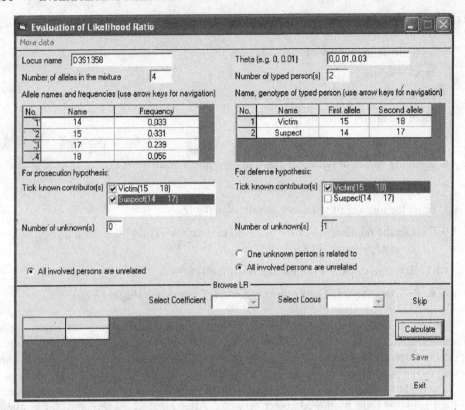

Figure 6.2 Captured input screen for running the EasyDNA_Mixture software for the Hong Kong case example with data given in Table 6.5.

(National Research Council 1996). In fact, two recommendations (Recommendations 4.1 and 4.2) have been suggested by the NRC II to deal with the departure from Hardy–Weinberg equilibrium. Recommendation 4.1 is also used by many forensic laboratories. In the following, we are going to provide the general formula for the interpretation of mixture under Recommendation 4.1.

Based on Equation (3.15) associated with the recommendation, we define

$$p_l * p_m = \begin{cases} p_l^2 + p_l(1 - p_l)\theta, & \text{if } l = m, \\ p_l p_m, & \text{otherwise.} \end{cases} \tag{6.13}$$

Then, the general formula for calculating $W(C)$ defined in Equation (6.7) can be expressed as

$$W(C) = \left(\sum_{A_l, A_m \in C} p_l * p_m \right)^{2x}. \tag{6.14}$$

The proof of Equation (6.14) is given in Section 6.9.5. See also Fung and Hu (2000a) for the details of the derivation of $W(C)$. Note that Equation (6.14) reduces to the Hardy–Weinberg equilibrium Equation (6.8) when $\theta = 0$. The match probability under Recommendation 4.1 can be evaluated after substituting Equation (6.14) into Equation (6.6).

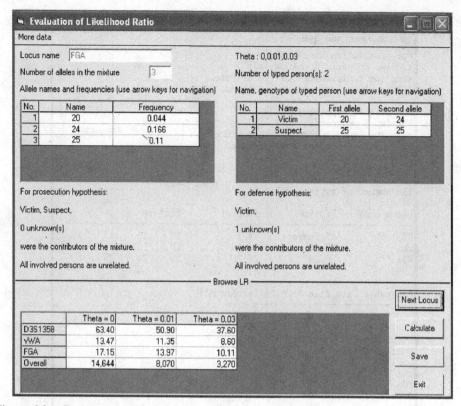

Figure 6.3   Captured screen for the results of the Hong Kong case example using the EasyDNA_Mixture software.

6.8.2   Multiple ethnic groups

In practice, in countries with multiple racial or ethnic groups such as the US, UK, New Zealand or Singapore, it is not uncommon that contributors to a mixed stain belong to different ethnic origins, as we discussed in Section 6.5. A well known example of this sort is the Simpson case introduced in Section 6.1. The general formula for evaluating the likelihood ratio when the contributors to a mixed stain belong to different ethnic groups, based on Recommendation 4.1 of the NRC II (National Research Council 1996), is exploited (Fung and Hu 2002a) as follows:

$$W(C) = \prod_{g \in G} \left(\sum_{A_l, A_m \in C} p_{gl} * p_{gm} \right)^{x_g}, \qquad (6.15)$$

where the asterisk operation $p_{gl} * p_{gm}$ is defined in Equation (6.13) with the measure of subdivision θ_g for the ethnic group $g \in G$. It is obvious that Equation (6.15) is an extension of Equation (6.14). The proof of Equation (6.15) is given in Section 6.9.5. See Table 6.12 for the notations used in Equation (6.15).

In the following, we consider the Hong Kong case example introduced in Section 6.2.4 to see the effect of Recommendation 4.1 on the statistical assessment of mixture. The victim and

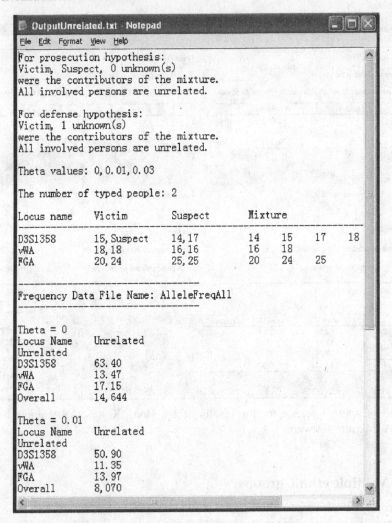

Figure 6.4 Captured screen for the output file of the Hong Kong case example with data given in Table 6.5, using the EasyDNA_Mixture software.

the suspect here were both Chinese and their genotypes are listed in Table 6.5. The prosecution and defense propositions are set as

H_p : the contributors to the mixture were the victim and suspect;

H_d : the contributors to the mixture were the victim and an unknown.

Since there are many Asians of different ethnic origins living in Hong Kong, the effects of different ethnic groups of contributors are considered, regarding the perpetrator being a Chinese, a Filipino or a Thai (they are in the sizes of millions, hundred thousands, and ten thousands, respectively). Allele frequencies of the corresponding groups (Pu *et al.* 1999; Wong *et al.* 2001) are presented in Table 6.15. It is noted that they are different across different ethnic groups. We may choose different θ values for different groups, but we take a common $\theta = 0.03$ for illustration.

Table 6.15   Allele frequencies of different ethnic groups for the Hong Kong case introduced in Section 6.2.4, from Fung and Hu (2002a). (Reproduced by permission of John Wiley & Sons, Ltd.)

Locus	Allele	Chinese	Filipino	Thai
D3S1358	14	0.033	0.026	0.048
	15	0.331	0.267	0.291
	17	0.239	0.286	0.281
	18	0.056	0.088	0.065
vWA	16	0.156	0.161	0.110
	18	0.160	0.225	0.240
FGA	20	0.044	0.048	0.069
	24	0.166	0.141	0.120
	25	0.110	0.088	0.069

The likelihood ratios calculated by Equation (6.15) are presented in Table 6.16. Taking different ethnic origins for the unknown contributor has effects on the likelihood ratio. For example, at locus D3S1358, the likelihood ratio, if the unknown contributor is a Thai, is 41 and 45% less than that if the unknown is a Chinese and a Filipino, respectively. Taking $\theta = 0.03$ makes the likelihood ratios smaller at all loci except D3S1358. The value of θ has no effect at locus D3S1358 because the victim and suspect are both heterozygous [see the asterisk operation introduced in Equation (6.13)]. The overall likelihood ratio drops from 14 721 to 13 434 when $\theta = 0.03$ is taken. The overall effect on the likelihood ratio due to different ethnic origins of the unknown is not large in this example. However, if the genotypes of the victim and suspect were interchanged, the overall likelihood ratio, if the unknown is a Chinese, is about double that if the unknown is a Filipino or a Thai (see the last row of Table 6.16). The ethnicity of the contributor has a larger effect in this situation.

The results in Table 6.16 demonstrate that the ethnicities of contributors have effects on the likelihood ratio. More importantly, the court would not be satisfied and the defendant attorney will strongly criticize if the single ethnic origin formula is applied to mixed stains with contributors from different ethnic origins.

Table 6.16   Likelihood ratios for the Hong Kong case in Section 6.2.4 with the unknown being a Chinese, a Filipino or a Thai, from Fung and Hu (2002a). (Reproduced by permission of John Wiley & Sons, Ltd.)

	Chinese		Filipino		Thai	
Locus	$\theta = 0$	0.03	0	0.03	0	0.03
D3S1358	63.4	63.4	67.2	67.2	37.1	37.1
vWA	13.5	13.0	10.2	9.8	15.4	14.7
FGA	17.2	16.3	24.4	23.0	32.4	30.5
Overall	14 721	13 434	16 724	15 085	18 511	16 633
Overall[a]	24 413	25 893	12 797	12 435	14 447	13 761

[a]The genotypes of the victim (V) and suspect (S) are interchanged.

Finally, let us consider the Simpson case introduced in Section 6.1 to investigate the effects of the ethnicities of unknown contributors on the evaluation of DNA mixtures, based on Recommendation 4.1 of NRC II (National Research Council 1996). The following two competing propositions are considered:

H_p : the contributors were the victim, suspect and m unknowns;
H_d : the contributors were n unknowns

The defendant and the victim were, respectively, an African American and a Caucasian. The unknown persons could be from various ethnic groups and they are taken to be African Americans (AA), Caucasians (CA) and/or Chinese (CH). See Section 6.5 for the population frequencies of alleles A_1, A_2, A_3 in ethnic groups AA, CA and CH, respectively.

The single-banded alleles are taken as true homozygous in the investigation of the effects of θ and different ethnic origins of contributors on the weight of DNA evidence. Table 6.17 lists the results for $n = 2$ and 3, and $m = 0$ and 1. A few things are noticed from the table. First, the likelihood ratio is highly affected by the different sets of propositions, and this is not unusual. Second, taking $\theta = 0.03$ often reduces the size of the likelihood ratio, in most cases by a few to about 20%. However, in some cases, the likelihood ratio increases slightly with θ (see scenario 2), indicating that Recommendation 4.1 is not always more conservative than the Hardy–Weinberg rule. Third, the ethnicity of the contributor has a large effect on the size of the likelihood ratio. For example, in scenario 1 with $\theta = 0.03$, the likelihood ratio when the unknowns in H_d are three Chinese is about five times that when the unknowns are three Caucasians. The other two scenarios also show a similar phenomenon.

The above example serves the purposes of illustrating the importance of taking the ethnicity of contributors into account in the evaluation of DNA evidence, and demonstrating the flexibility of the developed method in dealing with various situations (the theory is a

Table 6.17 Likelihood ratios of the Simpson case introduced in Section6.1 about H_p : the contributors were the victim, the suspect and m unknowns versus H_d: the contributors were n unknowns. Scenario 1, $m = 0$; scenario 2, $m = 1$ unknown of African American; scenario 3, $m = 1$ unknown of Caucasian, from Fung and Hu (2002a). (Reproduced by permission of John Wiley & Sons, Ltd.)

The numbers of unknowns			Scenario								
			1			2			3		
AA	CA	CH[a]	$\theta = 0$	0.03	$2p$	0	0.03	$2p$	0	0.03	$2p$
2	0	0	1 623	1 431	158	70	70	70	124	120	95
0	2	0	396	361	50	17	18	22	30	30	30
0	0	2	1 773	1 593	200	77	78	89	135	133	120
1	1	0	727	651	80	32	32	35	55	54	48
1	0	1	1 519	1 355	161	66	67	71	116	113	97
0	1	1	599	542	71	26	27	32	46	45	43
3	0	0	21 606	15 914	54	938	783	24	1645	1331	32
0	3	0	3 112	2 462	15	135	121	7	237	206	9
0	0	3	16 007	12 499	64	695	615	29	1218	1045	39

[a]AA: African American; CA: Caucasian; CH: Chinese

general one and the developed computer program can handle mixtures of up to 10 contributors). Forensic scientists can choose one or some of the likelihood ratios in Table6.17 that they found appropriate for their analysis. Alternatively, Triggs *et al.* (2000) suggested obtaining an overall likelihood ratio by averaging over different possibilities. In fact, considering various numbers of contributors to the DNA mixed stains was at the request order from the court for the Simpson case.

For the old RFLP technology, a '$2p$' rule is also used to deal with single-banded alleles (Budowle *et al.* 1991a; National Research Council 1996). A general formula in incorporating this rule in assessing mixture for a single ethnic group was provided by Weir *et al.* (1997), and Fung and Hu (2000a) gave proof to the formula. When the contributors to the mixed stain come from different ethnic groups, the corresponding general formula can be obtained from Equation (6.15) by just setting the homozygote match probability $p_l * p_l$ in Equation (6.13) to $2p_l$. When it is applied to the Simpson case, the corresponding results are shown in the columns under '$2p$' in Table 6.17. It is noticed that the '$2p$' rule can have a substantial effect on the evaluation of the likelihood ratio. The likelihood ratio can be reduced a few hundred times when the rule is taken (see the likelihood ratios in scenario 1). Consider a 'more reasonable' case with $m = 0, n = 2$ (row 1 of scenario 1); the likelihood ratio corresponding to the '$2p$' rule is only about one-tenth that when the Hardy–Weinberg rule or NRCII Recommendation4.1 is taken.

It is seen in the Simpson case example that Equation (6.15) not only applies to Recommendation4.1, but also to the '$2p$' rule when the $p_l * p_l$ term in Equation (6.13) is set to $2p_l$. Furthermore, if one prefers to use different formulas for $p_l * p_l$ and $p_l * p_m$ in Equation (6.13) such as $p_l^2 + 2p_l p_n$ for the former one where p_n is the null allele frequency, or Equation (6.13) that having a unit sum of the probabilities over all possible profiles, or other formulas as recommended by the NRCII report (National Research Council 1996), this can be done easily by just substituting these formulas in Equation (6.15). Thus, Equation (6.15) has a wider application than just being used for Recommendation4.1 of NRCII.

6.9 Proofs

The proofs in this section are mainly for mathematically oriented readers. They are provided in this last section, having little distraction to the flow of the main content in the text.

6.9.1 The proof of Equation (6.6)

First of all, we have

$$X \subset M = (U \subset X \subset M) \cup \left(\cup_{A_i \in U}(X \subset M \setminus \{A_i\})\right).$$

So,

$$P(M|K, H) = P(U \subset X \subset M|K)$$
$$= P(X \subset M|K) - P\left(\left(\cup_{A_i \in U}(X \subset M \setminus \{A_i\})\right)|K\right). \tag{6.16}$$

Let $B_i = X \subset M \setminus \{A_i\}$, $A_i \in U$, then $B_i B_j = X \subset M \setminus \{A_i, A_j\}$, $B_i B_j B_k = X \subset M \setminus \{A_i, A_j, A_k\}$, etc. By the principle of inclusion and exclusion

$$P(\cup_{A_i \in U} B_i | K) = \sum_{A_i \in U} P(B_i | K) - \sum_{A_i, A_j \in U} P(B_i B_j | K)$$

$$+ \sum_{A_i, A_j, A_k \in U} P(B_i B_j B_k | K) - \cdots$$

$$= \sum_{A_i \in U} W(M \setminus \{A_i\}) - \sum_{A_i, A_j \in U} W(M \setminus \{A_i, A_j\})$$

$$+ \sum_{A_i, A_j, A_k \in U} W(M \setminus \{A_i, A_j, A_k\})$$

$$- \cdots + (-1)^{|U|} W(M \setminus U), \tag{6.17}$$

where $M(C) = P(X \subset C | K)$ is defined for any subset of M satisfying $M \setminus U \subset C \subset M$. Substituting Equation (6.17) into Equation (6.16), we prove Equation (6.6).

6.9.2   The proof of Equation (6.8)

Considering the independence of genotypes amongst the people involved, we have

$$W(C) = P(X \subset M | K) = P(X \subset C).$$

For the x unrelated unknown contributors, let $A_{i_1} A_{j_1}, \ldots, A_{i_x} A_{j_x}$ denote the genotypes of the 1st, $\ldots$, x-th unknown contributors, respectively. It is easy to understand that $X \subset C$ if and only if $A_{i_1}, \ldots, A_{i_x} \in C$ and $A_{j_1}, \ldots, A_{j_x} \in C$. Further, we have

$$P(X \subset C) = \sum_{A_{i_1}, \ldots, A_{i_x} \in C; A_{j_1}, \ldots, A_{j_x} \in C} p_{i_1} p_{j_1} \cdots p_{i_x} p_{j_x} = \left(\sum_{A_l \in C} p_l \right)^{2x}.$$

So we prove Equation (6.8).

6.9.3   The proof of Equation (6.9)

Let X_a, X_b, $\ldots$, denote the genetic profiles of the x_a, x_b, x_c, $\ldots$, unknown contributors belonging to the ethnic groups a, b, c, $\ldots$, respectively. Note that $X \subset C$ if and only if $X_g \subset C$ for all $g \in G$ and $P(X_g \subset C) = \left(\sum_{A_l \in C} p_{gl} \right)^{2x_g}$. So

$$W(C) = \prod_{g \in G} P(X_g \subset C) = \prod_{g \in G} \left(\sum_{A_l \in C} p_{gl} \right)^{2x_g}.$$

6.9.4   The proofs of Equations (6.11) and (6.12)

In order to prove Equation (6.11), we first establish the following two lemmas which were first reported in Fung and Hu (2000b).

Lemma 6.9.1 *For any given real numbers p_1, p_2 and positive integers m, c_1, c_2, the following equation holds:*

$$(p_1 + p_2)^{(m)} (c_1 + c_2)$$

$$= p_1^{(m)}(c_1) + p_2^{(m)}(c_2) + \sum_{i=1}^{m-1} \binom{m}{i} p_1^{(i)}(c_1) p_2^{(m-i)}(c_2)$$

$$= \sum_{i_1+i_2=m} \binom{m}{i_1} p_1^{(i_1)}(c_1) p_2^{(i_2)}(c_2),$$

where $\binom{m}{i} = m!/[i!(m-i)!]$.

Proof. In the following, we prove Lemma 6.9.1 by induction for m. It is obvious that Lemma 6.9.1 holds for $m = 1$ from Equation (6.10). Assuming Lemma 6.9.1 holds for some integer $m \geq 1$, then we have, from Equation (6.10),

$$(p_1 + p_2)^{(m+1)} (c_1 + c_2)$$

$$= (p_1 + p_2)^{(m)} (c_1 + c_2) ((c_1 + c_2 + m)\theta + (1 - \theta)(p_1 + p_2))$$

$$= \sum_{i=0}^{m} \binom{m}{i} p_1^{(i)}(c_1) p_2^{(m-i)}(c_2) ((c_1 + i)\theta + (1 - \theta)p_1 + (c_2 + m - i)\theta + (1 - \theta)p_2)$$

$$= \sum_{i=0}^{m} \binom{m}{i} p_1^{(i+1)}(c_1) p_2^{(m-i)}(c_2) + \sum_{i=0}^{m} \binom{m}{i} p_1^{(i)}(c_1) p_2^{(m-i+1)}(c_2)$$

$$= p_1^{(m+1)}(c_1) + p_2^{(m+1)}(c_2)$$

$$+ \sum_{i=0}^{m-1} \binom{m}{i} p_1^{(i+1)}(c_1) p_2^{(m-i)}(c_2) + \sum_{i=1}^{m} \binom{m}{i} p_1^{(i)}(c_1) p_2^{(m+1-i)}(c_2)$$

$$= p_1^{(m+1)}(c_1) + p_2^{(m+1)}(c_2) + \sum_{i=1}^{m} \left[\binom{m}{i-1} + \binom{m}{i} \right] p_1^{(i)}(c_1) p_2^{(m+1-i)}(c_2)$$

$$= p_1^{(m+1)}(c_1) + p_2^{(m+1)}(c_2) + \sum_{i=1}^{m} \binom{m+1}{i} p_1^{(i)}(c_1) p_2^{(m+1-i)}(c_2).$$

Thus, Lemma 6.9.1 holds for $m + 1$. So Lemma 6.9.1 holds for any positive integer m.

As a special case, Lemma 6.9.1 is just the binomial expansion theorem of $(p_1 + p_2)^m$ when $\theta = 0$.

For given (p_1, p_2, p_3) and (c_1, c_2, c_3), using Lemma 6.9.1 twice, we have

$$(p_1 + p_2 + p_3)^{(m)}(c_1 + c_2 + c_3)$$

$$= (p_1 + (p_2 + p_3))^{(m)}(c_1 + (c_2 + c_3))$$

$$= \sum_{i_1=0}^{m} \binom{m}{i_1} p_1^{(i_1)}(c_1)(p_2 + p_3)^{(m-i_1)}(c_2 + c_3)$$

$$= \sum_{i_1=0}^{m} \sum_{i_2=0}^{m-i_1} \binom{m}{i_1} \binom{m-i_1}{i_2} p_1^{(i_1)}(c_1) p_2^{(i_2)}(c_2) p_3^{(m-i_1-i_2)}(c_3)$$

$$= \sum_{i_1+i_2+i_3=m} \frac{m!}{i_1! i_2! i_3!} p_1^{(i_1)}(c_1) p_2^{(i_2)}(c_2) p_3^{(i_3)}(c_3).$$

Simply using induction repeatedly, we can generalize Lemma 6.9.1 to

Lemma 6.9.2   *For any given real numbers $p_1, \ldots, p_n$ and non-negative integers m and $c_1, \ldots, c_n$ we have*

$$(p_1 + p_2 + \cdots + p_n)^{(m)} (c_1 + c_2 + \cdots + c_n)$$

$$= \sum_{i_1+i_2+\cdots+i_n=m} \frac{m!}{i_1! i_2! \cdots i_n!} \prod_{j=1}^{n} p_j^{(i_j)}(c_j). \tag{6.18}$$

In order to prove Equation (6.11), we first establish an elaborate probability model to calculate the probability that x people explain the mixed stain. The probability model is described as follows. There are $k + m(m \geq 2, k \geq 2)$ boxes and each box contains n balls labeled from 1 to n. Let $p_1, p_2, \ldots, p_n$ be n positive numbers satisfying $\sum_{1 \leq i \leq n} p_i = 1$. Now, we draw one ball from each box in sequence (not necessarily independent) and get $k + m$ balls at last. Let $G = [l_1, l_2, \ldots, l_m]$ denote the labels of the last m gained balls, which means that the ball labeled l_j is drawn from the $(k + j)$-th box, $1 \leq j \leq m$. Let K denote the labels of the first k balls and $P(G|K)$ denote the conditional probability of event G occurring given K. The probability $P(G|K)$ is calculated based on Equation (3.17). For instance, if $k = m = 4$, $K = [1, 2, 3, 4]$, then

$$P([1, 2, 2, 3]|K) = [\theta + (1 - \theta)p_1][\theta + (1 - \theta)p_2][2\theta + (1 - \theta)p_2][\theta + (1 - \theta)p_3]/1^{(4)}(4)$$

$$= p_1^{(1)}(1) p_2^{(2)}(1) p_3^{(1)}(1)/1^{(4)}(4),$$

$$P([1, 3, 3, 6]|K) = [\theta + (1 - \theta)p_1][\theta + (1 - \theta)p_3][2\theta + (1 - \theta)p_3](1 - \theta)p_6/1^{(4)}(4)$$

$$= p_1^{(1)}(1) p_3^{(2)}(1) p_6^{(1)}(0)/1^{(4)}(4),$$

and so on. It is not difficult to understand that the probability $P(G|K)$ is independent of the ordering of elements in G and K, e.g.

$$P([1, 2, 2, 3]|K) = P([1, 3, 2, 2]|K) = \cdots = p_1^{(1)}(1) p_2^{(2)}(1) p_3^{(1)}(1)/1^{(4)}(4).$$

Generally, let i_j denote the number of element j in G, $j = 1, 2, \ldots, n$, $\sum_{j=1}^{n} i_j = m$, and for given K, let c_j denote the number of element j in K, $j = 1, 2, \ldots, n$, $c = \sum_{j=1}^{n} c_j$, then

$$P(G|K) = \prod_{j=1}^{n} p_j^{(i_j)}(c_j) \bigg/ 1^{(m)}(c).$$

Of course, there are $m!/(i_1! i_2! \cdots i_n!)$ events which have the same probabilities as $P(G|K)$ due to multi-permutation. If we consider the summation of all combinations, then we have

$$\sum_{1\le l_1\le n,\dots,1\le l_m\le n} P([l_1, l_2, \dots, l_m]|K)$$

$$= \sum_{i_1+i_2+\cdots+i_n=m} \frac{m!}{i_1!i_2!\cdots i_n!} \prod_{j=1}^{n} p_j^{(i_j)}(c_j)/1^{(m)}(c),$$

which can be expressed from Equation (6.18) as

$$(p_1 + p_2 + \cdots + p_n)^{(m)}(c_1 + \cdots + c_n)/1^{(m)}(k) = 1.$$

This shows that $P(\cdot|K)$ is a probability. By analogy and from Equation (6.18), for any given subset C of set $\{1, 2, \dots, n\}$, we can have

$$\sum_{l_1,l_2,\dots,l_m\in C} P([l_1, l_2, \dots, l_m]|K) = \left(\sum_{l\in C} p_l\right)^{(m)} \left(\sum_{l\in C} c_l\right)/1^{(m)}(c). \qquad (6.19)$$

Letting $m = 2x$ leads immediately to Equation (6.11). Based on Equation (6.11) and employing the same principle as in the proof of Equation (6.9), we can prove Equation (6.12).

6.9.5   The proofs of Equations (6.14) and (6.15)

In fact, Equation (6.15) is an extension of Equation (6.14), so it is sufficient to prove Equation (6.15). For ethnic group g, since every person inherits two alleles at one locus from his/her parents, it is easy to understand that the probability of his/her alleles belonging to C can be expressed as $\sum_{A_l\in C} P(A_l A_l) + \sum_{l<m, A_l, A_m\in C} P(A_l A_m)$, where C is an arbitrary subset of M. According to Recommendation 4.1 of National Research Council (1996), $p_{gl}^2 + p_{gl}(1 - p_{gl})\theta$ is used to estimate the profile probability of a homozygote $A_l A_l$, while the profile probability of a heterozygote $A_l A_m$ remains the same as $2 p_{gl} p_{gm}$. Using the asterisk operation introduced in Equation (6.13), the probability that one's alleles belong to C can be expressed further as $\sum_{A_l\in C} p_{gl} * p_{gl} + 2\sum_{l<m, A_l, A_m\in C} p_{gl} * p_{gm} = \sum_{A_l, A_m\in C} p_{gl} * p_{gm}$. Generally, the probability that the alleles of x_g unknown contributors belong to set C is $\left(\sum_{A_l, A_m\in C} p_{gl} * p_{gm}\right)^{x_g}$. Since the alleles are independent across ethnic group, we find that the probability of the alleles of the x unknowns belonging to C is just the product of the probability of the alleles of the x_g unknowns belonging to C over all $g \in G$, i.e.

$$W(C) = P(X \subset C) = \prod_{g\in G} \left(\sum_{A_l, A_m\in C} p_{gl} * p_{gm}\right)^{x_g}.$$

6.10   Problems

1. Suppose that the mixture $M = \{A_1, A_2, A_3\}$, and the victim and the suspect are typed as $V = A_1 A_3$ and $S = A_2 A_2$. Calculate the likelihood ratio for the prosecution proposition H_p: the contributors were the victim and the suspect, versus the defense proposition H_d: the contributors were the victim and one unknown person. Hardy–Weinberg equilibrium is assumed.

2. For a crime DNA mixed sample of type $\{A_1, A_2\}$ and a suspect of type A_2A_2, calculate the likelihood ratio for the prosecution proposition H_p: the contributors were the suspect and one unknown, versus the defense proposition H_d: the contributors were two unknown persons. Hardy–Weinberg equilibrium is assumed.

3. Suppose that the DNA profiles for crime sample, victim and suspect are, respectively, $M = \{A_1, A_2, A_3\}$, $V = A_2A_3$ and $S = A_1A_3$. All involved people come from the same subdivided population with a population subdivision measure θ. Derive the likelihood ratio for the prosecution proposition H_p: the contributors were the victim and the suspect, versus the defense proposition H_d: the contributors were the victim and one unknown person.

4. Some crime sample contains DNA from more than one person, and there is only one suspect. Suppose that the mixture $M = \{A_1, A_2, A_3, A_4\}$, and the suspect is tested as $S = A_2A_4$. Calculate the likelihood ratio for the prosecution proposition H_p: the contributors were the suspect and one unknown X_1 (ethnic group a), versus the defense proposition H_d: the contributors were two unknown persons X_1 (ethnic group a) and X_2 (ethnic group b). Hardy–Weinberg equilibrium within each group is assumed.

5. Consider the following two suspects case. Suppose that the mixture $M = \{A_1, A_2, A_3, A_4\}$, and suspect 1 is tested as $S_1 = A_1A_2$ and suspect 2 is tested as $S_2 = A_3A_4$. Calculate the likelihood ratio for the prosecution proposition H_p: the contributors were the two suspects, versus the defense proposition H_d: the contributors were two unknown persons X_1 and X_2 for the three scenarios given below. All the involved persons may come from different ethnic groups with different population subdivision measures θ's.

    (a) The two unknowns and suspect S_1 come from ethnic group a, and suspect S_2 comes from ethnic group b.

    (b) The two unknowns come from ethnic group a, and the two suspects do not come from ethnic group a.

    (c) The first unknown X_1 comes from ethnic group a, the second unknown X_2 comes from ethnic group b, and the two tested suspects come from ethnic group c.

6. For a crime DNA mixed sample of type $\{A_1, A_2, A_3\}$, known to contain DNA from two contributors, the victim is tested as $V = A_1A_2$ and the suspect is tested as $S = A_3A_3$. Under Recommendation 4.1 of NRCII, calculate the likelihood ratio for the prosecution proposition H_p: the contributors were the victim and the suspect, versus the defense proposition H_d: the contributors were the victim and one unknown person.

7

Interpreting mixtures in the presence of relatives

It is not uncommon to have the situation in which the relatives of the suspect or the relatives of the typed persons are involved in a criminal offence. When there are two or more related people involved, it is more flexible to use the relatedness coefficients $(k_0, 2k_1, k_2)$ to describe the relationship between a pair of biologically related persons. When all the people involved come from the same subdivided population, the recursive formula in Equation (3.17) is employed to evaluate the weight of DNA mixture. The assessment of DNA mixture with the presence of relatives is discussed in this chapter. We focus on the derivation of the likelihood ratios, incorporating the relatedness coefficients into the evaluation, when there are a pair of relatives, or two pairs of relatives, when the population is in Hardy–Weinberg equilibrium or when it is not. The corresponding calculating formulas are given and the associated computer program is exhibited for demonstration. Several examples are reported to show the effect of relatedness on the evaluation of the likelihood ratios.

7.1   One pair of relatives: HWE

Consider a case of crime in which the stain is collected from the scene and the reference sample is gathered from the suspect, through a profiling system. The suspect cannot be excluded as a contributor of the stain if the reference sample matches the crime stain. If that is not the case, a suggestion may be made that one close relative of the suspect is a probable assailant when the suspect and crime stain share very rare alleles (Sjerps and Kloosterman 1999). Usually, a series of propositions will be raised to explain who the contributors were, and the likelihood ratio is an effective tool to assess the strength of the evidence. In this section, we shall first introduce a motivating example and then derive a general formula for the evaluation of DNA mixtures in the presence of a pair of relatives when the population is in Hardy–Weinberg equilibrium (Hu and Fung 2003b).

Statistical DNA Forensics: Theory, Methods and Computation   Wing Kam Fung and Yue-Qing Hu
© 2008 John Wiley & Sons, Ltd

7.1.1   Motivating example

In some situations, some person is suspected for the offence but his/her genotype is not available for analysis. A relative of his/hers, for example a full sibling, is, however, available. Also encountered is that in the defense proposition, one relative of the suspected person is claimed to be one of the contributors of the mixture.

Recall the case reported in Table 6.2 with mixture $M = \{A_1, A_2, A_3\}$, the victim's profile $V = A_1 A_2$ and the suspect's genotype $S = A_1 A_3$. The two competing propositions about who the contributors of the mixture were are listed below:

H_p :   the victim and the suspect were contributors;
H_d :   the victim and one unknown relative of the suspect were contributors.

Just as before, let $K = A_1 A_2, A_1 A_3$ denote the known genotypes and it is obvious that $P(M|K, H_p) = 1$. So we focus on the calculation of the denominator $P(M|K, H_d)$ of the likelihood ratio. Under the defense proposition H_d, it is noted that the unknown contributor, denoted by R, is related to the tested person S, so $P(M|K, H_d) = P(R|S = A_1 A_3)$. Since V and R are the only contributors of the mixture, it is concluded that R can take one of the following three genotypes: $A_1 A_3$, $A_2 A_3$, and $A_3 A_3$. Therefore,

$$P(M|K, H_d) = P(R = A_1 A_3 | S = A_1 A_3) + P(R = A_2 A_3 | S = A_1 A_3)$$
$$+ P(R = A_3 A_3 | S = A_1 A_3).$$

Let $(k_0, 2k_1, k_2)$ be the relatedness coefficients between the suspect S and the relative R. See Table 3.13 for the relatedness coefficients of commonly encountered relationships. Employing the results listed in Table 5.1, we have directly

$$P(R = A_1 A_3, S = A_1 A_3) = 4k_0 p_1^2 p_3^2 + 2k_1 p_1 p_3 (p_1 + p_3) + 2k_2 p_1 p_3,$$
$$P(R = A_2 A_3, S = A_1 A_3) = 4k_0 p_1 p_2 p_3^2 + 2k_1 p_1 p_2 p_3,$$
$$P(R = A_3 A_3, S = A_1 A_3) = 2k_0 p_1 p_3^3 + 2k_1 p_1 p_3^2,$$

and then

$$P(R = A_1 A_3 | S = A_1 A_3) = 2k_0 p_1 p_3 + k_1 (p_1 + p_3) + k_2,$$
$$P(R = A_2 A_3 | S = A_1 A_3) = 2k_0 p_2 p_3 + k_1 p_2,$$
$$P(R = A_3 A_3 | S = A_1 A_3) = k_0 p_3^2 + k_1 p_3.$$

So, we have

$$P(M|K, H_d) = k_0 p_3 (2p_1 + 2p_2 + p_3) + k_1 (p_1 + p_2 + 2p_3) + k_2, \tag{7.1}$$

and the likelihood ratio LR is one divided by this probability. To illustrate, we consider that R is a full sibling of the suspect S, then $k_0 = k_1 = k_2 = 1/4$. If $p_1 = p_2 = p_3 = 0.1$, we have $P(M|K, H_d) = 0.3625$ with $LR = 1/0.3625 = 2.76$.

Let us continue to see how the likelihood ratio is derived when the victim's genotype is changed to $A_1 A_1$ and the suspect's genotype is changed to $A_2 A_3$, and the others remain the same. Under the prosecution proposition H_p, $P(M|K, H_p) = 1$. Under the defense proposition H_d, the genotype of the unknown must be $G = A_2 A_3$. So $P(M|K, H_d) = P(G = A_2 A_3 | S = A_2 A_3)$. Considering the relatedness coefficients between the suspect S and the relative being

Table 7.1   Likelihood ratios for one victim, one suspect and one unknown case with H_p: the contributors were the victim and the suspect, and H_d: the contributors were the victim and one unknown relative of the suspect. The relatedness coefficients between the suspect and the relative are $(k_0, 2k_1, k_2)$.

Victim	Suspect	LR
$M = \{A_1, A_2\}$		
$A_1 A_1$	$A_1 A_2$	$1/[k_0 p_2 (2p_1 + p_2) + k_1 (p_1 + 2p_2) + k_2]$
	$A_2 A_2$	$1/[k_0 p_2 (2p_1 + p_2) + 2k_1 (p_1 + p_2) + k_2]$
$A_1 A_2$	$A_1 A_1$	$1/[k_0 (p_1 + p_2)^2 + 2k_1 (p_1 + p_2) + k_2]$
	$A_1 A_2$	$1/[k_0 (p_1 + p_2)^2 + 2k_1 (p_1 + p_2) + k_2]$
$M = \{A_1, A_2, A_3\}$		
$A_1 A_1$	$A_2 A_3$	$1/[2k_0 p_2 p_3 + k_1 (p_2 + p_3) + k_2]$
$A_1 A_2$	$A_1 A_3$	$1/[k_0 p_3 (2p_1 + 2p_2 + p_3) + k_1 (p_1 + p_2 + 2p_3) + k_2]$
	$A_3 A_3$	$1/[k_0 p_3 (2p_1 + 2p_2 + p_3) + 2k_1 (p_1 + p_2 + p_3) + k_2]$
$M = \{A_1, A_2, A_3, A_4\}$		
$A_1 A_2$	$A_3 A_4$	$1/[2k_0 p_3 p_4 + k_1 (p_3 + p_4) + k_2]$

$(k_0, 2k_1, k_2)$, we have

$$P(G = A_2 A_3 | S = A_2 A_3) = k_0 P(A_2 A_3) + k_1 P(A_2) + k_1 P(A_3) + k_2$$
$$= 2k_0 p_2 p_3 + k_1 (p_2 + p_3) + k_2.$$

So, $LR = 1/[2k_0 p_2 p_3 + k_1 (p_2 + p_3) + k_2]$. When the relative stated in the defense proposition is a full sibling of the suspect, i.e. $(k_0, 2k_1, k_2) = (1/4, 1/2, 1/4)$, the associated likelihood ratio is $LR = 4/(2p_2 p_3 + p_2 + p_3 + 1)$. Particularly, if $p_2 = 0.2$ and $p_3 = 0.3$, then $LR = 4/(2 \times 0.2 \times 0.3 + 0.2 + 0.3 + 1) = 2.47$.

Likelihood ratios for some specific combinations of M, V and S can be derived in a similar way and they are listed in Table 7.1 for easy reference.

7.1.2   A probability formula

Comparing the likelihood ratios in Tables 6.2 and 7.1, it is anticipated that it is more difficult to obtain the likelihood ratio under the general situation when the involved people are related. As before, let M denote the DNA profile of the mixture, K denote the collection of the known genotypes, H denote a proposition specifying the known contributors, unknown contributors, and the relationship amongst all the involved people, if any, x denote the number of unknown contributors stated in H, and $A_1, A_2, \ldots$, denote the alleles at an autosomal chromosome with corresponding population frequencies $p_1, p_2, \ldots$, respectively. As we know from Section 6.3, our focus is on the derivation of $P(M|K, H)$ defined there.

In order to give a concise representation of the calculating formula, we first define

$$Q(n, C) = \left(\sum_{A_l \in M} p_l \right)^n - \sum_{A_i \in C} \left(\sum_{A_l \in M \setminus \{A_i\}} p_l \right)^n + \sum_{A_i, A_j \in C} \left(\sum_{A_l \in M \setminus \{A_i, A_j\}} p_l \right)^n$$

$$- \cdots + (-1)^{|M \setminus C|} \left(\sum_{A_l \in M \setminus C} p_l \right)^n \tag{7.2}$$

for any set $C \subset M$ and non-negative integer n (Hu and Fung 2005a). It is noted that $Q(0, \phi) = 1$ and $Q(n, C) = 0$ for $n < |C|$. The calculation of $Q(n, C)$ by a computer program is straight-forward. From Equation (6.6), the quantity $Q(n, C)$ can be interpreted as the probability of n alleles taken from the set M that explain all the alleles in the set C. For example, we consider $n = 3$, $M = \{A_1, A_2, A_3\}$, $C = \{A_1, A_2\}$. From Equation (7.2), we have

$$Q(n, C) = (p_1 + p_2 + p_3)^3 - (p_2 + p_3)^3 - (p_1 + p_3)^3 + p_3^3$$

$$= p_1 p_2 (3p_1 + 3p_2 + 6p_3). \tag{7.3}$$

On the other hand, according to the interpretation of $Q(n, C)$ given above, it is concluded that all the combinations of $n = 3$ alleles (order is relevant) from $M = \{A_1, A_2, A_3\}$ explaining $C = \{A_1, A_2\}$ are given as follows: (A_2, A_1, A_1), (A_1, A_2, A_1), (A_1, A_1, A_2), (A_1, A_2, A_2), (A_2, A_1, A_2), (A_2, A_2, A_1), (A_1, A_2, A_3), (A_1, A_3, A_2), (A_2, A_1, A_3), (A_2, A_3, A_1), (A_3, A_1, A_2), (A_3, A_2, A_1). Summing over all the probabilities of these 12 combinations leads to

$$Q(n, C) = 3P(A_2, A_1, A_1) + 3P(A_1, A_2, A_2) + 6P(A_1, A_2, A_3)$$

$$= 3p_1^2 p_2 + 3p_1 p_2^2 + 6p_1 p_2 p_3$$

$$= p_1 p_2 (3p_1 + 3p_2 + 6p_3). \tag{7.4}$$

Comparing the two different approaches described in Equation (7.3) and Equation (7.4), the one based on Equation (7.2) seems to be simple and reliable.

7.1.3 Tested suspect with an unknown relative

Suppose that a suspect in a crime is typed with $S = s_1 s_2$ and the defense puts up the following proposition about the source contributors of the DNA mixture:

   H: one relative, R, of the suspect and other $x - 1$ unknowns were contributors,

where R is not typed. It should be pointed out that, for brevity, the known contributors are not specified in the proposition H. In practice, which tested persons are contributors of the DNA mixture is clear. The formula for calculating the $P(M|K, H)$ is given as follows:

$$P(M|K, H) = k_0 Q(2x, U)$$

$$+ k_1 [I_M(s_1) Q(2x - 1, U \setminus \{s_1\}) + I_M(s_2) Q(2x - 1, U \setminus \{s_2\})]$$

$$+ k_2 I_M(s_1) I_M(s_2) Q(2x - 2, U \setminus \{s_1\} \cup \{s_2\}). \tag{7.5}$$

The proof of Equation (7.5) is given in Section 7.4.2.

   Detailed expressions of $P(M|K, H)$ are given in Table 7.2 where the tested suspect S has nine different kinds of genotypes. Table 7.2 shows that the computation of $P(M|K, H)$ is

Table 7.2 Expressions for the conditional probability $P(M|K, H)$ for a tested suspect S with an unknown relative, who was one of the contributors of the mixture M stated in proposition H. The relatedness coefficients between S and the unknown relative are described by $(k_0, 2k_1, k_2)$.

Case	S^a	$P(M|K, H)$
1	$A_i A_i$	$k_0 Q(2x, U) + 2k_1 Q(2x - 1, U \setminus \{A_i\}) + k_2 Q(2x - 2, U \setminus \{A_i\})$
2	$A_i A_j$	$k_0 Q(2x, U) + k_1[Q(2x - 1, U \setminus \{A_i\}) + Q(2x - 1, U \setminus \{A_j\})]$
		$\quad + k_2 Q(2x - 2, U \setminus \{A_i, A_j\})$
3	$A_i A_k$	$k_0 Q(2x, U) + k_1[Q(2x - 1, U) + Q(2x - 1, U \setminus \{A_i\})]$
		$\quad + k_2 Q(2x - 2, U \setminus \{A_i\})$
4	$A_i A_m$	$k_0 Q(2x, U) + k_1 Q(2x - 1, U \setminus \{A_i\})$
5	$A_k A_k$	$k_0 Q(2x, U) + 2k_1 Q(2x - 1, U) + k_2 Q(2x - 2, U)$
6	$A_k A_l$	$k_0 Q(2x, U) + 2k_1 Q(2x - 1, U) + k_2 Q(2x - 2, U)$
7	$A_k A_m$	$k_0 Q(2x, U) + k_1 Q(2x - 1, U)$
8	$A_m A_m$	$k_0 Q(2x, U)$
9	$A_m A_n$	$k_0 Q(2x, U)$

$^a A_i, A_j \in U$; $A_k, A_l \in M \setminus U$; $A_m, A_n \in \overline{M}$ (complement of M)

rather simple for given relatedness coefficients $(k_0, 2k_1, k_2)$. In order to find the likelihood ratio using Equation (7.5) or Table 7.2, it is necessary to have a precise specification of the allele A_i out of the set U. For alleles in sets $M \setminus U$ and $\overline{M}$, solely the fact of being part of the set, not the precise specification of alleles, is of importance in the calculation of $P(M|K, H)$.

7.1.4 Unknown suspect with a tested relative

Suppose that the suspect S is unavailable for some reason in a crime case, but a relative of his/hers is typed instead and has genotype $R = r_1 r_2$. The proposition about the source contributors of the DNA mixture is:

H: the suspect S and the other $x - 1$ unknowns were contributors.

Then, the formula for calculating $P(M|K, H)$ is just the same as Equation (7.5), with the replacement of s_1 by r_1 and s_2 by r_2, respectively:

$$P(M|K, H) = k_0 Q(2x, U)$$
$$+ k_1[I_M(r_1)Q(2x - 1, U \setminus \{r_1\}) + I_M(r_2)Q(2x - 1, U \setminus \{r_2\})]$$
$$+ k_2 I_M(r_1) I_M(r_2) Q(2x - 2, U \setminus \{r_1\} \cup \{r_2\}). \tag{7.6}$$

Thus, the detailed expressions about the nine possible genotypes of R can also be referred to in Table 7.2, except S in the table is replaced by R.

Fukshansky and Bär (2000) discussed the evaluation of $P(M|K, H)$ in the situation of one unknown suspect with a tested relative under the Hardy–Weinberg law, where the relationships between the suspect and the relative are limited to child–parent, full siblings and half siblings. Their results are equivalent to Equation (7.5) when the relatedness coefficients are taken as the specified values of the relationships mentioned.

Turning back to the example introduced in Section 7.1.1 with $M = \{A_1, A_2, A_3\}$ and $V = A_1 A_2$ and $S = A_1 A_3$, we consider the following proposition about who the contributors were:

H_d : the victim and one unknown relative of the suspect were contributors.

It is easy to conclude under H_d that $x = 1$ and $U = \{A_3\}$. Regarding the two alleles A_1 and A_3 that the suspect carries, it is obvious that $A_1 \in M \setminus U$ and $A_3 \in U$. So, employing the results in case 3 in Table 7.2, we have

$$P(M|H, H_d) = k_0 Q(2, \{A_3\}) + k_1[Q(1, \{A_3\}) + Q(1, \phi)] + k_2 Q(0, \phi).$$

From Equation (7.2), we have

$$Q(0, \phi) = 1,$$

$$Q(1, \phi) = (p_1 + p_2 + p_3),$$

$$Q(1, \{A_3\}) = (p_1 + p_2 + p_3) - (p_1 + p_2) = p_3,$$

and

$$Q(2, \{A_3\}) = (p_1 + p_2 + p_3)^2 - (p_1 + p_2)^2 = p_3(2p_1 + 2p_2 + p_3).$$

Finally, it is concluded that

$$P(M|H, H_d) = k_0 p_3(2p_1 + 2p_2 + p_3) + k_1(p_1 + p_2 + 2p_3) + k_2.$$

This result coincides with that in Equation (7.1) obtained step-by-step in Section 7.1.1.

7.1.5   Two related persons were unknown contributors

Here, we consider the situation in which the genotypes of two related persons match with the profile of a mixture. The proposition can be written as

H: two biologically related persons X_1 and X_2, and $x - 2$ unknowns were contributors.

In this situation, it is shown in Section 7.4.3 that $P(M|K, H)$ has a simple form, which is given as

$$P(M|K, H) = k_0 Q(2x, U) + 2k_1 Q(2x - 1, U) + k_2 Q(2x - 2, U). \tag{7.7}$$

In this case, we do not need a table such as Table 7.2 for expressions on various possible combinations of genotypes.

The following is an example to illustrate the application of Equation (7.7). Change the defense proposition H_d in the example given in Section 7.1.1 to

H_d^*: two related unknown persons R_1 and R_2 were contributors.

Under H_d^*, $x = 2$ and $M = U = \{A_1, A_2, A_3\}$, so

$$P(M|K, H_d^*) = k_0 Q(4, U) + 2k_1 Q(3, U) + k_2 Q(2, U).$$

From Equation (7.2), we have

$$Q(4, U) = (p_1 + p_2 + p_3)^4 - (p_2 + p_3)^4 - (p_1 + p_3)^4 - (p_1 + p_2)^4 + p_1^4 + p_2^4 + p_3^4,$$

$$Q(3, U) = (p_1 + p_2 + p_3)^3 - (p_2 + p_3)^3 - (p_1 + p_3)^3 - (p_1 + p_2)^3 + p_1^3 + p_2^3 + p_3^3,$$

$$Q(2, U) = (p_1 + p_2 + p_3)^2 - (p_2 + p_3)^2 - (p_1 + p_3)^2 - (p_1 + p_2)^2 + p_1^2 + p_2^2 + p_3^2.$$

So, for given allele frequencies p_1, p_2, p_3, and relatedness coefficients $(k_0, 2k_1, k_2)$, it is not difficult to get the result of $P(M|K, H_d^*)$ and finally the likelihood ratio.

7.1.6   An application

Let us consider the Hong Kong case example introduced in Section 6.2.4. See Table 6.5 for the details of the mixture, tested persons at three loci and the allele population frequencies. The following two competing propositions are first considered:

H_p :   contributors were the victim and the suspect;
H_{d1} :   contributors were the victim and one relative of the suspect.

Here, the victim, the suspect and the unknown are assumed to come from the same local Chinese population. Table 7.3 lists the likelihood ratios for six commonly encountered relationships between the suspect and his/her relative, including the unrelated case. As we can see from this table, the effect of relatedness on the likelihood ratio is substantial. For example, at locus FGA, the maximum likelihood ratio value (17.15) is seven times the minimum one (2.36). Note that among those six relationships, the full siblings gives the smallest likelihood ratios at loci D3S1358, vWA and FGA.

If the evidence was collected from somewhere other than the victim's body (Fung and Hu 2000a), then another set of propositions should be raised:

H_p :   contributors were the victim and the suspect;
H_{d2} :   contributors were one relative of the suspect and one unknown.

The resultant likelihood ratios are listed in Table 7.3, which are larger than the corresponding one based on the preposition pair H_p and H_{d1}. However, the effect of relatedness on the likelihood ratio is not as large as before. The ratio of the maximum and minimum likelihood ratios is about 5. As in the previous case, the relatedness has the effect of giving a smaller likelihood ratio (compared with the unrelated situation), with the smallest likelihood ratio going to the full siblings relationship at loci D3S1358 and vWA, and going to the parent–child relationship at locus FGA.

Finally, we consider the following two competing propositions about who the source contributors of the mixed stain were:

H_p :   contributors were the victim and the suspect;
H_{d3} :   contributors were two related persons (relatives).

Equation (7.7) is used to evaluate the likelihood ratios for various relationships and the results are listed in Table 7.3. Unlike the other two earlier situations, under the current set of propositions, the likelihood ratio at locus D3S1358 for the full siblings relationship is the highest ($LR = 1140$), while that for the unrelated relationship is the lowest ($LR = 285$). However, the lowest likelihood ratios at loci vWA and FGA go to the full siblings ($LR = 37.75$) and the parent–child ($LR = 207.44$) relationships, respectively. The effect of relatedness is mixed

Table 7.3   The effect of relatedness on the likelihood ratios in the Hong Kong case example (see Table 6.5), in which the prosecution proposition is H_p: contributors were the victim and the suspect, and the defense proposition takes three different forms, i.e. H_{d1}: contributors were the victim and one relative of the suspect; H_{d2}: contributors were one relative of the suspect and one unknown; H_{d3}: contributors were two related persons (relatives), from Hu and Fung (2003b). (Reproduced by permission of Springer-Verlag.)

Defense proposition	Relationship	Likelihood ratios			Overall
		D3S1358	vWA	FGA	
H_{d1}	Parent–child	7.35	3.16	3.13	73
	Full siblings	3.11	2.34	2.36	17
	Half siblings[a]	13.18	5.12	5.29	357
	First cousins	21.82	7.42	8.08	1 309
	Second cousins	42.94	11.19	13.39	6 436
	Unrelated	63.40	13.47	17.15	14 644
H_{d2}	Parent–child	66.11	36.03	106.13	252 787
	Full siblings	56.47	28.62	109.48	176 943
	Half siblings[a]	107.33	54.82	159.91	940 898
	First cousins	155.94	74.17	214.16	2 476 984
	Second cousins	236.14	100.87	287.25	6 842 643
	Unrelated	285.01	114.63	324.13	10 589 598
H_{d3}	Parent–child[b]	—	42.26	207.44	—
	Full siblings	1140.04	37.75	314.31	13 525 658
	Half siblings[a]	570.02	61.76	252.98	8 905 310
	First cousins	380.01	80.27	284.17	8 667 933
	Second cousins	304.01	103.55	313.12	9 856 994
	Unrelated	285.01	114.63	324.13	10 589 598

[a] The same as the grandparent–child and the uncle–niece relationship
[b] The parent–child relationship is impossible for a mixture of four distinct alleles

under this particular set of propositions. Note that at locus D3S1358, the parent–child relationship is impossible for a mixture of four distinct alleles.

In the following, we use our developed computer software EasyDNA_Mixture to obtain the likelihood ratios about H_p versus H_{d1} for six commonly encountered relationships. Notice that we list in Section 6.7 the 12 steps in running the software where all persons involved are unrelated. In order to calculate the likelihood ratio when the defense proposition H_{d1} involves two related persons, we follow those 12 steps as below.

1 Select the appropriate allele frequency file

2 Input $\theta = 0$

3 Input 4, the number of alleles in the mixture for locus D3S1358

4 Input alleles 14, 15, 17 and 18 in this mixture

5 Input 2, the number of typed persons, i.e. the victim and the suspect

6 Input the genotypes of these two typed persons

7 Choose the victim and the suspect as the known contributors

8 Input 0 as the number of unknown contributors

9 Specify that all persons involved are unrelated

10 Choose the victim as the only known contributor

11 Input 1 as the number of unknown contributors

12 Specify that one unknown person is related to the suspect.

The entries in steps 7–9 constitute the prosecution proposition H_p, and the entries in steps 10-12 constitute the defense proposition H_d: the victim and one relative of the suspect were the contributors. After running these steps, we have the input screen as shown in Figure 7.1. By clicking the *Calculate* button, we can get the likelihood ratios for six kinds of relationships immediately. Clicking the *Next Locus* button leads to the process of calculating the likelihood

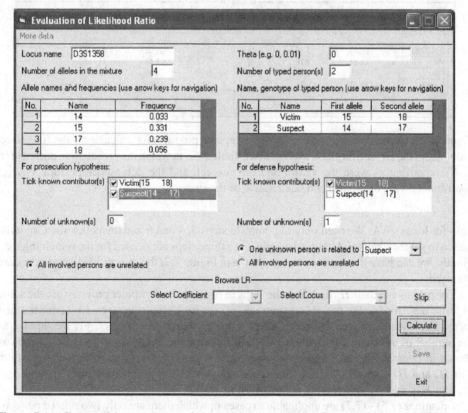

Figure 7.1 Captured input screen of the computer program for calculating the likelihood ratios about the Hong Kong case example (see Table 6.5), in which the prosecution proposition is H_p: contributors were the victim and the suspect, and the defense proposition is H_{d1}: contributors were the victim and one relative of the suspect.

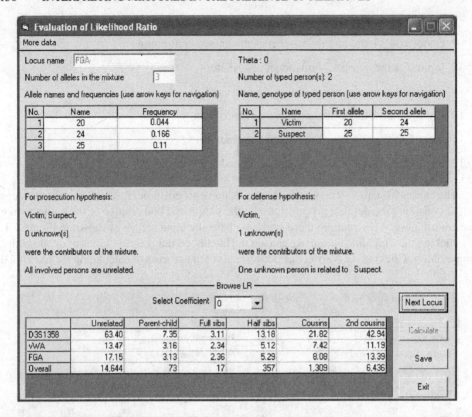

Figure 7.2 Captured result screen of the computer program for calculating the likelihood ratios about the Hong Kong case example (see Table 6.5), in which the prosecution proposition is H_p: contributors were the victim and the suspect, and the defense proposition is H_{d1}: contributors were the victim and one relative of the suspect.

ratio for locus vWA. We need only to complete steps 3, 4 and 6 and then click the *Calculate* button to get the likelihood ratio. Also only these three steps are needed for the remaining loci. Finally, we can have the result screen as shown in Figure 7.2; the overall likelihood ratios are obtained.

For proposition pair H_p and H_{d2}, the steps in running the computer program are the same as those described in the previous paragraph, except for changes in steps 10–11 for the first locus. Specifically, in step 10, there are no known contributors; in step 11, we input 2 as the number of unknown contributors. We have captured the input screen and result screen as shown in Figures 7.3 and 7.4, respectively. Similar steps can be conducted for proposition pair H_p and H_{d3} as well. All these likelihood ratio results for proposition pairs H_p and H_{d1}, H_p and H_{d2}, and H_p and H_{d3} are summarized in Table 7.3.

Equations (7.5)–(7.7) are applicable to cases in which there are only two related persons. We assume that the other unknown contributors are unrelated to the suspect and the population satisfies the Hardy–Weinberg law and linkage equilibrium. Besides Hu and Fung (2003b), who considered the evaluation of DNA evidence in the presence of a pair of relatives, the problem of how to assign the weight of the DNA evidence when one suspect's relative is involved in

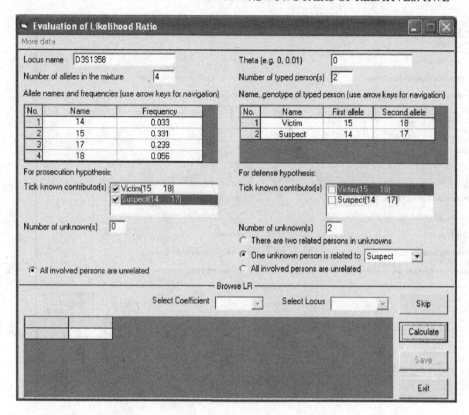

Figure 7.3   Captured input screen of the computer program for calculating the likelihood ratios about the Hong Kong case example (see Table 6.5), in which the prosecution proposition is H_p: contributors were the victim and the suspect, and the defense proposition is H_{d2}: contributors were one unknown and one relative of the suspect.

the pool of possible perpetrators has been discussed by several authors. For example, Evett (1992) established a formula for the likelihood ratio in a case in which the defense is 'It was my brother'; Brookfield (1994) evaluated the effect upon the likelihood ratio of the possibility that the suspect and the source of the crime-scene DNA are relatives; Donnelly (1995) quantified the effect of close relatives on the match probability; Belin *et al.* (1997) described a new methodology that summarized DNA evidence by addressing the possibility that a relative of the accused individual was the source of a crime sample; and Sjerps and Kloosterman (1999) discussed the assessment of DNA profiles for close relatives of an excluded suspect. These authors limited the effect of relatedness on the evaluation of match probability and likelihood ratio relating to a single source DNA sample. In the following section, we will discuss the evaluation of the DNA mixture when there are two pairs of relatives involved in the case.

7.2   Two pairs of relatives: HWE

In Section 7.1, we discussed the evaluation of the DNA mixture when there is a pair of relatives involved in a case. In some practical situations, we may face a more complicated

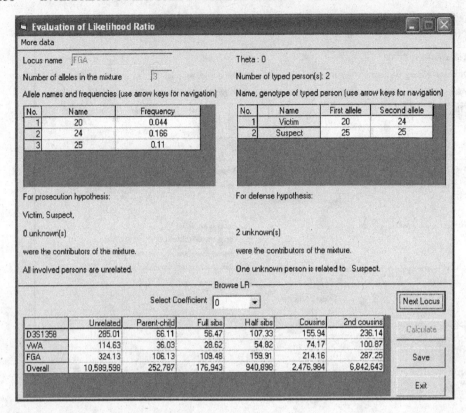

Figure 7.4   Captured result screen of the computer program for calculating the likelihood ratios about the Hong Kong case example (see Table 6.5), which the prosecution proposition is H_p: contributors were the victim and the suspect, and the defense proposition is H_{d2}: contributors were one unknown and one relative of the suspect.

scenario in which two pairs of relatives are involved, especially when the number of tested and untested persons is more than three. For example, if the number of unknown contributors is two, we may encounter the situation in which each unknown contributor is related to a single typed person. In other words, an unknown contributor X_1 is related to a typed person T_1, and independently, the other unknown contributor X_2 is related to another typed person T_2. If the number of unknown contributors is three, we may encounter the situation in which one unknown contributor is related to a typed person and the other two unknown contributors are related; that is, an unknown contributor X_1 is related to a typed person T_1, and X_2 and X_3 are two related unknown contributors. If the number of unknown contributors is four, we may have the situation in which two pairs of relatives, i.e. X_1 and X_2, are related unknown contributors and so are X_3 and X_4. These three cases will render calculations of likelihood ratios more difficult than those given in Section 7.1.

Denote $x > 1$ as the number of unknown contributors, $X_1, X_2, \ldots$ the unknown contributors, and $T_1, T_2, \ldots$ the typed persons. In this section, we consider the following three problems on the evaluation of the DNA mixture involving two pairs of relatives (Hu and Fung 2005a), under Hardy–Weinberg equilibrium:

(a) There are x ($x \geq 2$) unrelated unknown contributors, among which X_1 is related to T_1, and X_2 is related to T_2, and the other $x - 2$ unknown contributors are unrelated.

(b) There are x ($x \geq 3$) unknown contributors, among which X_1 is related to T_1, and X_2 and X_3 are related, and X_1 and the other $x - 3$ unknown contributors are unrelated.

(c) There are x ($x \geq 4$) unknown contributors, among which X_1 and X_2 are related, X_3 and X_4 are related, and the other $x - 4$ unknown contributors are unrelated.

We will focus on the derivation of $W(C)$ defined in Equation (6.7) for calculating the likelihood ratio for these three problems.

7.2.1 Two unknowns related respectively to two typed persons

Suppose that at least two persons are typed with genotypes $T_1 = t_{11}t_{12}$ and $T_2 = t_{21}t_{22}$, and the proposition about who the x ($x \geq 2$) unknown unrelated contributors are is

H : two of the x unknowns, X_1 and X_2, are related to T_1 and T_2, respectively.   (7.8)

Denote $(k_{10}, 2k_{11}, k_{12})$ as the relatedness coefficients between individuals X_1 and T_1, and $(k_{20}, 2k_{21}, k_{22})$ as the relatedness coefficients between X_2 and T_2; then, we have (Hu and Fung 2005a)

$$P(M|K, H) = (k_{10}, 2k_{11}, k_{12}) \begin{pmatrix} \sigma_{11} & \sigma_{12} & \sigma_{13} \\ \sigma_{21} & \sigma_{22} & \sigma_{23} \\ \sigma_{31} & \sigma_{32} & \sigma_{33} \end{pmatrix} \begin{pmatrix} k_{20} \\ 2k_{21} \\ k_{22} \end{pmatrix},$$ (7.9)

where

$\sigma_{11} = Q(2x, U),$

$\sigma_{12} = I_M(t_{21})Q(2x - 1, U \setminus \{t_{21}\})/2 + I_M(t_{22})Q(2x - 1, U \setminus \{t_{22}\})/2,$

$\sigma_{13} = I_M(t_{21})I_M(t_{22})Q(2x - 2, U \setminus \{t_{21}\} \cup \{t_{22}\}),$

$\sigma_{21} = I_M(t_{11})Q(2x - 1, U \setminus \{t_{11}\})/2 + I_M(t_{12})Q(2x - 1, U \setminus \{t_{12}\})/2,$

$\sigma_{22} = I_M(t_{11})I_M(t_{21})Q(2x - 2, U \setminus \{t_{11}\} \cup \{t_{21}\})/4$

$\qquad + I_M(t_{11})I_M(t_{22})Q(2x - 2, U \setminus \{t_{11}\} \cup \{t_{22}\})/4$

$\qquad + I_M(t_{12})I_M(t_{21})Q(2x - 2, U \setminus \{t_{12}\} \cup \{t_{21}\})/4$

$\qquad + I_M(t_{12})I_M(t_{22})Q(2x - 2, U \setminus \{t_{12}\} \cup \{t_{22}\})/4,$

$\sigma_{23} = I_M(t_{11})I_M(t_{21})I_M(t_{22})Q(2x - 3, U \setminus \{t_{11}\} \cup \{t_{21}\} \cup \{t_{22}\})/2$

$\qquad + I_M(t_{12})I_M(t_{21})I_M(t_{22})Q(2x - 3, U \setminus \{t_{12}\} \cup \{t_{21}\} \cup \{t_{22}\})/2,$

$\sigma_{31} = I_M(t_{11})I_M(t_{12})Q(2x - 2, U \setminus \{t_{11}\} \cup \{t_{12}\}),$

$\sigma_{32} = I_M(t_{11})I_M(t_{12})I_M(t_{21})Q(2x - 3, U \setminus \{t_{11}\} \cup \{t_{12}\} \cup \{t_{21}\})/2$

$\qquad + I_M(t_{11})I_M(t_{12})I_M(t_{22})Q(2x - 3, U \setminus \{t_{11}\} \cup \{t_{12}\} \cup \{t_{22}\})/2,$

$\sigma_{33} = I_M(t_{11})I_M(t_{12})I_M(t_{21})I_M(t_{22})Q(2x - 4, U \setminus \{t_{11}\} \cup \{t_{12}\} \cup \{t_{21}\} \cup \{t_{22}\}).$

The proof of Equation (7.9) is given in Section 7.4.4.

There are two particular relatedness coefficients to be noted. If $(k_{20}, 2k_{21}, k_{22}) = (0, 0, 1)$, i.e. $X_2 = T_2$, then the typed person T_2 becomes a known contributor and the proposition H in (7.8) becomes 'one of the $x - 1$ unknown contributors, X_1, is related to T_1'; if $(k_{10}, 2k_{11}, k_{12}) = (k_{20}, 2k_{21}, k_{22}) = (0, 0, 1)$, then both typed persons T_1 and T_2 become the known contributors and the proposition H in (7.8) becomes 'there are $x - 2$ unknown contributors'. It is thus concluded that the proposition H in (7.8) can cover a variety of propositions, which will be shown in the examples given in Section 7.2.4.

7.2.2   One unknown is related to a typed person and two other unknowns are related

Suppose that there are at least three unknown contributors involved in a proposition, among them, X_1 is related to a typed person T_1, and X_2 and X_3 are related. The relatedness coefficients between X_1 and T_1, and X_2 and X_3, are, respectively, $(k_{10}, 2k_{11}, k_{12})$ and $(k_{20}, 2k_{21}, k_{22})$. The proposition about who the contributors are is given as follows:

H :   one of the x (≥ 3) unknowns, X_1, is related to a typed person T_1
and two of the x unknowns, X_2 and X_3, are related. $\qquad$ (7.10)

In this situation, the corresponding formula for calculating $P(M|K, H)$ is (Hu and Fung 2005a)

$$P(M|K, H) = (k_{10}, 2k_{11}, k_{12}) \begin{pmatrix} \sigma_{11} & \sigma_{12} & \sigma_{13} \\ \sigma_{21} & \sigma_{22} & \sigma_{23} \\ \sigma_{31} & \sigma_{32} & \sigma_{33} \end{pmatrix} \begin{pmatrix} k_{20} \\ 2k_{21} \\ k_{22} \end{pmatrix}, \qquad (7.11)$$

where

$$\sigma_{11} = Q(2x, U),$$

$$\sigma_{12} = Q(2x - 1, U),$$

$$\sigma_{13} = Q(2x - 2, U),$$

$$\sigma_{21} = I_M(t_{11})Q(2x - 1, U \setminus \{t_{11}\})/2 + I_M(t_{12})Q(2x - 1, U \setminus \{t_{12}\})/2,$$

$$\sigma_{22} = I_M(t_{11})Q(2x - 2, U \setminus \{t_{11}\})/2 + I_M(t_{12})Q(2x - 2, U \setminus \{t_{12}\})/2,$$

$$\sigma_{23} = I_M(t_{11})Q(2x - 3, U \setminus \{t_{11}\})/2 + I_M(t_{12})Q(2x - 3, U \setminus \{t_{12}\})/2,$$

$$\sigma_{31} = I_M(t_{11})I_M(t_{12})Q(2x - 2, U \setminus \{t_{11}\} \cup \{t_{12}\}),$$

$$\sigma_{32} = I_M(t_{11})I_M(t_{12})Q(2x - 3, U \setminus \{t_{11}\} \cup \{t_{12}\}),$$

$$\sigma_{33} = I_M(t_{11})I_M(t_{12})Q(2x - 4, U \setminus \{t_{11}\} \cup \{t_{12}\}).$$

The proof of Equation (7.11) is outlined in Section 7.4.5. Note that if $t_{11}, t_{12} \in M \setminus U$, then $\sigma_{12} = \sigma_{21} = Q(2x - 1, U)$, $\sigma_{13} = \sigma_{22} = \sigma_{31} = Q(2x - 2, U)$, $\sigma_{23} = \sigma_{32} = Q(2x - 3, U)$ and $\sigma_{33} = Q(2x - 4, U)$, and the expression $P(M|K, H)$ can be simplified to

$$P(M|K, H)$$

$$= (k_{10}, 2k_{11}, k_{12}) \begin{pmatrix} Q(2x, U) & Q(2x - 1, U) & Q(2x - 2, U) \\ Q(2x - 1, U) & Q(2x - 2, U) & Q(2x - 3, U) \\ Q(2x - 2, U) & Q(2x - 3, U) & Q(2x - 4, U) \end{pmatrix} \begin{pmatrix} k_{20} \\ 2k_{21} \\ k_{22} \end{pmatrix}.$$

7.2.3 Two pairs of related unknowns

In the case of two pairs of relatives involved in the pool of contributors, we consider the proposition

H : amongst the x (≥ 4) unknowns contributors, X_1 and X_2 are related,

and X_3 and X_4 are related. $\qquad$ (7.12)

Denote $(k_{10}, 2k_{11}, k_{12})$ as the relatedness coefficients of X_1 and X_2, and $(k_{20}, 2k_{21}, k_{22})$ as the coefficients of X_3 and X_4. Under this proposition, we have (Hu and Fung 2005a)

$P(M|K, H)$

$$= (k_{10}, 2k_{11}, k_{12}) \begin{pmatrix} Q(2x, U) & Q(2x-1, U) & Q(2x-2, U) \\ Q(2x-1, U) & Q(2x-2, U) & Q(2x-3, U) \\ Q(2x-2, U) & Q(2x-3, U) & Q(2x-4, U) \end{pmatrix} \begin{pmatrix} k_{20} \\ 2k_{21} \\ k_{22} \end{pmatrix}.$$

$$(7.13)$$

See Section 7.4.6 for the proof of Equation (7.13).

We are interested in some particular cases of relatedness coefficients in Equation (7.13). If $(k_{20}, 2k_{21}, k_{22}) = (1, 0, 0)$ in Equation (7.13), i.e. there exists only one pair of related unknowns among the x unknowns, then the conditional probability $P(M|K, H)$ is simply $k_{10} Q(2x, U) + 2k_{11}Q(2x-1, U) + k_{12}Q(2x-2, U)$, which was reported in Equation (7.7) (Hu and Fung 2003b). If $(k_{20}, 2k_{21}, k_{22}) = (0, 0, 1)$, i.e. there exists only one pair of related unknowns among the $x-1$ unknowns, then the conditional probability $P(M|K, H)$ is $k_{10}Q(2x-2, U) + 2k_{11}Q(2x-3, U) + k_{12}Q(2x-4, U)$. If $(k_{20}, 2k_{21}, k_{22}) = (0, 1, 0)$, e.g. X_4 is the father of X_3, then the conditional probability $P(M|K, H)$ is simply $k_{10}Q(2x-1, U) + 2k_{11}Q(2x-2, U) + k_{12}Q(2x-3, U)$. In this situation, there is one and only one allele of the father X_4 which is ibd to one allele of child X_3, so only three alleles among those four alleles of X_3 and X_4 are not ibd and hence we regard the number of unknown contributors as $x - 1/2$. Thus, replacing x in the first case of this paragraph corresponding to $(k_{20}, 2k_{21}, k_{22}) = (1, 0, 0)$ by $x - 1/2$ will lead to the result. It is convenient to calculate the conditional probability given in Equation (7.13) by the computer program.

It is interesting to note that Equations (7.9) and (7.11) are equal when the two alleles of T_2 satisfy $t_{21}, t_{22} \in M \setminus U$, and Equations (7.11) and (7.13) are equal when the two alleles of T_1 satisfy $t_{11}, t_{12} \in M \setminus U$. We will see the latter case in the example of the next section.

7.2.4 Examples

The first example is taken from Stockmarr (2000). The DNA profile of the mixture was typed as $\{18, 24, 28, 31, 33, 36\}$ at locus D1S80 from a mixed stain recovered from a crime scene, and the DNA profile of the victim V was typed as $\{24, 33\}$. The population frequencies of these alleles are listed in Table 7.4. Stockmarr (2000) considered two propositions, namely 'the victim and $n - 1$ unknowns are contributors' versus 'n unknowns are contributors', with a range of values of n. In the following analysis, we fix n at 4 and investigate two competing

Table 7.4   Alleles and allele frequencies at locus D1S80.

Mixture (M)	Victim (V)	Frequency
18		0.2487
24	24	0.3622
28		0.0657
31		0.0738
33	33	0.0044
36		0.0077

propositions:

H'_p : the victim and three unknowns are contributors; among these three unknowns, one unknown is related to the victim, and the other two are related;

H'_d : the four unknowns are contributors; among them, two unknowns are related, and the other two are also related.

Since there can be various sorts of relationships, for simplicity, we consider only the following two particular propositions:

H_p : the victim V, one untyped relative R of the victim, and two untyped full siblings are contributors;

H_d : two related unknowns X_1 and X_2, and two untyped full siblings are contributors.

Equation (7.11) is used to calculate the likelihood ratio, i.e. $P(M|K, H_p)/P(M|K, H_d)$. Under the prosecution proposition H_p, the number of unknown contributors x is three, $U = \{18, 28, 31, 36\}$, $M = \{18, 24, 28, 31, 33, 36\}$, the relatedness coefficients of full siblings are $(1/4, 1/2, 1/4)$, and the two alleles of typed victim V satisfy $24, 33 \in M \setminus U$; so, from Equation (7.11), after simplification, we have

$$P(M|K, H_p) = (k_{10}, 2k_{11}, k_{12}) \begin{pmatrix} Q(6, U) & Q(5, U) & Q(4, U) \\ Q(5, U) & Q(4, U) & Q(3, U) \\ Q(4, U) & Q(3, U) & Q(2, U) \end{pmatrix} \begin{pmatrix} 1/4 \\ 1/2 \\ 1/4 \end{pmatrix},$$

where $(k_{10}, 2k_{11}, k_{12})$ are the relatedness coefficients of individuals R and V specified in H_p. Under the defense proposition H_d, $x = 4$ and $U = \{18, 24, 28, 31, 33, 36\}$; using Equation (7.13), we can find

$$P(M|K, H_d) = (k_{20}, 2k_{21}, k_{22}) \begin{pmatrix} Q(8, U) & Q(7, U) & Q(6, U) \\ Q(7, U) & Q(6, U) & Q(5, U) \\ Q(6, U) & Q(5, U) & Q(4, U) \end{pmatrix} \begin{pmatrix} 1/4 \\ 1/2 \\ 1/4 \end{pmatrix},$$

where $(k_{20}, 2k_{21}, k_{22})$ are the relatedness coefficients of individuals X_1 and X_2 specified in H_d. So, we can obtain the likelihood ratio $P(M|K, H_p)/P(M|K, H_d)$ for different biological relationships between R and V, and X_1 and X_2.

The seven most common relationships including unrelated and monozygotic (MZ) twins are considered, and the corresponding 7×7 likelihood ratios are shown in Table 7.5. The relationship is ordered from the most to the least related, i.e. monozygotic twins, parent–child, full siblings, ..., unrelated. The following three points are observed (Hu and Fung 2005a):

Table 7.5   Likelihood ratios for the propositions 'the victim V, one untyped relative R of the victim, and two untyped full siblings are contributors' versus 'two related unknowns X_1 and X_2, and two untyped full siblings are contributors' about the criminal case. Different relationships for R and V, and for X_1 and X_2 are considered, from Hu and Fung (2005a). (Reproduced by permission of Springer-Verlag.)

				(X_1, X_2)			
(R, V)	MZ twins	Parent –child	Full siblings	Half siblings	First cousins	Second cousins	Unrelated
MZ twins	20.92	4.48	3.94	2.69	2.24	1.99	1.92
Parent–child	100.87	21.61	19.02	12.97	10.81	9.61	9.27
Full siblings	115.88	24.82	21.85	14.90	12.42	11.04	10.65
Half siblings	170.87	36.60	32.21	21.98	18.32	16.28	15.70
First cousins	205.87	44.09	38.81	26.48	22.07	19.62	18.92
Second cousins	232.12	49.72	43.76	29.86	24.88	22.12	21.33
Unrelated	240.86	51.59	45.41	30.98	25.82	22.96	22.14

(a) The looser the relationship between R and V in H_p, the larger the likelihood ratio. Within each column, the largest likelihood ratio (unrelated case) is about 10 times the lowest likelihood ratio (MZ twins case) and 2 times the second lowest (parent–child case).

(b) The looser the relationship between X_1 and X_2 in H_d, the smaller the likelihood ratio. Within each row, the smallest likelihood ratio (unrelated case) is about one-tenth of the largest likelihood ratio (MZ twins case) and half of the second largest likelihood ratio (parent–child case).

(c) Excluding the case of MZ twins, the effect of relationship of R and V, or X_1 and X_2 on the likelihood ratio is not large; it only has at most double or half the likelihood ratio value of unrelated relationships.

The second example is a group rape investigated by Fukshansky and Bär (1998), in which three persons, namely the victim, the suspect S_1 and the suspect S_2, were typed at three loci DQa, FES and F13A1. See Table 7.6 for the details of the DNA profiles for the mixed stain, victim and two suspects at those three loci. The mixed stain was assumed to be contributed by the victim and two assailants. The prosecution proposition is taken as

$H_p : S_1$ and S_2 are both contributors to the mixed stain.

Fukshansky and Bär (1998) considered three different sets of defense propositions in which all involved people are assumed to be unrelated. When there is one pair of related people involved, we can employ the result in Section 7.1 for weighting the DNA evidence. Hu *et al.* (2005) considered seven different defense propositions to investigate the effect of various propositions on the evaluation of DNA evidence. In the following, we consider a particular defense proposition involving two pairs of related persons:

$H_d : R_1$, one relative of S_1, and R_2, one relative of S_2, are both contributors to the mixed stain.

Table 7.6 Mixed DNA stain and single person tests for the victim V and two suspects S_1 and S_2 as well as frequencies of alleles found for the three systems, from Fukshansky and Bär (1998). (Reproduced by permission of Springer-Verlag.)

Locus	Mixture (M)	Victim (V)	Suspect 1 (S_1)	Suspect 2 (S_2)	Frequency
DQa	1.1	1.1		1.1	0.134
	1.2		1.2		0.170
	1.4	1.4	1.4	1.4	0.324
FES	10			10	0.327
	11	11	11		0.396
	12	12			0.224
	13			13	0.032
F13A1	3	3			0.082
	5			5	0.174
	6	6		6	0.314
	7		7		0.341
	15		15		0.026

Under the prosecution proposition H_p, all the alleles in the mixture are explained by the victim and the two known contributors S_1 and S_2, so $P(M|K, H_p) = 1$ for each locus. Using Equation (7.9), we can find the likelihood ratio $1/P(M|K, H_d)$ for each of the three loci separately and then the overall one by multiplication. Table 7.7 shows the overall likelihood ratios when R_1 and S_1, and R_2 and S_2 take 49 possible combinations of commonly encountered relationships including unrelated and monozygotic twins. For example, when R_1 and S_1 are half siblings and R_2 and S_2 are full siblings, the likelihood ratio is 112, and when R_1 and S_1 are second cousins and R_2 and S_2 are first cousins, the likelihood ratio is 1604. It is noted

Table 7.7 Overall likelihood ratios for the propositions 'S_1 and S_2 are contributors' versus 'R_1, one relative of S_1, and R_2, one relative of S_2, are contributors' about the case of a group rape, from Hu and Fung (2005a). (Reproduced by permission of Springer-Verlag.)

(R_1, S_1)	MZ twins	Parent –child	Full siblings	Half siblings	First cousins	Second cousins	Unrelated
				(R_2, S_2)			
MZ twins	1	16	7	46	101	254	410
Parent–child	14	66	50	153	281	550	754
Full siblings	6	44	30	110	213	432	596
Half siblings	35	135	112	297	521	949	1245
First cousins	74	243	209	513	872	1533	1972
Second cousins	187	495	444	980	1604	2710	3425
Unrelated	319	713	650	1350	2154	3562	4464

that the first row of Table 7.7 corresponds to the likelihood ratios about the two completing hypotheses:

H_p: the victim and two suspects were contributors;
H_d: the victim, the suspect S_1, and one relative of the suspect S_2 were the contributors.

The first column of Table 7.7 corresponds to the likelihood ratios about another pair of hypotheses:

H_p: the victim and two suspects were contributors;
H_d: the victim, the suspect S_2, and one relative of the suspect S_1 were the contributors.

It can be observed from Table 7.7 that the difference among the likelihood ratios of different biological relationships can be very large. For example, the likelihood ratio for both parent–child relationships is 66, which is only 1.48% of the highest likelihood ratio 4464, corresponding to both unrelated relationships.

7.2.5   Extension

It is noted that the results in Sections 7.2.1 – 7.2.3 extend those in Section 7.1 to the situation of two pairs of relatives and thus widens the scope of the application. Although the expressions, e.g. Equation (7.9), for calculating likelihood ratios look complex, they are in essence just linear combinations of $Q(\cdot, \cdot)$. Moreover, the implementation of $Q(\cdot, \cdot)$ by a computer program is not difficult.

The idea shown in Sections 7.2.1–7.2.3 can be used to tackle more complex problems involving more than two pairs of relatives. For example, if there are three pairs of related unknowns among the x unknown contributors with corresponding relatedness coefficients $(K_{i0}, K_{i1}, K_{i2}) = (k_{i0}, 2k_{i1}, k_{i2})$, $i = 1, 2, 3$, then the conditional probability can be expressed as

$$P(M|K, H) = \sum_{i,j,k=0,1,2} K_{1i} K_{2j} K_{3k} Q(2x - i - j - k, U),$$

which is an extension of Equation (7.13).

The Hardy–Weinberg equilibrium is assumed in Sections 7.1 and 7.2. This independence assumption of alleles may be relaxed in the next section to allow for the possible existence of population subdivision.

7.3   Related people from the same subdivided population

In this section, we continue to consider the mixture problem when the relative of the suspect is involved in the pool of possible perpetrators or the suspect is unavailable for typing and his/her one relative is typed instead. In contrast to Sections 7.1 and 7.2, the Hardy–Weinberg law is not assumed in this section, and the involved people come from a subdivided population with the degree of subdivision θ.

7.3.1   Introductory example

We first consider a simple case in which the mixed stain M is $\{A_1, A_2, A_3, A_4\}$, and the suspect S is of type $A_1 A_3$. So, the typed genotype in this example is $K = S = A_1 A_3$. The two competing propositions on the source of the mixed stain are formulated as follows:

H_p: the suspect and one unknown person were contributors;
H_d: a relative of the suspect, R, and one unknown person were contributors.

Under H_p, from the DNA profiles of the mixture and known contributors, the genotype G of the unknown must be of A_2A_4. So

$$P(M|K, H_p) = P(G = A_2A_4|S = A_1A_3).$$

Under H_d, we partition the mixture contributed by R, a relative of the suspect, and an unknown G into six possible sets of genotypes:

$$G_1 = (R = A_1A_2, G = A_3A_4), \quad G_2 = (R = A_1A_3, G = A_2A_4),$$

$$G_3 = (R = A_1A_4, G = A_2A_3), \quad G_4 = (R = A_2A_3, G = A_1A_4),$$

$$G_5 = (R = A_2A_4, G = A_1A_3), \quad G_6 = (R = A_3A_4, G = A_1A_2).$$

So

$$P(M|K, H_d) = \sum_{i=1}^{6} P(G_i|S = A_1A_3).$$

Thus, the likelihood ratio is

$$LR = \frac{P(G = A_2A_4|S = A_1A_3)}{\sum_{i=1}^{6} P(G_i|S = A_1A_3)}. \tag{7.14}$$

After passing the genotype to the set of alleles and taking account of whether the genotype is heterozygous or homozygous, the numerator of the likelihood ratio in Equation (7.14) can be evaluated using Equation (3.17) successively, as follows:

$$P(G = A_2A_4|S = A_1A_3) = 2P(A_2, A_4|A_1, A_3)$$

$$= 2P(A_2|A_1, A_3)P(A_4|A_1, A_2, A_3)$$

$$= 2\left[\frac{(1-\theta)p_2}{1+\theta}\right]\left[\frac{(1-\theta)p_4}{1+2\theta}\right].$$

In the following, we show the details in the evaluation of the first term of the denominator in Equation (7.14), i.e. $P(G_1|S = A_1A_3) = P(R = A_1A_2, G = A_3A_4|S = A_1A_3)$.

It can be seen from the genotypes of R and S, i.e. $R = A_1A_2$ and $S = A_1A_3$, that the ibd alleles between R and S, denoted by $IBDA$, can take two possible values: $IBDA = $ none and $IBDA = A_1$. Using the relatedness coefficients $(k_0, 2k_1, k_2)$, we can have

$$P(R = A_1A_2, G = A_3A_4, IBDA = \text{none}|S = A_1A_3)$$

$$= 4k_0 P(A_1, A_2, A_3, A_4|S = A_1A_3),$$

$$P(R = A_1A_2, G = A_3A_4, IBDA = A_1|S = A_1A_3)$$

$$= 2k_1 P(A_2, A_3, A_4|S = A_1A_3).$$

Using the law of total probability introduced in Section 2.3 and applying Equation (3.17) recursively, we have

$$P(G_1|S = A_1A_3)$$

$$= 4k_0 P(A_1, A_2, A_3, A_4 | A_1, A_3) + 2k_1 P(A_2, A_3, A_4 | A_1, A_3)$$

$$= 4k_0 \frac{[\theta + (1-\theta)p_1][\theta + (1-\theta)p_3](1-\theta)p_2(1-\theta)p_4}{(1+\theta)(1+2\theta)(1+3\theta)(1+4\theta)}$$

$$+ 2k_1 \frac{[\theta + (1-\theta)p_3](1-\theta)p_2(1-\theta)p_4}{(1+\theta)(1+2\theta)(1+3\theta)}.$$

The derivation of $P(G_i | S = A_1 A_2)$, $i = 2, \ldots, 6$, can be done in a similar way and so we omit the details.

This example shows the way of evaluating the match probabilities in a simple mixed stain problem. The expression for the likelihood ratio is rather complicated when the involved people come from a subdivided population. It is desired to derive a compact general formula for evaluating the match probabilities.

7.3.2   A simple case with one victim, one suspect and one relative

We consider the situation in which only one victim, one suspect and a relative of the suspect are involved and the two competing propositions are, respectively,

H_p: the contributors were the victim and the suspect;
H_d: the contributors were the victim and a relative of the suspect,

where all the involved people are coming from the same subdivided population.

Suppose we consider $M = \{A_1, A_2, A_3\}$, $V = A_1 A_1$, and $S = A_2 A_3$. Under the prosecution proposition H_p, $P(M|K, H_p) = 1$. Under the defense proposition H_d, the genotype of the unknown must be $G = A_2 A_3$. So, $P(M|K, H_d) = P(G = A_2 A_3 | V = A_1 A_1, S = A_2 A_3)$. Considering the relatedness coefficients $(k_0, 2k_1, k_2)$ between the suspect S and the relative and using the recursive formula given in Equation (3.17), we have

$$P(M|K, H_d) = 2k_0 P(A_2, A_3 | V = A_1 A_1, S = A_2 A_3)$$

$$+ k_1 P(A_3 | V = A_1 A_1, S = A_2 A_3)$$

$$+ k_1 P(A_2 | V = A_1 A_1, S = A_2 A_3) + k_2$$

$$= 2k_0 \left[\frac{\theta + (1-\theta)p_2}{1+3\theta} \right] \left[\frac{\theta + (1-\theta)p_3}{1+4\theta} \right] + k_1 \left[\frac{\theta + (1-\theta)p_3}{1+3\theta} \right]$$

$$+ k_1 \left[\frac{\theta + (1-\theta)p_2}{1+3\theta} \right] + k_2$$

$$= 2k_0 \frac{[\theta + (1-\theta)p_2][\theta + (1-\theta)p_3]}{(1+3\theta)(1+4\theta)} + k_1 \left[\frac{2\theta + (1-\theta)(p_2+p_3)}{1+3\theta} \right] + k_2.$$

So, the likelihood ratio is just the reciprocal of $P(M|K, H_d)$. The other likelihood ratios can be derived similarly and they are listed in Table 7.8.

7.3.3   General formulas

The examples shown in Sections 7.3.1 and 7.3.2 reveal a way of obtaining a formula for the conditional probability $P(M|K, H)$ when there are two biologically related individuals amongst the involved people who come from the same subdivided population. In order to give

Table 7.8 Likelihood ratio for one victim, one suspect and one unknown case with H_p: the contributors were the victim and the suspect, and H_d: the contributors were the victim and a relative of the suspect. The relatedness coefficients between the suspect and the relative are $(k_0, 2k_1, k_2)$. All involved people come from the same subdivided population with the degree of subdivision θ.

Victim	Suspect	LR
$M = \{A_1, A_2\}$		
A_1A_1	A_1A_2	$\left\{ k_0 \dfrac{[\theta + (1-\theta)p_2][8\theta + (1-\theta)(2p_1 + p_2)]}{(1+3\theta)(1+4\theta)} + k_1 \dfrac{5\theta + (1-\theta)(p_1 + 2p_2)}{1+3\theta} + k_2 \right\}^{-1}$
	A_2A_2	$\left\{ k_0 \dfrac{[2\theta + (1-\theta)p_2][7\theta + (1-\theta)(2p_1 + p_2)]}{(1+3\theta)(1+4\theta)} + 2k_1 \dfrac{4\theta + (1-\theta)(p_1 + p_2)}{1+3\theta} + k_2 \right\}^{-1}$
A_1A_2	A_1A_1	$\left\{ k_0 \dfrac{[4\theta + (1-\theta)(p_1 + p_2)][5\theta + (1-\theta)(p_1 + p_2)]}{(1+3\theta)(1+4\theta)} + 2k_1 \dfrac{4\theta + (1-\theta)(p_1 + p_2)}{1+3\theta} + k_2 \right\}^{-1}$
	A_1A_2	$\left\{ k_0 \dfrac{[4\theta + (1-\theta)(p_1 + p_2)][5\theta + (1-\theta)(p_1 + p_2)]}{(1+3\theta)(1+4\theta)} + 2k_1 \dfrac{4\theta + (1-\theta)(p_1 + p_2)}{1+3\theta} + k_2 \right\}^{-1}$
$M = \{A_1, A_2, A_3\}$		
A_1A_1	A_2A_3	$\left\{ k_0 \dfrac{2[\theta + (1-\theta)p_2][\theta + (1-\theta)p_3]}{(1+3\theta)(1+4\theta)} + k_1 \dfrac{2\theta + (1-\theta)(p_2 + p_3)}{1+3\theta} + k_2 \right\}^{-1}$
A_1A_2	A_1A_3	$\left\{ k_0 \dfrac{[\theta + (1-\theta)p_3)][8\theta + (1-\theta)(2p_1 + 2p_2 + p_3)]}{(1+3\theta)(1+4\theta)} + k_1 \dfrac{5\theta + (1-\theta)(p_1 + p_2 + 2p_3)}{1+3\theta} + k_2 \right\}^{-1}$
	A_3A_3	$\left\{ k_0 \dfrac{[2\theta + (1-\theta)p_3][7\theta + (1-\theta)(2p_1 + 2p_2 + p_3)]}{(1+3\theta)(1+4\theta)} + 2k_1 \dfrac{4\theta + (1-\theta)(p_1 + p_2 + p_3)}{1+3\theta} + k_2 \right\}^{-1}$
$M = \{A_1, A_2, A_3, A_4\}$		
A_1A_2	A_3A_4	$\left\{ k_0 \dfrac{2[\theta + (1-\theta)p_3][\theta + (1-\theta)p_4]}{(1+3\theta)(1+4\theta)} + k_1 \dfrac{2\theta + (1-\theta)(p_3 + p_4)}{1+3\theta} + k_2 \right\}^{-1}$

a concise expression of $P(M|K, H)$, we introduce (Fung and Hu 2004)

$$Q(n, C, \theta) = \sum_{M \setminus C \subset D \subset M} (-1)^{|M \setminus D|} q(n, D)$$

$$= q(n, M) - \sum_{A_i \in C} q(n, M \setminus \{A_i\}) + \sum_{A_i, A_j \in C} q(n, M \setminus \{A_i, A_j\})$$

$$- \cdots + (-1)^{|C|} q(n, M \setminus C), \tag{7.15}$$

for any integer-valued n and allele subset C of the mixture M, where

$$q(n, C) = \left(\sum_{A_l \in C} p_l \right)^{(n)} \left(\sum_{A_l \in C} c_l, \theta \right) / 1^{(n)}(c, \theta), \tag{7.16}$$

c is the count of total alleles present in K, which is twice the number of tested persons, c_l is the count of allele A_l present in K, which gives rise to the sum $\sum_l c_l = c$ (see Table 6.6 for more details of notations), and $r^{(n)}(k, \theta)$ is defined in Equation (6.10). Notice that $Q(0, \phi, \theta) = 1$, $Q(n, C, \theta) = 0$ for all $n < |C|$, and $Q(n, C, 0)$ is just the quantity of $Q(n, C)$ defined in Equation (7.2).

Note that $q(n, C)$ in Equation (7.15) is just the conditional probability that n alleles belong to set C given the total alleles in K, and $Q(n, C, \theta)$ is the conditional probability that n alleles coming from set M explain the alleles in set C given the total alleles in K. These two quantities make the expression of $P(M|K, H)$ more concise.

Now, we consider a criminal case with mixture M, typed genotypes K, and $T = t_1 t_2$ being one of the typed persons. The proposition about who the unknown contributors to the mixed stain were is given as follows:

> H: one relative, R, of the typed T and $x - 1$ other unrelated unknowns were
> contributors.   (7.17)

Notice that, in this case, the individual R is an unknown contributor, since, in some situations, the person concerned may refuse to cooperate or cannot be approached for various reasons including death, and a relative is tested instead. The formula for calculating $P(M|K, H)$ is given as follows (Fung and Hu 2004):

$$P(M|K, H) = k_0 Q(2x, U, \theta)$$

$$+ k_1 [I_M(t_1) Q(2x - 1, U \setminus \{t_1\}, \theta) + I_M(t_2) Q(2x - 1, U \setminus \{t_2\}, \theta)]$$

$$+ k_2 I_M(t_1) I_M(t_2) Q(2x - 2, U \setminus \{t_1\} \cup \{t_2\}, \theta). \tag{7.18}$$

The proof of Equation (7.18) is given in Section 7.4.7. Note that Equation (7.18) is applicable to the situations in which the suspect is unavailable but one of his/her relatives is tested instead, or a relative of the tested suspect is a potential contributor to the mixture.

For the case in which two related unknown persons (e.g. two siblings) were the source contributors to the mixed stain, the proposition of interest becomes

> H: two related persons, X_1 and X_2, and $x - 2$ other unrelated unknowns were
> contributors.   (7.19)

In this situation, we have

$$P(M|K, H) = k_0 Q(2x, U, \theta) + 2k_1 Q(2x - 1, U, \theta) + k_2 Q(2x - 2, U, \theta). \qquad (7.20)$$

The proof of Equation (7.20) is given in Section 7.4.7.

It is necessary for a proposition H to specify the known contributors to the mixture M and then the set U can be determined, although we omit such details for propositions (7.17) and (7.19) for brevity. Equations (7.18) and (7.20) show that $P(M|K, H)$ are linear combinations of $Q(\cdot, \cdot, \cdot)$ and so the implementation of $P(M|K, H)$ via a computer program is easy. When the involved persons in a crime case belong to the same subdivided population but are all biologically unrelated, both Equations (7.18) and (7.20) reduce to the same equation as $P(M|K, H) = Q(2x, U)$ due to $k_0 = 1$ and $k_1 = k_2 = 0$, which was reported in Fung and Hu (2000b).

7.3.4   An example analyzed by the software

The Hong Kong case example as described in Table 6.5 is considered. We study the following two competing propositions:

H_p: the victim and the suspect were contributors of the mixed stain;
H_{d1}: the victim and one relative of the suspect were contributors.

The victim was biologically unrelated to the suspect and the relative of the suspect. The purpose of this example is mainly for illustration, and so we consider six commonly encountered relationships between the suspect and his relative: parent–child, full siblings, half siblings, first cousins, second cousins and unrelated. The relatedness coefficients for these relationships can be referred to in Table 3.13.

For locus vWA, from Table 6.5, we have $M = \{16, 18\}$ and $K = 16/16, 18/18$. Under the prosecution proposition H_p, the alleles in M are explained by the known contributors, the victim and the suspect, so $P(M|K, H_p) = 1$. Under the defense proposition, the number of unknown contributors x is 1, and $U = \{16\}$ is concluded from the mixture and the genotypes of known contributors. So, $P(M|K, H_d) = k_0 Q(2, U, \theta) + 2k_1 Q(1, U, \theta) + k_2 Q(0, U, \theta)$.

Table 7.9 shows the corresponding likelihood ratios with $\theta = 0, 0.01$ and 0.03, respectively. The likelihood ratio for the full siblings case is the lowest for any of the θ values. When $\theta = 0$, the overall likelihood ratio for the unrelated case is more than 800 times higher than that for the full siblings case. The genetic evidence is strong for the unrelated case, but it is rather weak if the full siblings proposition is chosen. It is clear that the effect of relatedness on the likelihood ratio is substantial. When the population structure is taken into account, i.e. $\theta > 0$, all the likelihood ratios drop. The highest and the lowest drops correspond to the unrelated and full siblings cases, respectively. The ratios of the highest and the lowest overall likelihood ratios are about 500 when $\theta = 0.01$ and 250 when $\theta = 0.03$.

Suppose that the evidence was collected from somewhere other than the victim's body; then, the defense proposition could be

H_{d2}: one relative of the suspect and one unrelated unknown were contributors,

while the prosecution proposition H_p remains unchanged. The likelihood ratios are shown in Table 7.10. They are all larger than those in the previous set of propositions. The likelihood ratios at D3S1358 and vWA both have the smallest values in the full siblings relationship,

Table 7.9 The effects of relatedness and population structure on the likelihood ratios for a DNA mixture in the Hong Kong case example, in which the prosecution and defense propositions are H_p: the victim and the suspect were contributors of the mixed stain, and H_{d1}: the victim and one relative of the suspect were contributors, respectively, from Fung and Hu (2004). (Reproduced by permission of Blackwell Publishing.)

θ	Relationship	Likelihood ratios			
		D3S1358	vWA	FGA	Overall
0	Parent–child	7.35	3.16	3.13	73
	Full siblings	3.11	2.34	2.36	17
	Half siblings[a]	13.18	5.12	5.29	357
	Cousins	21.82	7.42	8.08	1 309
	Second cousins	42.94	11.19	13.39	6 436
	Unrelated	63.40	13.47	17.15	14 644
0.01	Parent–child	7.12	2.92	2.89	60
	Full siblings	3.08	2.26	2.27	16
	Half siblings[a]	12.49	4.64	4.79	278
	First cousins	20.06	6.59	7.13	943
	Second cousins	36.77	9.61	11.27	3 983
	Unrelated	50.90	11.35	13.97	8 070
0.03	Parent–child	6.73	2.56	2.53	44
	Full siblings	3.02	2.11	2.12	13
	Half siblings[a]	11.42	3.94	4.05	182
	First cousins	17.52	5.40	5.78	548
	Second cousins	29.22	7.49	8.52	1 865
	Unrelated	37.60	8.60	10.11	3 270

[a] The same as the grandparent–child and the uncle–niece relationship

while the likelihood ratio is the lowest in the parent–child relationship for locus FGA. In general, the effect of relatedness on the likelihood ratios is smaller than that in H_p versus H_{d1}.

Finally, while keeping the same H_p, we consider a third kind of defense proposition:

H_{d3}: two related unknown persons were contributors.

Unlike that of the other two sets of propositions, the likelihood ratio at locus D3S1358 for the full siblings case is the highest, while that for the unrelated case is the lowest (Table 7.11). When $\theta = 0$, the smallest likelihood ratios at loci vWA and FGA go to the full siblings and half siblings cases, respectively. If we compare $\theta = 0$ and $\theta = 0.01/0.03$, the largest likelihood ratio at FGA shifts from the unrelated to the full siblings relationship. The effect of either relatedness or θ on the likelihood ratio is mixed under this particular set of propositions.

All the results listed in Tables 7.9, 7.10 and 7.11 were obtained using our developed software. For proposition pairs H_p and H_{d1}, and H_p and H_{d2}, all the steps are the same as described in Section 7.1.6, except in step 2, where multiple values of θ, i.e. 0, 0.01 and 0.03 are input here. For proposition pair H_p and H_{d3}, the procedure of running the computer software is very similar, except in step 12, where the option *there are two related persons in*

Table 7.10   The effects of relatedness and population structure on the likelihood ratios for a DNA mixture in the Hong Kong case example, in which the prosecution and defense propositions are H_p: the victim and the suspect were contributors of the mixed stain, and H_{d2}: one relative of the suspect and one unrelated unknown were contributors, respectively, from Fung and Hu (2004). (Reproduced by permission of Blackwell Publishing.)

| | | Likelihood ratios | | | |
θ	Relationship	D3S1358	vWA	FGA	Overall
0	Parent–child	66.11	36.03	106.13	252 787
	Full siblings	56.47	28.62	109.48	176 943
	Half siblings[a]	107.33	54.82	159.91	940 898
	Cousins	155.94	74.17	214.16	2 476 984
	Second cousins	236.14	100.87	287.25	6 842 643
	Unrelated	285.01	114.63	324.13	10 589 598
0.01	Parent–child	69.23	27.12	79.40	149 053
	Full siblings	58.99	22.69	84.55	113 144
	Half siblings[a]	108.63	40.03	115.74	503 255
	First cousins	151.85	52.53	150.08	1 197 177
	Second cousins	216.42	68.61	193.04	2 866 279
	Unrelated	252.16	76.40	213.41	4 111 306
0.03	Parent–child	75.78	17.35	51.30	67 460
	Full siblings	64.39	15.55	56.77	56 827
	Half siblings[a]	113.11	24.40	70.88	195 607
	First cousins	150.07	30.61	87.59	402 436
	Second cousins	198.81	37.84	106.41	800 602
	Unrelated	222.94	41.08	114.62	1 049 659

[a] The same as the grandparent–child and the uncle–niece relationship

unknowns is chosen. Figure 7.5 shows the captured input screen when all the entries are input for locus D3S1358. When we complete the steps for subsequent loci vWA and FGA, we have the individual and overall likelihood ratios for different θ values and various relationships, as shown in Figure 7.6.

7.4   Proofs

The proofs in this section are mainly for mathematically oriented readers. They are provided in this last section, having little distraction to the flow of the main content in the text.

7.4.1   Preliminary

First of all, we give the following lemma to calculate the joint genotype probability of $X = x_1 x_2$ and $Y = y_1 y_2$, whose seven detailed expressions are given in Table 5.1:

Table 7.11   The effects of relatedness and population structure on the likelihood ratios for a DNA mixture in the Hong Kong case example, in which the prosecution and defense propositions are H_p: the victim and the suspect were contributors of the mixed stain, and H_{d3}: two related unknown persons were contributors, respectively, from Fung and Hu (2004). (Reproduced by permission of Blackwell Publishing.)

θ	Relationship[a]	Likelihood ratios			
		D3S1358	vWA	FGA	Overall
0	Full siblings	1140.04	37.75	314.31	13 525 658
	Half siblings[b]	570.02	61.76	252.98	8 905 310
	Cousins	380.01	80.27	284.17	8 667 933
	Second cousins	304.01	103.55	313.12	9 856 994
	Unrelated	285.01	114.63	324.13	10 589 598
0.01	Full siblings	854.51	30.06	228.22	5 861 232
	Half siblings[b]	427.26	45.42	180.07	3 494 270
	First cousins	284.84	56.97	195.33	3 169 537
	Second cousins	227.87	70.40	208.58	3 345 913
	Unrelated	213.63	76.40	213.41	3 483 050
0.03	Full siblings	574.47	20.68	140.32	1 667 192
	Half siblings[b]	287.24	27.92	107.44	861 744
	First cousins	191.49	33.25	110.92	706 134
	Second cousins	153.19	38.79	113.67	675 531
	Unrelated	143.62	41.08	114.62	676 204

[a] The parent–child relationship is impossible for a mixture of four distinct alleles at locus D3S1358, assuming no mutation

[b] The same as the grandparent–child and the uncle–niece relationship

Lemma 7.4.1   *For any two persons* $X = x_1 x_2$ *and* $Y = y_1 y_2$,

$$P(X = x_1 x_2, Y = y_1 y_2)$$
$$= k_0 P(X) P(Y) + k_1 (2 - \delta_{x_1 x_2})[I_{\{y_1\} \cup \{y_2\}}(x_1) p_{x_2} + I_{\{y_1\} \cup \{y_2\}}(x_2) p_{x_1}] p_{y_1} p_{y_2}$$
$$+ k_2 P(Y) \delta_{XY}$$
$$= k_0 P(X) P(Y) + k_1 (2 - \delta_{y_1 y_2})[I_{\{x_1\} \cup \{x_2\}}(y_1) p_{y_2} + I_{\{x_1\} \cup \{x_2\}}(y_2) p_{y_1}] p_{x_1} p_{x_2}$$
$$+ k_2 P(Y) \delta_{XY}, \tag{7.21}$$

where $(k_0, 2k_1, k_2)$ *are the relatedness coefficients between* X *and* Y, $\{x_1\} \cup \{x_2\}$ *is the genetic profile comprising the two alleles that* X *carries, which is a singleton for homozygous* X, $\{y_1\} \cup \{y_2\}$ *is defined similarly for individual* Y, I *is the indicator function,* δ *is the Kronecker delta function defined by* $\delta_{XY} = 1$ *if individuals* X *and* Y *have the same genotype,* 0 *otherwise. Note that the second equality in Equation (7.21) follows the symmetry of* X *and* Y.

Proof.   Suppose individual X has alleles a and b and Y has alleles c and d at some autosomal locus, where alleles a and c are of paternal and alleles b and d are of maternal (Evett and

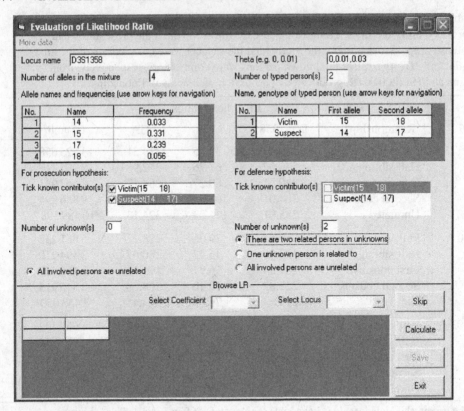

Figure 7.5 Captured input screen for analyzing the Hong Kong case example about two alternative propositions H_p: the victim and the suspect were the contributors of the mixed stain versus H_{d3}: two biologically related unknown contributors were the contributors. All people involved come from the same subdivided population.

Weir 1998). It is noted that alleles a and b take a unique value for a homozygous X and two values for a heterozygous X, and also for Y. Then, the relatedness coefficients $(k_0, 2k_1, k_2)$ defined in Equation (3.18) can be expressed as $k_0 = P(\text{no ibd allele})$, $2k_1 = P(a \equiv c, b \not\equiv d) + P(a \equiv d, b \not\equiv c) + P(b \equiv c, a \not\equiv d) + P(b \equiv d, a \not\equiv c)$, and $k_2 = P(a \equiv c, b \equiv d) + P(a \equiv d, b \equiv c)$, where the equivalence sign $\equiv$ is used to indicate an ibd relationship.

Let $IBDA$ denote the ibd alleles between the two individuals $X = x_1 x_2$ and $Y = y_1 y_2$; then, all the possibilities for $IBDA$ are: $IBDA = \text{none}$, $IBDA = x_1$, $IBDA = x_2$ (if $x_2 \neq x_1$), and $IBDA = x_1, x_2$. It is obvious that

$$P(X = x_1 x_2, Y = y_1 y_2, IBDA = \text{none}) = k_0 P(X) P(Y). \tag{7.22}$$

For two identical homozygous X and Y where $X = Y = A_i A_i$, we have

$$P(X = A_i A_i, Y = A_i A_i, IBDA = A_i, A_i)$$

$$= P(a = A_i, b = A_i; c = A_i, d = A_i, IBDA = A_i, A_i)$$

$$= P(a = A_i, b = A_i; c = A_i, d = A_i, a \equiv c, b \equiv d)$$

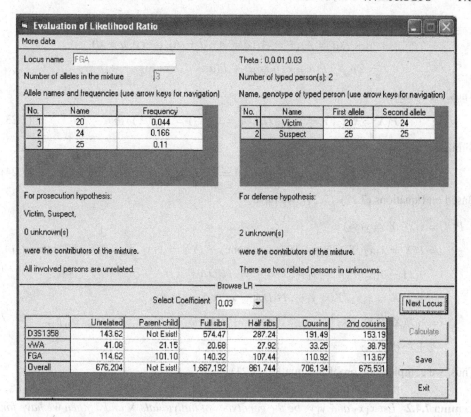

Figure 7.6 Captured result screen for analyzing the Hong Kong case example about two alternative propositions H_p: the victim and the suspect were the contributors of the mixed stain versus H_{d3}: two biologically related unknown contributors were the contributors. All people involved come from the same subdivided population.

$$+ P(a = A_i, b = A_i; c = A_i, d = A_i, a \equiv d, b \equiv c)$$

$$= \left[P(a \equiv c, b \equiv d) + P(a \equiv d, b \equiv c) \right] p_i^2.$$

For two identical heterozygous X and Y where $X = Y = A_i A_j$, we have

$$P(X = A_i A_j, Y = A_i A_j, IBDA = A_i, A_j)$$

$$= P(a = A_i, b = A_j; c = A_i, d = A_j, IBDA = A_i, A_j)$$

$$+ P(a = A_j, b = A_i; c = A_i, d = A_j, IBDA = A_i, A_j)$$

$$+ P(a = A_i, b = A_j; c = A_j, d = A_i, IBDA = A_i, A_j)$$

$$+ P(a = A_j, b = A_i; c = A_j, d = A_i, IBDA = A_i, A_j)$$

$$= P(a = A_i, b = A_j; c = A_i, d = A_j, a \equiv c, b \equiv d)$$

$$+ P(a = A_j, b = A_i; c = A_i, d = A_j, a \equiv d, b \equiv c)$$

$$+ P(a = A_i, b = A_j; c = A_j, d = A_i, a \equiv d, b \equiv c)$$
$$+ P(a = A_j, b = A_i; c = A_j, d = A_i, a \equiv c, b \equiv d)$$
$$= 2 p_i p_j \left[P(a \equiv c, b \equiv d) + P(a \equiv d, b \equiv c) \right].$$

Thus, we obtain

$$P(X = x_1 x_2, Y = y_1 y_2, IBDA = x_1, x_2) = k_2 P(X) \delta_{XY}. \tag{7.23}$$

Similarly, we have

$$P(X = x_1 x_2, Y = y_1 y_2, IBDA = x_1) = 2 k_1 I_{\{y_1\} \cup \{y_2\}}(x_1) p_{x_2} p_{y_1} p_{y_2}. \tag{7.24}$$

Based on Equations (7.22)–(7.24), we have

$$P(X = x_1 x_2, Y = y_1 y_2)$$
$$= P(X = x_1 x_2, Y = y_1 y_2, IBDA = \text{none}) + P(X = x_1 x_2, Y = y_1 y_2, IBDA = x_1)$$
$$+ (1 - \delta_{x_1 x_2}) P(X = x_1 x_2, Y = y_1 y_2, IBDA = x_2)$$
$$+ P(X = x_1 x_2, Y = y_1 y_2, IBDA = x_1, x_2)$$
$$= k_0 P(X) P(Y) + k_1 \left[2 I_{\{y_1\} \cup \{y_2\}}(x_1) p_{x_2} + 2(1 - \delta_{x_1 x_2}) I_{\{y_1\} \cup \{y_2\}}(x_2) p_{x_1} \right] p_{y_1} p_{y_2}$$
$$+ k_2 P(Y) \delta_{XY}.$$

Thus, we complete the proof of Equation (7.21).

Lemma 7.4.2 *Let $x_1 x_2$ and $y_1 y_2$ be the genotypes of individuals X and Y, then we have for any set C of alleles*

$$\sum_{x_1, x_2 \in C} P(X) = \left(\sum_{A_l \in C} p_l \right)^2, \tag{7.25}$$

$$\sum_{x_1, x_2 \in C} I_{\{x_1\} \cup \{x_2\}}(y_1) p_{x_1} p_{x_2} = I_C(y_1) p_{y_1} \sum_{A_l \in C} p_l, \tag{7.26}$$

$$\sum_{x_1, x_2 \in C} \delta_{XY} = I_C(y_1) I_C(y_2). \tag{7.27}$$

Proof.   Note that Equations (7.25) and (7.27) are straightforward. For $x_1, x_2 \in C$, the genotype X may be homozygous or heterozygous, viz. $X = x_1 x_1$ or $X = x_1 x_2$ ($x_1 \neq x_2$). When $I_{\{x_1\} \cup \{x_2\}}(y_1) = 1$, we can assume $x_1 = y_1$ without loss of generality. So

$$\sum_{x_1, x_2 \in C} I_{\{x_1\} \cup \{x_2\}}(y_1) p_{x_1} p_{x_2} = I_C(y_1) \left(p_{y_1}^2 + \sum_{A_l \neq y_1, A_l \in C} p_{y_1} p_l \right)$$
$$= I_C(y_1) p_{y_1} \sum_{A_l \in C} p_l$$

and Equation (7.26) holds.
  Based on Equation (7.21), we have further

Lemma 7.4.3 *For any subset C of the mixture M and $X = x_1 x_2$ and $Y = y_1 y_2$ that*

$$P(x_1, x_2 \in C | Y = y_1 y_2)$$

$$= k_0 \left(\sum_{A_l \in C} p_l \right)^2 + k_1 [I_C(y_1) + I_C(y_2)] \sum_{A_l \in C} p_l + k_2 I_C(y_1) I_C(y_2), \qquad (7.28)$$

$$P(y_1, y_2 \in C | X = x_1 x_2)$$

$$= k_0 \left(\sum_{A_l \in C} p_l \right)^2 + k_1 [I_C(x_1) + I_C(x_2)] \sum_{A_l \in C} p_l + k_2 I_C(x_1) I_C(x_2), \qquad (7.29)$$

$$P(x_1, x_2, y_1, y_2 \in C) = \left(\sum_{A_l \in C} p_l \right)^2 \left[k_0 \left(\sum_{A_l \in C} p_l \right)^2 + 2k_1 \sum_{A_l \in C} p_l + k_2 \right].$$

$$(7.30)$$

Proof. According to Equation (7.21), we first find the summation of joint genotype probabilities $P(X, Y)$ over all $x_1, x_2 \in C$ for any given set C. It is observed from Equation (7.21) that the summation comes down to finding the summation corresponding to the coefficients of k_0, k_1 and k_2 therein over all $x_1, x_2 \in C$, designated as a_0, a_1, a_2, respectively. From Equations (7.25) – (7.27), we have

$$a_0 = P(Y) \sum_{x_1, x_2 \in C} P(X) = P(Y) \left(\sum_{A_l \in C} p_l \right)^2,$$

$$a_1 = \sum_{x_1, x_2 \in C} (2 - \delta_{x_1 x_2})[I_{\{y_1\} \cup \{y_2\}}(x_1) p_{x_2} + I_{\{y_1\} \cup \{y_2\}}(x_2) p_{x_1}] p_{y_1} p_{y_2}$$

$$= \sum_{x_1, x_2 \in C} (2 - \delta_{y_1 y_2})[I_{\{x_1\} \cup \{x_2\}}(y_1) p_{y_2} + I_{\{x_1\} \cup \{x_2\}}(y_2) p_{y_1}] p_{x_1} p_{x_2}$$

$$= (2 - \delta_{y_1 y_2}) p_{y_1} p_{y_2} [I_C(y_1) + I_y(s_2)] \sum_{A_l \in C} p_l$$

$$= P(Y)[I_C(y_1) + I_C(y_2)] \sum_{A_l \in C} p_l,$$

$$a_2 = P(Y) \sum_{x_1, x_2 \in C} \delta_{XY} = P(Y) I_C(y_1) I_C(y_2).$$

So, we have

$$\sum_{x_1, x_2 \in C} P(X, Y)$$

$$= k_0 P(Y) \left(\sum_{A_l \in C} p_l \right)^2 + k_1 P(Y)[I_C(y_1) + I_C(y_2)] \sum_{A_l \in C} p_l + k_2 P(Y) I_C(y_1) I_C(y_2),$$

and

$$P(x_1, x_2, y_1, y_2 \in C)$$

$$= \sum_{x_1, x_2 \in C} \sum_{y_1, y_2 \in C} P(X, Y)$$

$$= k_0 \left(\sum_{A_l \in C} p_l \right)^2 \sum_{y_1, y_2 \in C} P(Y) + k_1 \sum_{A_l \in C} p_l \sum_{y_1, y_2 \in C} P(Y)[I_C(y_1) + I_C(y_2)]$$

$$+ k_2 \sum_{y_1, y_2 \in C} P(Y) I_C(y_1) I_C(y_2)$$

$$= k_0 \left(\sum_{A_l \in C} p_l \right)^2 \left(\sum_{A_l \in C} p_l \right)^2 + 2k_1 \sum_{A_l \in C} p_l \left(\sum_{A_l \in C} p_l \right)^2 + k_2 \left(\sum_{A_l \in C} p_l \right)^2.$$

Thus, Equation (7.30) holds.

Furthermore,

$$P(x_1, x_2 \in C | Y) = \sum_{x_1, x_2 \in C} P(X, Y) / P(Y)$$

$$= k_0 \left(\sum_{A_l \in C} p_l \right)^2 + k_1 [I_C(y_1) + I_C(y_2)] \sum_{A_l \in C} p_l + k_2 I_C(y_1) I_C(y_2).$$

This is just Equation (7.29). Equation (7.30) follows from the interchanging of X and Y in Equation (7.29).

In the following, we provide two more lemmas which are used in the subsequent proofs.

Lemma 7.4.4 *For any allele set $U \subset M$, and any pairwise distinct alleles a, b, c and $d \in U$,*

$$Q(n, U \setminus \{a\}) = \sum_{M \setminus U \subset C \subset M} I_C(a)(-1)^{|M \setminus C|} \left(\sum_{A_l \in C} p_l \right)^n, \tag{7.31}$$

$$Q(n, U \setminus \{a, b\}) = \sum_{M \setminus U \subset C \subset M} I_C(a) I_C(b)(-1)^{|M \setminus C|} \left(\sum_{A_l \in C} p_l \right)^n, \tag{7.32}$$

$$Q(n, U \setminus \{a, b, c\}) = \sum_{M \setminus U \subset C \subset M} I_C(a) I_C(b) I_C(c)(-1)^{|M \setminus C|} \left(\sum_{A_l \in C} p_l \right)^n, \tag{7.33}$$

$$Q(n, U \setminus \{a, b, c, d\}) = \sum_{M \setminus U \subset C \subset M} I_C(a) I_C(b) I_C(c) I_C(d)(-1)^{|M \setminus C|} \left(\sum_{A_l \in C} p_l \right)^n.$$

$$\tag{7.34}$$

Proof. It is sufficient to note that for $M \setminus U \subset C \subset M$, $a \in U$,

$$I_C(a) = 1 \Leftrightarrow a \in C \Leftrightarrow (M \setminus U) \cup \{a\} \subset C \subset M \Leftrightarrow M \setminus (U \setminus \{a\}) \subset C \subset M,$$

so

$$\sum_{M \setminus U \subset C \subset M} I_C(a)(-1)^{|M \setminus C|} \left(\sum_{A_l \in C} p_l \right)^n = \sum_{M \setminus (U \setminus \{a\}) \subset C \subset M} (-1)^{|M \setminus C|} \left(\sum_{A_l \in C} p_l \right)^n$$

$$= Q(n, U \setminus \{a\}),$$

from Equation (7.2).

Similarly,

$$I_C(a)I_C(b) = 1 \Leftrightarrow a, b \in C \Leftrightarrow (M \setminus U) \cup \{a, b\} \subset C \subset M$$
$$\Leftrightarrow M \setminus (U \setminus \{a, b\}) \subset C \subset M.$$

So, Equation (7.32) holds from Equation (7.2).

$$I_C(a)I_C(b)I_C(c) = 1 \Leftrightarrow a, b, c \in C \Leftrightarrow (M \setminus U) \cup \{a, b, c\} \subset C \subset M$$
$$\Leftrightarrow M \setminus (U \setminus \{a, b, c\}) \subset C \subset M.$$

So, Equation (7.33) holds from Equation (7.2).

$$I_C(a)I_C(b)I_C(c)I_C(d) = 1 \Leftrightarrow a, b, c, d \in C \Leftrightarrow (M \setminus U) \cup \{a, b, c, d\} \subset C \subset M$$
$$\Leftrightarrow M \setminus (U \setminus \{a, b, c, d\}) \subset C \subset M.$$

So, Equation (7.34) holds from Equation (7.2).

Lemma 7.4.5 *For any $U \subset M$, and any alleles a, b, c and d, we have*

$$\sum_{M \setminus U \subset C \subset M} I_C(a)(-1)^{|M \setminus C|} \left(\sum_{A_l \in C} p_l \right)^n$$
$$= I_M(a)Q(n, U \setminus \{a\}), \tag{7.35}$$

$$\sum_{M \setminus U \subset C \subset M} I_C(a)I_C(b)(-1)^{|M \setminus C|} \left(\sum_{A_l \in C} p_l \right)^n$$
$$= I_M(a)I_M(b)Q(n, U \setminus \{a\} \cup \{b\}), \tag{7.36}$$

$$\sum_{M \setminus U \subset C \subset M} I_C(a)I_C(b)I_C(c)(-1)^{|M \setminus C|} \left(\sum_{A_l \in C} p_l \right)^n$$
$$= I_M(a)I_M(b)I_M(c)Q(n, U \setminus \{a\} \cup \{b\} \cup \{c\}), \tag{7.37}$$

$$\sum_{M \setminus U \subset C \subset M} I_C(a)I_C(b)I_C(c)I_C(d)(-1)^{|M \setminus C|} \left(\sum_{A_l \in C} p_l \right)^n$$
$$= I_M(a)I_M(b)I_M(c)I_M(d)Q(n, U \setminus \{a\} \cup \{b\} \cup \{c\} \cup \{d\}). \tag{7.38}$$

Proof. If allele a is not in the mixture M, then both sides of Equation (7.35) are zero; if $a \in M \setminus U$, then Equation (7.35) is just Equation (7.2); if $a \in U$, then Equation (7.35) is just Equation (7.31). Thus, Equation (7.35) holds.

If alleles a and b are identical, then Equation (7.36) is just Equation (7.35). Next, we consider $a \neq b$. If a or b is not in M, then both sides of Equation (7.36) are zero; if $a, b \in U$, then Equation (7.36) is just Equation (7.32); if $a \in U$ and $b \in M \setminus U$, then Equation (7.36) is just Equation (7.35); if $a, b \in M \setminus U$, then Equation (7.36) is just Equation (7.2). Thus, we have Equation (7.36) by the symmetry of a and b.

If two of alleles a, b and c are identical, then Equation (7.37) is just Equation (7.36). So, we consider that a, b and c are all distinct. If one of a, b and c is not in M, then both sides of Equation (7.37) are zero; if $a, b, c \in U$, then Equation (7.37) is just Equation (7.33); if $a, b \in$

U and $c \in M \setminus U$, then Equation (7.37) is just Equation (7.36); if $a \in U$ and $b, c \in M \setminus U$, then Equation (7.37) is just Equation (7.35); if $a, b, c \in M \setminus U$, then Equation (7.37) is just Equation (7.2). By the symmetry of a, b and c, Equation (7.37) is hence proved.

If two of alleles a, b, c and d are identical, then Equation (7.38) is just Equation (7.37). So, we assume a, b, c and d are all distinct. If one of a, b, c and d is not in M, then both sides of Equation (7.38) are zero; if $a, b, c, d \in U$, then Equation (7.38) is just Equation (7.34); if $a, b, c \in U$ and $d \in M \setminus U$, then Equation (7.38) is just Equation (7.37); if $a, b \in U$ and $c, d \in M \setminus U$, then Equation (7.38) is just Equation (7.36); if $a \in U$ and $b, c, d \in M \setminus U$, then Equation (7.38) is just Equation (7.35); if $a, b, c, d \in M \setminus U$, then Equation (7.38) is just Equation (7.2). Thus, we prove Equation (7.38) by the symmetry of a, b, c and d.

7.4.2   The proof of Equation (7.5)

Under proposition H, the suspect $S = s_1 s_2$ is a tested man and $R = r_1 r_2$ is an unknown contributor. So, we can write K as (S, K_0) and $X = \{r_1\} \cup \{r_2\} \cup X_0$, where K_0 is the collection of genotypes of the typed person(s) except S, X_0 is the genetic profile of the unknown contributor(s) except R. We have from Equation (7.29) for any $M \setminus U \subset C \subset M$,

$$P(X \subset C | K)$$

$$= P(\{r_1\} \cup \{r_2\} \cup X_0 \subset C | S, K_0)$$

$$= P(r_1, r_2 \in C | S) P(X_0 \subset C)$$

$$= \left(\sum_{A_l \in C} p_l \right)^{2(x-1)} \left\{ k_0 \left(\sum_{A_l \in C} p_l \right)^2 + k_1 [I_C(s_1) + I_C(s_2)] \sum_{A_l \in C} p_l + k_2 I_C(y_1) I_C(y_2) \right\}.$$

$$(7.39)$$

Substituting Equation (7.39) into Equation (6.6) and using the notation $Q(\cdot, \cdot)$ defined in Equation (7.2), we have Equation (7.5), for a given proposition H, after simplification using the fact that $I_C(s_1)$ is always 0 for any $s_1 \notin M$, $I_C(s_1)$ is always 1 for any $s_1 \in M \setminus U$, and $I_C(s_1)$ may take value 0 or 1 if $s_1 \in U$.

7.4.3   The proof of Equation (7.7)

Under proposition H, there are two biologically related $X_1 = x_{11} x_{12}$ and $X_2 = x_{21} x_{22}$ amongst x unknown contributors. So we can write X, the genetic profile of the x unknowns, as $\{x_{11}\} \cup \{x_{12}\} \cup \{x_{21}\} \cup \{x_{22}\} \cup X_0$, where X_0 is the genetic profile of the other $x - 2$ unknown contributors. From Equation (7.30), we have for any $M \setminus U \subset C \subset M$ that

$$P(X \subset C | K) = P(X_0 \subset C) P(x_{11}, x_{12}, x_{21}, x_{22} \in C)$$

$$= \left(\sum_{A_l \in C} p_l \right)^{2x-2} \left[k_0 \left(\sum_{A_l \in C} p_l \right)^2 + 2k_1 \sum_{A_l \in C} p_l + k_2 \right]. \qquad (7.40)$$

Substituting Equation (7.40) into Equation (6.6) and using the notation $Q(\cdot, \cdot)$ defined in Equation (7.2), we immediately have Equation (7.7), for a given proposition H.

7.4.4   The proof of Equation (7.9)

Under the proposition specified in Equation (7.8), the only related individuals are X_1 and T_1, and X_2 and T_2. Let $x_{11}x_{12}$ and $x_{21}x_{22}$ be the genotypes of the two unknown contributors; X_1 and X_2, respectively, and X_0 be the genetic profiles of the other $x - 2$ unknown contributor; then, we have $X = \{x_{11}\} \cup \{x_{12}\} \cup \{x_{21}\} \cup \{x_{22}\} \cup X_0$ and further, from Equation (6.7),

$$W(C) = P(x_{11}, x_{12}, x_{21}, x_{22} \in C, X_0 \subset C | K)$$

$$= P(x_{11}, x_{12} \in C | T_1) P(x_{21}, x_{22} \in C | T_2) P(X_0 \subset C). \tag{7.41}$$

Using Equation (7.29) for the first two items on the right-hand side of Equation (7.41), $P(X_0 \subset C) = (\sum_{A_l \in C} p_l)^{2(x-2)}$, and the results of Lemma 7.4.5, we can have Equation (7.9) from Equation (6.6) after some matrix manipulation.

7.4.5   The proof of Equation (7.11)

Under the proposition specified in Equation (7.10), the only related individuals are X_1 and T_1, and X_2 and X_3. Let $x_{11}x_{12}$, $x_{21}x_{22}$, and $x_{31}x_{32}$ be the genotypes of the two unknown contributors X_1, X_2 and X_3, respectively, and X_0 be the genetic profiles of the other $x - 3$ unknown contributors; then, we have $X = \{x_{11}\} \cup \{x_{12}\} \cup \{x_{21}\} \cup \{x_{22}\} \cup \{x_{31}\} \cup \{x_{32}\} \cup X_0$ and further, from Equation (6.7),

$$W(C) = P(x_{11}, x_{12} \in C | T_1) P(x_{21}, x_{22}, x_{31}, x_{32} \in C) P(X_0 \subset C). \tag{7.42}$$

Substituting Equations (7.30), (7.29) and $P(X_0 \subset C) = (\sum_{A_l \in C} p_l)^{2(x-3)}$ into the expression of $W(C)$ in Equation (7.42) and then using Lemma 7.4.5, we can have Equation (7.11) from Equation (6.6) after some matrix manipulation.

7.4.6   The proof of Equation (7.13)

Under the proposition specified in Equation (7.12), the only related individuals are X_1 and X_2, and X_3 and X_4. Let $x_{11}x_{12}$, $x_{21}x_{22}$, $x_{31}x_{32}$, and $x_{41}x_{42}$ be the genotypes of the two unknown contributors X_1, X_2, X_3, and X_4, respectively, and X_0 be the genetic profiles of the other $x - 4$ unknown contributors; then, we have $X = \{x_{11}\} \cup \{x_{12}\} \cup \{x_{21}\} \cup \{x_{22}\} \cup \{x_{31}\} \cup \{x_{32}\} \cup \{x_{41}\} \cup \{x_{42}\} \cup X_0$ and further, from Equation (6.7),

$$W(C) = P(x_{11}, x_{12}, x_{21}, x_{22} \in C) P(x_{31}, x_{32}, x_{41}, x_{42} \in C) P(X_0 \subset C). \tag{7.43}$$

Substituting Equation (7.30) and $P(X_0 \subset C) = (\sum_{A_l \in D} p_l)^{2(x-4)}$ into Equation (7.43) and then using Lemma 7.4.5, we have Equation (7.13) from Equation (6.6) after some matrix manipulation.

7.4.7   The proofs of Equations (7.18) and (7.20)

Suppose that the relatedness coefficients between two individuals $X = x_1x_2$ and $Y = y_1y_2$ are $(k_0, 2k_1, k_2)$. Let Z denote the persons who are biologically unrelated to X and Y, and X, Y, Z come from the same subdivided population with the degree of subdivision θ. Then

$$P(X = x_1 x_2, Y = y_1 y_2, Z)$$

$$= k_0 (2 - \delta_{x_1 x_2})(2 - \delta_{y_1 y_2}) P(x_1, x_2, y_1, y_2, Z)$$

$$+ k_1 (2 - \delta_{x_1 x_2}) \left[I_{\{y_1\} \cup \{y_2\}}(x_1) P(x_2, y_1, y_2, Z) + I_{\{y_1\} \cup \{y_2\}}(x_2) P(x_1, y_1, y_2, Z) \right]$$

$$+ k_2 (2 - \delta_{y_1 y_2}) P(y_1, y_2, Z) \delta_{XY}. \tag{7.44}$$

It is noted that each probability of a mixture of alleles and genotypes, e.g. $P(x_1, x_2, y_1, y_2, Z)$, on the right-hand side of Equation (7.44) can be found using Equation (3.17) successively, since there is no more ibd relationship among alleles x_1, x_2, y_1, y_2, and those in Z.

Since Z is biologically unrelated to X and Y, there is no ibd allele between Z and (X, Y). It is necessary to make clear which allele(s) of X and Y is (are) ibd. Let $IBDA$ be the ibd alleles of $X = x_1 x_2$ and $Y = y_1 y_2$. The possible values of $IBDA$ are: $IBDA = $ none, $IBDA = x_1$, $IBDA = x_2$ (if $x_1 \neq x_2$), and $IBDA = x_1, x_2$. It is straightforward that

$$P(X, Y, Z, IBDA = \text{none}) = k_0 (2 - \delta_{x_1 x_2})(2 - \delta_{y_1 y_2}) P(x_1, x_2, y_1, y_2, Z). \tag{7.45}$$

If $IBDA = x_1, x_2$, X and Y would need to share two alleles, i.e. $X = Y$. It can then be concluded that

$$P(X, Y, Z, IBDA = x_1, x_2) = k_2 \delta_{XY} P(Y, Z)$$

$$= k_2 (2 - \delta_{y_1 y_2}) P(y_1, y_2, Z) \delta_{XY}. \tag{7.46}$$

If $IBDA = x_1$, X and Y would need to share the allele x_1. Taking account of the two possibilities that allele x_1 may be paternal or maternal for each of X and Y, it results in four combinations with the total probability being $2k_1$ about which alleles, paternal or maternal, for each of X and Y are ibd. So

$$P(X, Y, Z, IBDA = x_1) = 2k_1 I_{\{y_1\} \cup \{y_2\}}(x_1) P(x_2, y_1, y_2, Z). \tag{7.47}$$

Based on Equations (7.45)–(7.47) and using the law of total probability, it follows that

$$P(X, Y, Z)$$

$$= P(X, Y, Z, IBDA = \text{none}) + P(X, Y, Z, IBDA = x_1)$$

$$+ (1 - \delta_{x_1 x_2}) P(X, Y, Z, IBDA = x_2) + P(X, Y, Z, IBDA = x_1, x_2)$$

$$= k_0 (2 - \delta_{x_1 x_2})(2 - \delta_{y_1 y_2}) P(x_1, x_2, y_1, y_2, Z)$$

$$+ 2k_1 I_{\{y_1\} \cup \{y_2\}}(x_1) P(x_2, y_1, y_2, Z) + 2(1 - \delta_{x_1 x_2}) k_1 I_{\{y_1\} \cup \{y_2\}}(x_2) P(x_1, y_1, y_2, Z)$$

$$+ k_2 (2 - \delta_{y_1 y_2}) P(y_1, y_2, Z) \delta_{XY}.$$

Thus, we have Equation (7.44) after simplification. Note that Equation (7.44) is an extension of Equation (7.21).

Lemma 7.4.6 *Suppose the relatedness coefficients between individuals $X = x_1 x_2$ and $Y = y_1 y_2$ are $(k_0, 2k_1, k_2)$, and Z denotes persons who are biologically unrelated to X and Y; then*

$$\sum_{x_1, x_2 \in C} P(X, Y, Z) = k_0 \sum_{x_1, x_2 \in C} P(x_1, x_2, Y, Z)$$

$$+ k_1 [I_C(y_1) + I_C(y_2)] \sum_{x_1 \in C} P(x_1, Y, Z) + k_2 I_C(y_1) I_C(y_2) P(Y, Z), \tag{7.48}$$

where C is a set of alleles.

Proof.   By simple algebraic manipulation, we can have

$$\sum_{x_1, x_2 \in C} (2 - \delta_{x_1 x_2})(2 - \delta_{y_1 y_2}) P(x_1, x_2, y_1, y_2, Z) = \sum_{x_1, x_2 \in C} P(x_1, x_2, Y, Z) \qquad (7.49)$$

and

$$\sum_{x_1, x_2 \in C} (2 - \delta_{y_1 y_2}) P(y_1, y_2, Z) \delta_{XY} = I_C(y_1) I_C(y_2) P(Y, Z). \qquad (7.50)$$

In order to find the summation of the coefficient of k_1 in Equation (7.44) over $x_1, x_2 \in C$, which is denoted by a_1 hereafter, we should distinguish whether $Y = y_1 y_2$ is homozygous or heterozygous.

When $y_2 = y_1$,

$$a_1 = \sum_{x_1, x_2 \in C} (2 - \delta_{x_1 x_2}) \left[I_{\{y_1\} \cup \{y_2\}}(x_1) P(x_2, y_1, y_1, Z) + I_{\{y_1\} \cup \{y_2\}}(x_2) P(x_1, y_1, y_1, Z) \right]$$

$$= I_C(y_1) \sum_{x_1 = x_2 = y_1} 2P(y_1, y_1, y_1, Z) + I_C(y_1) \sum_{x_2 = y_1; x_1 \neq y_1, x_1 \in C} 2P(x_1, y_1, y_1, Z)$$

$$= 2I_C(y_1) \sum_{x_1 \in C} P(x_1, y_1, y_1, Z).$$

When $y_2 \neq y_1$, $a_1 = 0$, if $y_1 \notin C$ and $y_2 \notin C$;

$$a_1 = \sum_{x_1 = x_2 = y_1} 2P(y_1, y_1, y_2, Z) + \sum_{x_2 = y_1; x_1 \neq y_1, x_1 \in C} 2P(x_1, y_1, y_2, Z)$$

$$= 2 \sum_{x_1 \in C} P(x_1, y_1, y_2, Z),$$

if $y_1 \in C$ and $y_2 \notin C$; similarly,

$$a_1 = 2 \sum_{x_1 \in C} P(x_1, y_1, y_2, Z),$$

if $y_1 \notin C$ and $y_2 \in C$; and

$$a_1 = \sum_{x_1 = x_2 = y_1} 2P(y_1, y_1, y_2, Z) + \sum_{x_1 = x_2 = y_2} 2P(y_2, y_1, y_2, Z)$$

$$+ \sum_{x_1 = y_1; x_2 = y_2} [2P(y_1, y_1, y_2, Z) + 2P(y_2, y_1, y_2, Z)]$$

$$+ \sum_{x_2 = y_1; x_1 \in C, x_1 \neq y_1, y_2} 2P(x_1, y_1, y_2, Z) + \sum_{x_2 = y_2; x_1 \in C, x_1 \neq y_1, y_2} 2P(x_1, y_1, y_2, Z)$$

$$= 4 \sum_{x_1 \in C} P(x_1, y_1, y_2, Z),$$

if $y_1 \in C$ and $y_2 \in C$.

Thus, a_1 can be unified as

$$T = \sum_{x_1, x_2 \in C} (2 - \delta_{x_1 x_2}) \left[I_{\{y_1\} \cup \{y_2\}}(x_1) P(x_2, y_1, y_2, Z) + I_{\{y_1\} \cup \{y_2\}}(x_2) P(x_1, y_1, y_2, Z) \right]$$

$$= (2 - \delta_{y_1 y_2})[I_C(y_1) + I_C(y_2)] \sum_{x_1 \in C} P(x_1, y_1, y_2, Z)$$

$$= [I_C(y_1) + I_C(y_2)] \sum_{x_1 \in C} P(x_1, Y, Z). \tag{7.51}$$

Finally, Equations (7.49) – (7.51) lead to Equation (7.48).

Lemma 7.4.7 *For any alleles* $a \in U, b \in U, a \neq b, U \subset M,$

$$Q(n, U \setminus \{a\}, \theta) = \sum_{M \setminus U \subset C \subset M} I_C(a)(-1)^{|M \setminus C|} q(n, C), \tag{7.52}$$

$$Q(n, U \setminus \{a, b\}, \theta) = \sum_{M \setminus U \subset C \subset M} I_C(a) I_C(b)(-1)^{|M \setminus C|} q(n, C). \tag{7.53}$$

Proof. It is sufficient to note that for $M \setminus U \subset C \subset M, a \in U,$

$$I_C(a) = 1 \Leftrightarrow a \in C \Leftrightarrow (M \setminus U) \cup \{a\} \subset C \subset M \Leftrightarrow M \setminus (U \setminus \{a\}) \subset C \subset M,$$

so

$$\sum_{M \setminus U \subset C \subset M} I_C(a)(-1)^{|M \setminus C|} q(n, C) = \sum_{M \setminus (U \setminus \{a\}) \subset C \subset M} (-1)^{|M \setminus C|} q(n, C).$$

Thus, Equation (7.52) follows immediately from Equation (7.15). The derivation of Equation (7.53) is similar and then omitted.

Proof of Equation (7.18). For the proposition H in Equation (7.17), the genotypes of the tested persons, K, can be expressed as (T, K_0), where K_0 constitutes the genotypes of the tested persons except T. Write $X = \{r_1\} \cup \{r_2\} \cup X_0$, where X_0 is the genetic profile of those $x - 1$ unknown contributors whose genotypes are denoted by G_0. Substituting (G_0, K_0) for Z in Equation (7.48), we have that

$$\sum_{r_1, r_2 \in C, X_0 \subset C} P(R, T, G_0, K_0)$$

$$= k_0 \sum_{r_1, r_2 \in C, X_0 \subset C} P(r_1, r_2, G_0 | T, K_0) P(T, K_0)$$

$$+ k_1 [I_C(t_1) + I_C(t_2)] \sum_{r_1 \in C, X_0 \subset C} P(r_1, G_0 | T, K_0) P(T, K_0)$$

$$+ k_2 I_C(t_1) I_C(t_2) \sum_{X_0 \subset C} P(G_0 | T, K_0) P(T, K_0),$$

and then

$$W(C) = \sum_{r_1, r_2 \in C, X_0 \subset C} P(R, G_0 | T, K_0)$$

$$= k_0 q(2x, C) + k_1 [I_C(t_1) + I_C(t_2)] q(2x - 1, C)$$

$$+ k_2 I_C(t_1) I_C(t_2) q(2x - 2, C)$$

from Equation (6.19). Substituting the above equation into Equation (6.6) gives

$$P(M | K, H) = k_0 Q(2x, U) + k_1 (T_{11} + T_{12}) + k_2 T_2, \tag{7.54}$$

where

$$T_{11} = \sum_{M \setminus U \subset C \subset M} I_C(t_1)(-1)^{|M \setminus C|} q(2x - 1, C),$$

$$T_{12} = \sum_{M \setminus U \subset C \subset M} I_C(t_2)(-1)^{|M \setminus C|} q(2x - 1, C),$$

$$T_2 = \sum_{M \setminus U \subset C \subset M} I_C(t_1) I_C(t_2)(-1)^{|M \setminus C|} q(2x - 2, C).$$

In the following, the expressions for T_{11}, T_{12} and T_2 can be simplified further. Note that $t_1 \notin M \Rightarrow I_C(t_1) = 0$ for all $M \setminus U \subset C \subset M$, so $T_{11} = 0$; $t_1 \in M \setminus U \Rightarrow I_C(t_1) = 1$ for all $M \setminus U \subset C \subset M$, so $T_{11} = Q(2x - 1, U)$ from Equation (7.15); $t_1 \in U \Rightarrow T_{11} = Q(2x - 1, U \setminus \{t_1\})$ from Equation (7.52). Thus

$$T_{11} = I_M(t_1) Q(2x - 1, U \setminus \{t_1\}). \tag{7.55}$$

Similarly, we can have

$$T_{12} = I_M(t_2) Q(2x - 1, U \setminus \{t_2\}). \tag{7.56}$$

Meanwhile, if $t_1 \notin M$ or $t_2 \notin M$, then $I_C(t_1)I_C(t_2) = 0$ and $T_2 = 0$; if $t_1 \in M \setminus U$ and $t_2 \in M \setminus U$, then $T_2 = Q(2x - 2, U)$; if $t_1 \in U$ and $t_2 \in M \setminus U$, then $I_C(t_1)I_C(t_2) = I_C(t_1)$ and $T_2 = Q(2x - 2, U \setminus \{t_1\})$ from Equation (7.52); if $t_1 \in M \setminus U$ and $t_2 \in U$, then $I_C(t_1)I_C(t_2) = I_C(t_2)$ and $T_2 = Q(2x - 2, U \setminus \{t_2\})$ from Equation (7.52); if $t_1 \in U, t_2 \in U$, and $t_1 \neq t_2$, then $I_C(t_1)I_C(t_2) = 1 \Leftrightarrow M \setminus (U \setminus \{t_1, t_2\}) \subset C \subset M$, so $T_2 = Q(2x - 2, U \setminus \{t_1, t_2\})$ from Equation (7.53); if $t_1 \in U, t_2 \in U$, and $t_1 = t_2$, then $I_C(t_1)I_C(t_2) = 1 \Leftrightarrow M \setminus (U \setminus \{t_1\}) \subset C \subset M$, so $T_2 = Q(2x - 2, U \setminus \{t_1\})$ from Equation (7.52). Finally, we have

$$T_2 = I_M(t_1) I_M(t_2) Q(2x - 2, U \setminus \{t_1\} \cup \{t_2\}). \tag{7.57}$$

Substituting Equations (7.55), (7.56) and (7.57) into Equation (7.54) yields Equation (7.18).

Proof of Equation (7.20).   For the proposition H listed in Equation (7.19), we can express the genetic profile of the x unknown contributors as $X = \{x_{11}\} \cup \{x_{12}\} \cup \{x_{21}\} \cup \{x_{22}\} \cup X_0$, where $x_{11}x_{12}$ and $x_{21}x_{22}$ are the genotypes of the two related persons X_1 and X_2, respectively, and X_0 is the genetic profile of the $x - 2$ unknown contributors, whose genotypes are denoted by G_0. Substituting $X_1, X_2, (G_0, K)$ for X, Y, Z, respectively, in Equation (7.48) and from Equation (6.19), we have

$$\sum_{x_{11}, x_{12}, x_{21}, x_{22} \in C, X_0 \subset C} P(X_1, X_2, G_0, K)$$

$$= k_0 \sum_{x_{11}, x_{12}, x_{21}, x_{22} \in C, X_0 \subset C} P(x_{11}, x_{12}, x_{21}, x_{22}, G_0, K)$$

$$+ 2k_1 \sum_{x_{11}, x_{21}, x_{22} \in C, X_0 \subset C} P(x_{11}, x_{21}, x_{22}, G_0, K)$$

$$+ k_2 \sum_{x_{21}, x_{22} \in D, X_0 \subset C} P(x_{21}, x_{22}, G_0, K)$$

$$= P(K)[k_0 q(2x, C) + 2k_1 q(2x - 1, C) + k_2 q(2x - 2, C)].$$

So

$$W(C) = \sum_{x_{11}, x_{12}, x_{21}, x_{22} \in C, X_0 \subset C} P(X_1, X_2, G_0 | K)$$

$$= k_0 q(2x, C) + 2k_1 q(2x - 1, C) + k_2 q(2x - 2, C).$$

Substituting the above equation into Equation (6.6) and from Equation (7.15), Equation (7.20) follows immediately.

7.5   Problems

1. Suppose that the DNA profiles for the crime DNA mixed sample, victim and suspect are, respectively, $M = \{A_1, A_2, A_3, A_4\}$, $V = A_1 A_3$, and $S = A_2 A_4$. Derive the likelihood ratio for the prosecution proposition H_p: the contributors were the victim and the suspect, versus the defense proposition H_d: the contributors were the victim and one relative of the suspect. The relatedness coefficients between the relative and the suspect are $(k_0, 2k_1, k_2)$ and the population is in Hardy–Weinberg equilibrium.

2. For a crime DNA mixed sample of type $\{A_1, A_2, A_3, A_4\}$, a suspect of type $A_2 A_4$ and the victim of type $A_1 A_3$, derive the likelihood ratio for the prosecution proposition H_p: the contributors were the victim and the suspect, versus the defense proposition H_d: the contributors were two related unknown persons. The relatedness coefficients between these two related unknowns are $(k_0, 2k_1, k_2)$ and the population is in Hardy–Weinberg equilibrium.

3. For a crime DNA mixed sample of type $\{A_1, A_2, A_3, A_4\}$, known to contain DNA from two contributors, the victim is of type $A_2 A_3$ and the suspect is of type $A_1 A_4$. Derive the likelihood ratio for the prosecution proposition H_p: the contributors were the victim and the suspect, versus the defense proposition H_d: the contributors were the victim and one relative of the suspect. The relatedness coefficients between the relative and the suspect are $(k_0, 2k_1, k_2)$ and all the involved people come from the same subdivided population with degree of subdivision θ.

4. Consider the situation in which the crime sample was contributed by two persons. Suppose $M = \{A_1, A_2, A_3, A_4\}$, $V = A_1 A_3$, $S = A_2 A_4$. Derive the likelihood ratio for the prosecution proposition H_p: the contributors were the victim and the suspect, versus the defense proposition H_d: the contributors were two related unknown persons. The relatedness coefficients between these two related unknowns are $(k_0, 2k_1, k_2)$ and all the involved people come from the same subdivided population with degree of subdivision θ.

5. Using Equation (7.18), check the results of the likelihood ratio listed in the Table 7.8 in the case of $M = \{A_1, A_2, A_3\}$, $V = A_1 A_2$ and $S = A_1 A_3$.

8

Other issues

8.1 Lineage markers

Besides autosomal markers, which are most commonly used nowadays for forensic investigation, Y chromosome STR (Gill *et al.* 2001) and mitochondrial DNA (mtDNA) (Carracedo *et al.* 2000) analyses are also employed in some circumstances. These two kinds of markers are particularly useful for lineage and genealogy studies.

Y chromosomes are transmitted from fathers alone to sons only. So each male has only one Y chromosome, and a female does not possess any. Barring mutation, a Y-STR profile is identical for all paternally related males. The Y chromosome is relatively short and it is approximately 60 Mb in length. About 95% of the length of the Y chromosome cannot recombine. The Y-STR markers which reside on this nonrecombining region are therefore genetically linked.

Y-STR haplotypes may be shared by many individuals such as brothers and other paternally related males, and so they do not allow individualization to the extent that autosomal markers do. However, Y-STR profiling is found to be applicable in many situations, such as violent crime and sexual offenses, in which the majority of the offenders are males. The usefulness of Y-STRs has been recognized in cases in which the autosomal markers fail to provide clear information. For example, in some sexual offences having DNA mixtures with the major components coming from the females, the autosomal STR profiles of the males cannot be shown clearly and, under these circumstances, the genetic information of the Y-STRs would be particularly relevant and useful.

Since Y-STR markers are linked, the usual product rule based on the multiplication of allele frequencies across markers cannot be applied. The Y-STR haplotype frequency is considered instead, which is commonly determined by the counting method. Suppose that there is a population database of size n with the database count x for a particular haplotype. The haplotype frequency can be estimated by the sample proportion, when $x > 0$,

$$\hat{p} = x/n, \tag{8.1}$$

Statistical DNA Forensics: Theory, Methods and Computation   Wing Kam Fung and Yue-Qing Hu
© 2008 John Wiley & Sons, Ltd

and the approximate 95% confidence interval (Holland and Parsons 1999) may also be used

$$\hat{p} \pm 1.96\sqrt{\frac{\hat{p}(1 - \hat{p})}{n}}. \tag{8.2}$$

Nowadays, many databases are often of the size of a few hundreds, and so some possible haplotypes may not be observed. In that situation, the 95% confidence limit for the frequency (Holland and Parsons 1999), when $x = 0$,

$$1 - 0.05^{1/n}, \tag{8.3}$$

can then be employed. It is to be noticed that the approximation in Equation (8.2) may not be good if x is too small.

An alternative method given below was suggested by Balding and Nichols (1994):

$$\hat{p} = \frac{x + 2}{n + 2}, \tag{8.4}$$

where both the crime scene and the defendant haplotypes are included in the population database for estimation.

A comparison has been made between Equation (8.4) and each of Equations (8.2) and (8.3) (Tully *et al.* 2001). The former equation is often found to be more conservative, i.e. giving a smaller estimate for the frequency, but the difference between the estimates based on different equations is not really that substantial.

It is of interest to consider the probability of a random match of the crime scene Y-STR haplotype A_i with that of the defendant's under a subdivided population having a degree of subdivision θ. This conditional match probability, according to Equation (3.17), can be obtained as

$$P(A_i \mid A_i) = \theta + (1 - \theta)p_i, \tag{8.5}$$

where p_i is the frequency for haplotype A_i, which can be estimated using some of the methods given earlier. Note that the conditional match probability is always great than θ, the measure of degree of subdivision in the population. The effect of θ on the conditional probability can be large if p_i is very small. The values of θ have been found to be less than 0.01 among European populations (Roewer *et al.* 2000).

Y chromosomes are inherited paternally alone, and that limits their diversity, which can only be accumulated by mutational processes. In addition, due to the fact that half of the human population is male and the Y chromosome only constitutes half of the sex chromosome pair, the effective population size of the Y chromosome is only a quater of that of the autosomes. As in autosomal STR loci, mutations have been observed in Y-STRs. The average mutation rate for Y-STRs is found to be about 0.2–0.3% (Heyer *et al.* 1997; Kayser *et al.* 2000). The effects of mutations have to be taken into account (Gill *et al.* 2001; Gusmão *et al.* 2006) for paternity testing, identity and kinship analyses involving male relatives. Rolf *et al.* (2001) suggested a method incorporating the mutation rates across multiple Y-STR loci to analyse data with apparent exclusions caused by mutation.

Unlike nuclear DNA, mtDNA resides outside the nucleus of the cell, which is a circular molecule of about 16.5 Kb in length. Sequence analysis of mtDNA is being used widely to characterize forensic specimens, particularly when there are insufficient nuclear DNA samples ·for typing (Carracedo *et al.* 2000). MtDNA profiles can be obtained from bones, teeth, hairs and other samples that are severely decomposed. Some more well known applications of mtDNA analysis include the identification of the Russian Tsar, Nicholas II (Gill *et al.* 1994), and of the unknown soldier remains in the Vietnam War (Lidor 2002) [see also Holland and Parsons (1999) for applications to forensic casework].

MtDNA is almost entirely maternally inherited, i.e. only the mtDNA of the mother will be transmitted to the offspring. It is very rare, if at all, to have mtDNA recombination (Wiuf 2001). The mutation rate for a mtDNA genome is higher than that for the nuclear genome. Excluding mutations, an mtDNA sequence is identical for all maternally linked relatives. MtDNA samples have been widely used to infer aspects of human female population histories (Jobling *et al.* 2004).

Two portions within the noncoding control region in the mtDNA, called hypervariable regions I and II (HVI and HVII), are found to have the highest degree of variation among individuals. Currently, mtDNA is the only DNA type for which sequencing is used as the method of profiling. A mtDNA type usually refers to the entire sequence of one or both of the hypervariable regions and is treated as a single locus. A specific feature of mtDNA typing is its heteroplasmy characteristic: the existence of more than one mtDNA type within an individual. Several ways of heteroplasmy may be observed (Carracedo *et al.* 2000): (1) individuals may have more than one mtDNA type in a single tissue; (2) individuals may exhibit one mtDNA type in one tissue and a different type in another issue; and/or (3) individuals may be heteroplasmic in one tissue sample and homoplasmic in another tissue sample. Balding (2005) considered some methods to deal with heteroplasmy [see also Tully *et al.* (2001) and Buckleton *et al.* (2005)].

As in Y chromosome profiling, mtDNA profiling essentially types the haplotype, too. Thus, the estimates for the frequency of mtDNA haplotype can be constructed based on the same formulas as in Equations (8.1)–(8.4) used for the Y chromosome. Moreover, Equation (8.5) can be employed for evaluating the conditional match probability of mtDNA profiles in a subdivided population.

8.2 Haplotypic genetic markers for mixture

Chapters 6 and 7 focus on the evaluation of DNA mixtures at an autosomal locus. In practice, DNA profiles at multiple loci are investigated. Many of the commonly used STR loci are located at different chromosomes, and so they may be regarded as in linkage equilibrium. If two loci are located at the same chromosome, then the distances between the markers are usually far enough such that alleles at different markers can be regarded as statistically independent. So, the overall likelihood ratio can be obtained by multiplication of likelihood ratios for individual loci. Besides the autosomal markers, more and more countries have begun to build their databases of haplotypes in the sex-chromosome, for example the database of European Y chromosomal STR haplotypes (Roewer *et al.* 2001) and databases of Y chromosomal STR haplotypes for US populations (Kayser *et al.* 2002). These databases are more often used now in forensic science. Y chromosomal genetic markers represent a useful tool to resolve cases of criminal sexual offence, since female contamination of a given trace can usually be excluded in such instances. The features of Y chromosomal genetic markers as introduced in the previous section, principally haploidy and the absence of recombination, provide a number of advantages but also limitations, both being problem-dependent. The major difference between the autosomal marker and haplotypic genetic marker is that the autosomal data across loci are essentially statistically independent, while the haplotypic data

Table 8.1   Profiles of the mixture, the victim and two suspects at three linked loci.

Locus	Mixture	Victim	Suspect 1	Suspect 2
a	A_1	A_1	A_1	A_1
b	B_1, B_2	B_1	B_2	B_2
c	C_1, C_2, C_3	C_1	C_2	C_3

are highly linked and therefore dependent. The limited number of Y chromosomal genetic markers makes the tool less discriminating than a battery of autosomal markers.

Regarding haplotypic genetic markers, the likelihood ratio introduced in Equation (2.27) is again used to measure the weight of DNA evidence. Fukshansky and Bär (2005) established a statistical framework based on the testing of statistical hypothesis and provided a recursive formula to calculate the likelihood ratio in the evaluation of DNA mixtures of haplotypic data. In the following, we give an illustrative example to look at this issue and the general approach is referred to in Fukshansky and Bär (2005). Wolf *et al.* (2005) also derived a general formula for forensic interpretation of Y chromosomal DNA mixtures.

Let $A_1, A_2, \ldots$ denote the alleles at locus a, $B_1, B_2, \ldots$ denote the alleles at locus b, and $C_1, C_2, \ldots$ denote the alleles at locus c. Then, the haplotype at these three loci is of $A_i B_j C_k$ and its frequency is denoted simply as p_{ijk}, which is usually known. Suppose that the profile of a mixed stain is a triple of $(A_1, B_1 B_2, C_1 C_2 C_3)$, which means that there are one, two and three alleles detected at loci a, b and c, respectively. It is concluded that the number of contributors, known or unknown, is at least three. For simplicity, we regard that there are three contributors to the mixed stain in the subsequent analysis. Now, the victim and two suspects are typed and their haplotypes are respectively $A_1 B_1 C_1$, $A_1 B_2 C_2$, and $A_1 B_2 C_3$ (see Table 8.1 for details). The prosecution proposition about the donors of the mixed stain is

H_p: contributors were the victim and two suspects.

Several different defense propositions can be raised in this situation, such as:

H_{d1}: contributors were the victim, suspect 1 and one unknown;
H_{d2}: contributors were the victim and two unknowns;
H_{d3}: contributors were three unknowns.

Recall the notations introduced in Chapter 6, and it is easy to understand that $P(M|K, H_p) = 1$. Under H_{d1}, we consider which alleles in the profile of the mixed stain the unknown can carry at these three loci separately. From the profiles of the mixture at these three loci a, b and c, it is concluded that the allele of the unknown at locus a must be A_1, the allele of the unknown is either B_1 or B_2 at locus b, and must be C_3 at locus c. It implies that $P(M|K, H_{d1}) = P(A_1 B_1 C_3) + P(A_1 B_2 C_3) = p_{113} + p_{123}$.

Under H_{d2}, the situation becomes more complex than the above. It is necessary to make clear which alleles the two unknowns X_1 and X_2 can carry at these three loci. At locus a, the alleles of X_1 and X_2 must be A_1, since the profile of the mixed stain at this locus has only one allele, A_1. At locus b, the two alleles of X_1 and X_2 must explain B_2, so there are a total of three possibilities: (B_1, B_2), (B_2, B_1), and (B_2, B_2). At locus c, the alleles of X_1 and X_2 must explain C_2 and C_3 and therefore there are two combinations: (C_2, C_3) and (C_3, C_2). Considering these three loci jointly, the haplotypes of the two unknowns could be

$(A_1B_1C_2, A_1B_2C_3)$, $(A_1B_1C_3, A_1B_2C_2)$, ..., or $(A_1B_2C_3, A_1B_2C_2)$, and so we have

$$P(M|K, H_{d2}) = P(A_1B_1C_2)P(A_1B_2C_3) + P(A_1B_1C_3)P(A_1B_2C_2)$$
$$+ P(A_1B_2C_2)P(A_1B_1C_3) + P(A_1B_2C_3)P(A_1B_1C_2)$$
$$+ P(A_1B_2C_2)P(A_1B_2C_3) + P(A_1B_2C_3)P(A_1B_2C_2)$$
$$= 2p_{112}p_{123} + 2p_{113}p_{122} + 2p_{122}p_{123}.$$

Under H_{d3}, there are a total of three unknown contributors. We can also enumerate all the possible combinations of the three unknowns at each locus and then consider them jointly. For locus a, it is unique that the allele of unknowns X_1, X_2 and X_3 must be A_1. For locus b, the three alleles of the three unknowns must explain both B_1 and B_2, so the possible combinations of these three alleles among the unknowns are given as follows: (B_1, B_1, B_2), (B_1, B_2, B_1), (B_2, B_1, B_1), (B_1, B_2, B_2), (B_2, B_1, B_2), (B_2, B_2, B_1). For locus c, the alleles of X_1, X_2 and X_3 must be a permutation of $C_1C_2C_3$ and therefore there are $3! = 6$ kinds of combinations: (C_1, C_2, C_3), (C_1, C_3, C_2), (C_2, C_1, C_3), (C_2, C_3, C_1), (C_3, C_1, C_2), (C_3, C_2, C_1). So, finally, there are $1 \times 6 \times 6 = 36$ kinds of combinations of the haplotypes of X_1, X_2 and X_3, and $P(M|K, H_d)$ is a summation of probabilities over all these 36 combinations:

$$P(M|K, H_d) = P(A_1B_1C_1)P(A_1B_1C_2)P(A_1B_2C_3) + \cdots$$

which, after simplification, can be expressed as

$$P(M|K, H_d) = 6p_{111}p_{112}p_{123} + 6p_{111}p_{113}p_{122} + 6p_{111}p_{122}p_{123}$$
$$+ 6p_{112}p_{113}p_{121} + 6p_{112}p_{121}p_{123} + 6p_{113}p_{121}p_{122}.$$

Note that the general algorithm reported in Fukshansky and Bär (2005) and Wolf *et al.* (2005) employs a recursive relationship over the unknown contributors and is computationally efficient when the number of such contributors is small.

8.3 Bayesian network

Bayesian network, also called Bayes net, is one diagrammatic approach that uses graphical probabilistic methods to assist forensic scientists and jurists to understand the dependencies which may exist between different aspects of evidence and to deal with the formal analysis of decision making. Bayesian network has been found to provide an aid in the representation of the relationship between characteristics of interest in situations of uncertainty, unpredictability or imprecision (Aitken and Taroni 2004). Some examples of the applications of the Bayesian network in forensic science are referred to in Dawid *et al.* (2002), Evett *et al.* (2002), Garbolino and Taroni (2002), Aitken et al. (2003) and Mortera *et al.* (2003).

The two fundamental elements in constructing a Bayesian network are nodes and arrows, which are combined to form what is known as a directed acyclic graph. A node represents an uncertainty state variable and an arrow is used to link two nodes when these two nodes represent either causal or evidential relationships. A node is called a source or parent node if it has no entering arrows, and is called a child node if it receives arrows from other nodes. There are three basic types of connections amongst nodes in a Bayesian network: serial, diverging and converging connections.

It there is an arrow from node A to B, from node B to C, but no arrow from A to C, then there is a serial connection linking three nodes A, B and C (Figure 8.1(i)). This relationship

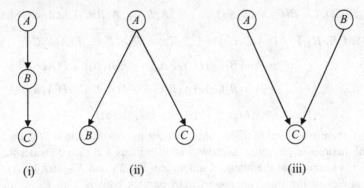

Figure 8.1   Three basic types of connections in Bayesian networks: (i) serial, (ii) diverging and (iii) converging.

can be expressed in the context of probability as $P(A|B, C) = P(A|B)$, which means that if the value of B is known, then A and C are independent. For example, let A, B and C denote the genotypes of the grandfather, father and child, respectively; then, A and C are independent if B is known and there is a serial connection linking A, B and C.

A diverging connection (Figure 8.1(ii)) linking three nodes A, B and C can be interpreted, in the context of probability, as $P(B|A, C) = P(B|A)$ and $P(C|A, B) = P(C|A)$, which means that B and C are independent if A is known. A diverging connection is used to present the spurious correlation amongst several variables.

Figure 8.1(iii) gives an example of a converging connection linking nodes A, B and C. Suppose that A, B and C denote the genotypes of the mother, father and child, respectively; then, A and B are independent if C is unknown and are dependent if C is known.

So a Bayesian network provides a compact representation of uncertain relationships among parameters involved. The key feature of a Bayesian network is the fact that it provides a method for decomposing a joint probability distribution of many variables into a set of local distributions, each having a few variables. This facilitates the investigation of relationships amongst the variables in the context of a particular case. The intellectually difficult task of organizing and arraying complex sets of evidence to exhibit dependencies and independencies can also be made visual and intuitive.

The population allele frequencies that we commonly use are often estimated from a database of a few hundred individuals. These frequency estimates contain sampling variation and uncertainty, which may need to be taken into account. By using a Bayesian model in which the frequencies of alleles were treated as random variables, Balding and Donnelly (1995) investigated the effect of frequency parameter uncertainty on the simplest identification cases [see also Balding (1995) and Foreman *et al.* (1997)]. They found that the strength of the evidence may become weaker if the database size is too small, and so it may be conservative and favorable to the defendant.

Corradi *et al.* (2003) investigated the effect of frequency parameter uncertainty on the identification problems in which two pedigrees corresponding to the prosecution and defense propositions are required for comparison. A Dirichlet prior distribution was assigned for the population parameters. A graphical model (Lauritzen 1996) was used to describe clearly the relatedness of individuals involved in which population parameters are treated as unobserved vertices. One general formula for calculating the weight of evidence was reported therein. The formula was applied to three illustrative examples selected from the literature. One example was taken from Brenner (1997) in which the profiles of the mother, the child and the alleged father were obtained for a paternity testing case. Corradi *et al.* (2003) found numerically that the weight of evidence was monotonically increasing as the sample size increased and their method provided a more conservative evaluation of the weight of evidence.

A common feature found in the reanalysis of case studies from the literature is that a greater difference is observed between the approach taking account of population parameters uncertainty and not, if rare alleles in the population are found in the alleged persons and in the alleged person's relatives (Corradi *et al.* 2003). In criminal cases, this could be a positive feature, since the court might prefer to avoid the mistake of identifying an innocent person rather than the mistake of not identifying the culprit.

In the evaluation of the conditional probability $P(M|K, H)$ or equivalently $P(M, K|H)$ that we discussed in the previous two chapters, the allele frequencies are treated as constant. But they are in fact estimated from a sample D of size n taken from a population with the degree of subdivision θ. So the uncertainty is naturally raised in the process of estimating allele frequencies, as the sample size n is usually not very large. By intuition, the uncertainty of the estimated allele frequencies will decrease when the sample size n increases. In order to take account of that uncertainty, let $x_\theta = (x_{\theta 1}, x_{\theta 2}, \ldots,)$ ($\sum_l x_{\theta l} = 1$) denote the allele frequency vector at an autosomal locus, which is distributed as the Dirichlet (see Section 3.5) prior distribution with parameter $\alpha = (\alpha_1, \alpha_2, \ldots,)$, i.e. the corresponding probability density function is

$$\text{Dir}(x_\theta|\alpha) = \frac{\Gamma(\alpha_.)}{\prod_l \Gamma(\alpha_l)} \prod_l x_{\theta l}^{\alpha_l - 1}, \quad x_{\theta l} \geq 0, l = 1, 2, \ldots, \quad \sum_l x_{\theta l} = 1$$

where $\alpha_. = \sum_l \alpha_l$. Figure 8.2 shows a network representing that the mixture M is contributed by the unknown persons X and some known persons in K, where the uncertainty of allele frequencies are taken into account. In this situation, the evaluation of $P(M, K|H)$ can be evaluated as

$$P(M, K, D|H) = \int_{\chi_\theta} P(M, K, D|x_\theta, H)\text{Dir}(x_\theta|\alpha)\, dx_\theta,$$

where the integration region χ_θ is the sample space of parameter x_θ, to take account of the sampling uncertainty. The likelihood ratio based on two such probabilities is expected to be conservative and so is more favorable to the defendant.

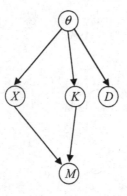

Figure 8.2   Mixture interpretation network.

Bayesian networks have also been applied to solve parentage and mixture problems (Dawid *et al.* 2002; Mortera *et al.* 2003). Generally, the networks are often complex and difficult to comprehend by forensic scientists. Little work is found in applying Bayesian networks in subdivided populations in the literature.

8.4   Peak information

Suppose that we observe a DNA mixture of $\{A_1, A_2, A_3, A_4\}$ which is presumably contributed by two unknown persons. There are a total of six possible combinations of the genotypes G_1 and G_2 of the two unknowns. The first two columns in Table 8.2 show three combinations of G_1 and G_2 and the other three combinations follow immediately from the interchange of G_1 and G_2. These six combinations are assumed to be equally likely to occur in the analysis of DNA mixtures in Chapters 6 and 7. However, in some situations, the peak height and area may provide additional information on the choice of these possible combinations.

The current technology makes it relatively simple to collect not only qualitative, but also quantitative, information such as the peak height and peak area. For simplicity, the term 'peak information' is used to refer to the quantitative peak data. Sometimes, it is possible to separate the major and minor components of a simple mixture (originally from two heterozygous individuals) by visual examination, particularly if the different contributors are in the proportion of less than 1:5 (Gill *et al.* 1998). For example, for the four-allele mixture $\{A_1, A_2, A_3, A_4\}$ consisting of two contributors as depicted in Figure 8.3, it may be relatively easy to decompose such mixture by an expert with visual judgement. Clearly, A_1 and A_2 are major components and A_3 and A_4 are minor components. Specifically, this mixture may be contributed by one

Table 8.2   All possible combinations of genotypes G_1 and G_2 of two individuals comprising the mixture $\{A_1, A_2, A_3, A_4\}$, and the corresponding gene matrix G.

G_1	G_2	G
A_1A_2	A_3A_4	$\begin{bmatrix} 1 & 0 \\ 1 & 0 \\ 0 & 1 \\ 0 & 1 \end{bmatrix}$
A_1A_3	A_2A_4	$\begin{bmatrix} 1 & 0 \\ 0 & 1 \\ 1 & 0 \\ 0 & 1 \end{bmatrix}$
A_1A_4	A_2A_3	$\begin{bmatrix} 1 & 0 \\ 0 & 1 \\ 0 & 1 \\ 1 & 0 \end{bmatrix}$

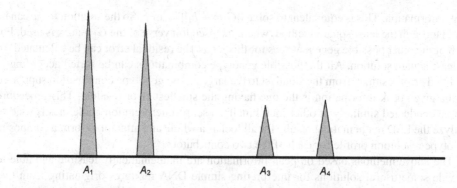

Figure 8.3   A mixture of two individuals comprising alleles A_1, A_2 and A_3, A_4.

contributor with genotype $A_1 A_2$ and the other one with $A_3 A_4$. The other possible combinations $(A_1 A_3, A_2 A_4)$ and $(A_1 A_4, A_2 A_3)$ seem more unlikely and may be excluded in the consideration. As the proportion approaches 1:1, or if the mixture comprises contributors from three or more individuals, or when there is a contamination, then the interpretation becomes increasingly problematical.

In the PCR amplification of a mixture, the amount of each PCR product scales roughly in proportion to the relative weighting of each component DNA template. Evett *et al.* (1998) established a framework to assess mixtures taking account of peak areas and to estimate the ratio of the component genotypes of a mixture using the quantitative information available. A computer model was constructed by Gill *et al.* (1998) which estimates the proportion of the components of a simple mixture of two individuals, and then proceeds to rank the genotype combinations that give the highest likelihoods. This model may be used to guide the reporting officer to interpret simple mixtures, especially by highlighting those combinations for which the data are highly unlikely.

Perlin and Szabady (2001) presented a linear mixture analysis using STR data from all the loci simultaneously for greater robustness. Its mathematical linearity permits easy computer calculation. The principle used in Perlin and Szabady (2001) can be summarized as follows. For any locus i, let b_i be the observed vector consisting of the peak information of alleles present in the mixture, $w = (w_j)$ and $G_i = (g_{ijk})$, where w_j is the weighting in the mixture of individual j's proportion, and g_{ijk} is the number of kth allele in the mixture that individual j carries, that is the contribution of the genotype of individual j to the mixture. For example, when $M = \{A_1, A_2, A_3\}$ at locus i, then $(g_{ijk}) = [2, 0, 0]$ if individual j is homozygous $A_1 A_1$, and $(g_{ijk}) = [1, 0, 1]$ if individual j is heterozygous $A_1 A_3$. See also the last column of Table 8.2 for the four-allele mixture. Once the vector b_i and matrix G_i are assigned for all loci, we construct a high-dimensional peak information vector b and gene matrix G by stacking vertically all b_i and G_i one by one. Note that different combinations of genotypes comprising mixtures lead to different gene matrices G. The final step is to find the gene matrix G such that $||Gw - b|| = \min$, where $|| \cdot ||$ is the Euclidian distance defined as the sum of the squares of all components of a vector.

Recently, Wang *et al.* (2006) proposed a least-square deconvolution (LSD) in resolving STR mixtures. LSD operates on the peak-data information of each locus separately, independently of all other loci for interpreting two-contributors STR mixture samples using the peak information. This is equivalent to solve $||G_i w - b_i|| = \min$. So the solution for w can be found through the least-square method, where the pseudoinverse of the G_i matrix is used. For each of the other possible gene matrices for this locus, the residual error can be calculated for its least-square solution. All the possible genotype combinations can be sorted according to the fitted error residual, from the smallest to the largest. The genotype combination supported by the given peak information is the one having the smallest error residual. This procedure can be conducted similarly at other loci. Finally, a set of interpretation guidelines is used to analyze the LSD mathematical results for all loci as a whole and attempt to form a composite genotype resolution profile for each of the two contributors.

The above methods based on peak information are mathematically feasible and able to provide some useful solutions for interpreting simple DNA mixtures originating from two contributors. However, when there are three or more contributors and/or contaminations in the mixed samples, etc., the problems would be much more complicated due to the high variability, uncertainty and ambiguity in DNA mixtures. A widely acceptable general approach is yet to be sought.

8.5   Mass disaster

Besides the major applications that we have discussed in early chapters, DNA profiling is also found to be a useful tool for the identification of victim and human remains in mass disasters. However, as summarized in Buckleton *et al.* (2005), there are still some difficulties in body identification by genetic means in a mass disaster situation. First, a cataclysmic physical event causes severe fragmentation of the bodies and so to reunify fragmentary remains is a key part of the identification process. Second, it is difficult to obtain DNA in satisfactory concentrations and of sufficient quality. Third, a number of individuals from the same family are thought to be the victims, so they are biologically related and, in turn, the genetic information via surviving relatives may be insufficient. Lastly, the sheer scale of the exercise may present difficulties.

The following are some examples of mass disaster: 1996 Spitzebergen crash (Ballantyne 1997), which involved 141 victims; Cebu Pacific Flight 387 on February 2, 1998 (Goodwin *et al.* 1999); Crash of Swissair Flight 111 on September 2, 1998 (Leclair *et al.* 2000); the terrorist attacks on the World Trade Center on September 11, 2001 (Brenner and Weir 2003); China Airlines crash on May 25, 2002 (Dornheim 2002); Indian Ocean tsunami on December 26, 2004 (Tsokos *et al.* 2006).

Brenner and Weir (2003) and Vastag (2002) identified the following three steps in the identification process. The first step – 'Collapsing' – refers to the association of like profiles to condense the amount of data; the second step – 'Screening' – refers to the comparison of every victim profile in the collapsed list with every missing person profile, and the final step – 'Testing' – is the confirming calculation of likelihood ratios and was undertaken as described in the equations and tables listed in Chapter 5.

The closed set matching was described in detail by Buckleton *et al.* (2005) for a comparison of the bodies and a list of missing persons. The term 'closed set' matching means to match a finite number of bodies or body parts to a finite set of missing people. This approach was demonstrated in Egeland *et al.* (2000) on the nine bodies found in the grave in Ekaterinburg and thought to include most of the Russian royal family. The issue when the pedigree information is not available for some missing persons was also discussed in Buckleton *et al.* (2005). The closed set matching is briefly described in the following.

Suppose there are n persons associated with a mass disaster. The genotypes of the bodies are denoted by $G_1, \ldots, G_n$. In addition, for each person, a sample known to be from them (say a toothbrush, hair, a database sample, or some pedigree information) is available. Let $P_1, \ldots, P_n$ denote the known sample or pedigree information. Assume, without loss of generality, that the first m bodies can be assigned without error to missing people after direct match comparisons between bodies, body parts and complete profiles of missing people. For the remaining $n - m$ unassigned bodies, there are $(n - m)!$ possible assignments: $S_1, \ldots, S_{(n-m)!}$. Given $G_{m+1}, \ldots, G_n$ and $P_{m+1}, \ldots, P_n$, we can find the posterior probability using the Bayes' Theorem:

$$P(S_i|G_{m+1}, \ldots, G_n, P_{m+1}, \ldots, P_n)$$
$$= \frac{P(G_{m+1}, \ldots, G_n|P_{m+1}, \ldots, P_n, S_i)P(S_i)}{\sum\limits_{j=1}^{(n-m)!} P(G_{m+1}, \ldots, G_n|P_{m+1}, \ldots, P_n, S_j)P(S_j)}$$

for each possible assignment S_i, $1 \le i \le (n - m)!$. The prior probabilities $P(S_i)$ can be assigned from a physical examination of the bodies, location or other information (Buckleton *et al.* 2005). Egeland *et al.* (2000) provided advice on how to assign prior probabilities in an elegant manner. After the posterior probability on each member of the possible set of assignments is assessed, we can evaluate the posterior probability for each assignment of a certain body to a certain missing person. This posterior probability can be obtained by summing the terms $P(S_i|G_{m+1}, \ldots, G_n, P_{m+1}, \ldots, P_n)$ for those assignment S_i that contain this pairing (Buckleton *et al.* 2005).

8.6   Database search

In previous discussions, we regard the suspect as being identified based on non-DNA evidence, such as witness report. When the suspect is selected by a database search comparing two profiles, the evaluation of the weight of DNA evidence requires a different formulation. Nowadays, many countries and places such as the US, UK, Hong Kong and many European countries have built up their (offender) DNA databases. Some of those databases contain samples of DNA profiles from a few million people. The samples in the database may be collected during the investigation of unsolved criminal cases, from convicted felons and other kinds of criminals, etc. The DNA database search has become an important tool in identifying the suspects for different sorts of offences.

Suppose that a crime was committed and a blood stain, presumably left by the perpetrator, was recovered at the crime scene. The profile of the blood is A and the population frequency of profile A is denoted by $p = p_A$. There is no other evidence to suspect the perpetrator. A database search is thus conducted and it turns out that only Mr Smith matches the profile A.

If we ignore the manner of Mr Smith being suspected and consider the following two competing propositions

H_{p1}: Smith is the contributor of the blood;
H_{d1}: one unknown person is the contributor of the blood,

then the likelihood ratio in the probable cause case, defined by Balding and Donnelly (1996) as the setting in which the suspect has been identified on other grounds and subsequently subjected to DNA profiling, is simply as $LR_0 = 1/p$ (Balding and Donnelly 1995; Dawid and Mortera 1996). If we consider the fact that Smith is identified through a database search, the likelihood ratio of the case against the suspect Smith is then $LR_1 = (1 - \delta)/[p(1 - \pi)]$, where δ is the prior probability that Smith left the crime stain and π is the prior probability that someone in the database left the crime stain. It has been argued that the evidential strength is slightly larger in a database search case than in a probable cause case (Balding and Donnelly 1995), while Stockmarr (1999) reached a different conclusion.

Stockmarr (1999) argued that the propositions set of H_{p1} and H_{d1} are data-independent, which means that the proposition is proposed after the database search. Alternatively, he proposed the following general pair of propositions:

H_{p2}: the true perpetrator is amongst the suspects identified from the database;
H_{d2}: the profile of the true perpetrator is stochastically independent of the profiles in the database.

Then, the corresponding likelihood ratio is $LR = \delta/(\pi p)$. In the case of all people in the population being equally likely to be the criminal, i.e. $\delta = 1/N$ and $\pi = n/N$, where n and N are the sizes of the database and the population, respectively, the likelihood ratio is induced to $LR_2 = 1/(np)$, which differs from the likelihood ratio LR_0 in a probable cause case by a factor of n. The figure LR_2 supports Recommendation 5.1 in NRC II (National Research Council 1996), which suggests dividing the likelihood ratio LR_0 by the number n of people in the database. The above likelihood ratio findings imply that $LR_0 > LR_1 > LR_2$. The figure LR_2 indicates that the larger the database, the weaker the DNA evidence. It is also noted that different pairs of propositions about the donor of the crime stain lead to completely different likelihood ratios.

In the following, we consider the posterior odds, the product of the likelihood ratio and the prior odds, instead of the likelihood ratio itself. The prior odds of H_{p1} versus H_{d1} are $\delta/(1 - \delta)$, so the posterior odds are

$$\frac{1 - \delta}{p(1 - \pi)} \frac{\delta}{1 - \delta} = \frac{\delta}{p(1 - \pi)}.$$

Similarly, the prior odds of H_{p2} versus H_{d2} are $\pi/(1 - \pi)$, so the posterior odds are

$$\frac{\delta}{p\pi} \frac{\pi}{1 - \pi} = \frac{\delta}{p(1 - \pi)}.$$

The posterior odds derived above are the same (Meester and Sjerps 2003).

It is concluded that when a scientific expert has to assess the weight of DNA evidence, the manner in which both the suspect was selected and the propositions were set is crucial in the calculation of the likelihood ratio. Although different pairs of propositions lead to different likelihood ratios, the posterior odds remain the same. The reason is that the proposition pairs are conditionally equivalent; that is, they are logically equivalent given the evidence (Dawid 2001). The likelihood ratio is referred to as a measure of the strength of the evidence and the posterior odds are referred to as an indication of the strength of the case (Meester and Sjerps 2003).

It is commented that the database controversy is a false controversy and there is no dilemma at all (Meester and Sjerps 2003). In the database search, the posterior odds are more meaningful than a likelihood ratio (Dawid 2001). Thus, when a forensic expert interprets a match in a database search, a good approach might be to provide the juror with a table exhibiting the relationship between the prior odds and the posterior odds (see such a table in Table 4.4 for a parentage testing case). The juror can then see to what posterior odds his or her prior odds lead (Meester and Sjerps 2003).

Solutions to problems

Solutions to Chapter 2

1. (a) $P(A \cup B) = P(A) + P(B) - P(AB)$

$$= 0.2 + 0.3 - 0.1$$

$$= 0.4.$$

(b) $P(B|A) = \dfrac{P(AB)}{P(A)} = \dfrac{0.1}{0.2} = 0.5.$

$P(A|C) = \dfrac{P(AC)}{P(C)} = \dfrac{0.1}{0.4} = 0.25.$

(c) From $P(BC) = 0$, we have $P(ABC) = 0$. So

$$P(A \cup B \cup C) = P(A) + P(B) + P(C) - P(AB) - P(AC) - P(BC)$$

$$+ P(ABC)$$

$$= 0.2 + 0.3 + 0.4 - 0.1 - 0.1$$

$$= 0.7.$$

2. Let $R_1 =$ 'the first ball drawn is red',

$\bar{R}_1 =$ 'the first ball drawn is yellow',

$R_2 =$ 'the second ball drawn is red',

$\bar{R}_2 =$ 'the second ball drawn is yellow',

(a) $P(R_1 \bar{R}_2 \text{ or } \bar{R}_1 R_2) = P(R_1 \bar{R}_2) + P(\bar{R}_1 R_2)$

$$= \frac{8}{12} \times \frac{4}{11} + \frac{4}{12} \times \frac{8}{11} = \frac{16}{33}.$$

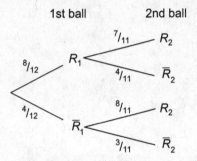

1st ball   2nd ball

(b) $P(R_2) = \dfrac{8}{12} \times \dfrac{7}{11} + \dfrac{4}{12} \times \dfrac{8}{11} = \dfrac{2}{3}.$

(c) $P(R_1|R_2) = \dfrac{P(R_1 R_2)}{P(R_2)}$

$$= \left(\dfrac{2}{3} \times \dfrac{7}{11}\right) \Big/ \left(\dfrac{2}{3}\right) = \dfrac{7}{11}.$$

3. Using the binomial probability,

$$P(X = 4) = \binom{6}{4} \times 0.1^4 \times (1 - 0.1)^2$$

$$= \dfrac{6!}{4!2!} \times 0.0001 \times 0.81$$

$$= 15 \times 0.000081 = 0.001215.$$

4. Let X_1, X_2 and X_3 be the numbers of people having genotypes AA, Aa and aa, respectively. By the multinomial distribution,

$$P(X_1 = 1, X_2 = 2, X_3 = 4) = \dfrac{7!}{1!2!4!} \times 0.09^1 \times 0.42^2 \times 0.49^4$$

$$= \dfrac{7 \times 6 \times 5}{2 \times 1} \times 0.09 \times 0.1764 \times 0.05764801$$

$$= 0.096.$$

5. $X \sim N(4, 10^2) \Longrightarrow Z = \dfrac{X - 4}{10} \sim N(0, 1).$

(a) $P(X > 6) = P\left(\dfrac{X - 4}{10} > \dfrac{6 - 4}{10}\right)$

$= P(Z > 0.2)$

$= 0.5 - 0.0793$, from the normal table in Appendix A

$= 0.4207.$

(b) $P(-2 < X < 8) = P\left(\dfrac{-2-4}{10} < \dfrac{X-4}{10} < \dfrac{8-4}{10}\right)$

$= P(-0.6 < Z < 0.4)$

$= P(-0.6 < Z < 0) + P(0 \leq Z < 0.4)$

$= P(0 < Z < 0.6) + P(0 \leq Z < 0.4)$

$= 0.2257 + 0.1554$, from the normal table in Appendix A

$= 0.3811.$

(c) $P(X \not> x) = P\left(\dfrac{X-4}{10} > \dfrac{x-4}{10}\right) = P\left(Z > \dfrac{x-4}{10}\right)$

We want this probability equal to 0.025. From the normal table in Appendix A, we know that $P(Z > 1.96) = 0.025$. So, we have

$$\dfrac{x-4}{10} = 1.96,$$

$$x = 10 \times 1.96 + 4 = 23.6.$$

6. The hypotheses of interest are

H_0 : the coin is balanced;
H_1 : the coin is not balanced.

Under H_0, the expected numbers of heads and tails in 300 flips are both 150. So, the goodness-of-fit test statistic is

$$T = \dfrac{(145-150)^2}{150} + \dfrac{(155-150)^2}{150}$$

$$= \dfrac{50}{150} = \dfrac{1}{3}.$$

The critical value of $\chi^2(1)$ at the 5% level of significance is 3.84. Since $1/3 < 3.84$, we accept H_0 and conclude that the coin is balanced.

7. $\bar{x} = \dfrac{1}{9}\sum_{i=1}^{9} x_i = 11.793,$

$$\hat{\sigma} = \sqrt{\dfrac{1}{9-1}\sum_{i=1}^{9}(x_i - \bar{x})^2} = 8.354.$$

$\hat{\sigma}_{\bar{x}} = \hat{\sigma}/\sqrt{9} = 2.785.$
The 95% confidence interval for the mean μ of the population is
$(\bar{x} - 1.96\hat{\sigma}_{\bar{x}}, \bar{x} + 1.96\hat{\sigma}_{\bar{x}}) = (6.34, 17.25).$
The 99% confidence interval for the mean μ of the population is
$(\bar{x} - 2.575\hat{\sigma}_{\bar{x}}, \bar{x} + 2.575\hat{\sigma}_{\bar{x}}) = (4.62, 18.96).$

Solutions to Chapter 3

1. (a) The frequencies of alleles A and a:

$$\hat{p}_A = \dfrac{2 \times 18 + 8}{2 \times 30} = \dfrac{44}{60} = \dfrac{11}{15},$$

$$\hat{p}_a = \frac{2 \times 4 + 8}{2 \times 30} = \frac{16}{60} = \frac{4}{15}.$$

(b) From Section 3.2.1, the observed heterozygosity is

$$OH = 1 - \sum_i \hat{p}_{ii}$$

$$= 1 - \frac{18}{30} - \frac{4}{30}$$

$$= \frac{8}{30} = \frac{4}{15} = 0.267.$$

The estimate of expected heterozygosity is

$$EH = 1 - \sum_i \hat{p}_i^2$$

$$= 1 - \left(\frac{11}{15}\right)^2 - \left(\frac{4}{15}\right)^2$$

$$= 1 - \frac{121}{225} - \frac{16}{225}$$

$$= \frac{225 - 121 - 16}{225}$$

$$= \frac{88}{225}$$

$$= 0.391.$$

(c) The hypotheses of interest are:

H_0 : population is in Hardy-Weinberg equilibrium at the locus;
H_1 : population is not in Hardy-Weinberg equilibrium at the locus.

Under H_0 of Hardy–Weinberg equilibrium, the expected counts for genotypes AA, Aa and aa are, respectively,

$$E_{AA} = n\hat{p}_A^2 = 30 \times \left(\frac{11}{15}\right)^2 = 16.13,$$

$$E_{Aa} = 2n\hat{p}_A\hat{p}_a = 2 \times 30 \times \frac{11}{15} \times \frac{4}{15} = 11.73,$$

$$E_{aa} = n\hat{p}_a^2 = 30 \times \left(\frac{4}{15}\right)^2 = 2.14.$$

So the chi-square test statistic is

$$T = \sum \frac{(\text{Observed} - \text{Expected})^2}{\text{Expected}}$$

$$= \frac{(18 - 16.13)^2}{16.13} + \frac{(8 - 11.73)^2}{11.73} + \frac{(4 - 2.14)^2}{2.14}$$

$$= 3.02,$$

which is smaller than the critical value 3.84 of the χ^2 distribution with $2(2-1)/2 = 1$ degree of freedom. The 5% critical value is obtained from the χ^2 table given in Appendix B. We accept H_0 that Hardy–Weinberg equilibrium holds. Notice that the usual rule-of-five is not satisfied in this example, but we expect the χ^2 distribution approximation is still acceptable [see Fienberg (1979)].

(d) The standard error for the estimate of expected heterozygosity is

$$SE = \left[\frac{EH(1-EH)}{n}\right]^{1/2} = \left[\frac{0.391 \times 0.609}{30}\right]^{1/2} = 0.0891.$$

We have

$$\frac{EH - OH}{SE} = \frac{0.391 - 0.267}{0.0891} = 1.39,$$

which is less than 1.96 or 2. So we accept the null hypothesis H_0 of Hardy–Weinberg equilibrium.

2. There are totally $n = n_{11} + n_{12} + n_{13} + n_{22} + n_{23} + n_{33} = 100$. The frequencies for alleles A_1, A_2 and A_3 are, respectively,

$$p_1 = \frac{2n_{11} + n_{12} + n_{13}}{2n} = \frac{2 \times 14 + 18 + 22}{200} = \frac{68}{200} = 0.34,$$

$$p_2 = \frac{2n_{22} + n_{12} + n_{23}}{2n} = \frac{2 \times 12 + 18 + 20}{200} = \frac{62}{200} = 0.31,$$

$$p_3 = \frac{2n_{33} + n_{13} + n_{23}}{2n} = \frac{2 \times 14 + 22 + 20}{200} = \frac{70}{200} = 0.35.$$

The probability of identity, as seen in Section 3.3.2, is

$$PI = \sum p_i^4 + 4 \sum_{i<j} p_i^2 p_j^2$$

$$= (0.34)^4 + (0.31)^4 + (0.35)^4 + 4 \times (0.34)^2 \times (0.31)^2 + 4 \times (0.34)^2 \times (0.35)^2$$
$$+ 4 \times (0.31)^2 \times (0.35)^2$$

$$= 0.1858.$$

So, the power of discrimination is

$$PD = 1 - PI = 1 - 0.1858 = 0.8142.$$

3. (a) Based on Equations (3.10) and (3.16), the likelihood ratios are

Locus	HWE	Subdivided population
THO1	$\dfrac{1}{p_8^2}$	$\dfrac{(1+\theta)(1+2\theta)}{[2\theta + (1-\theta)p_8][3\theta + (1-\theta)p_8]}$
TPOX	$\dfrac{1}{2p_8 p_9}$	$\dfrac{(1+\theta)(1+2\theta)}{2[\theta + (1-\theta)p_8][\theta + (1-\theta)p_9]}$

(b) Plugging in $p_8 = 0.053$ at THO1, $p_8 = 0.545$ and $p_9 = 0.1$ at TPOX, $\theta = 0$ and $\theta = 0.03$ into formulas of the table in (a), we obtain the following likelihood ratios:

| Locus | HWE | Subdivided population | |
		$\theta = 0$	$\theta = 0.03$
THO1	356	356	69.3
TPOX	9.17	9.17	7.69
Overall	3265	3265	533

4. Without loss of generality, we consider Equation (3.17) with $i = 1$. Based on the third law of probability for dependent events, we obtain

$$P(A_1 | y \ A_1 \text{ alleles among } n \text{ alleles}) = \frac{P(A_1^{y+1} A_2^{m_2} A_3^{m_3} \cdots)}{P(A_1^y A_2^{m_2} A_3^{m_3} \cdots)},$$

which, according to Equation (3.14), can be expressed as

$$\frac{\frac{\Gamma(\gamma)}{\Gamma(\gamma+n+1)} \frac{\Gamma(\gamma_1+y+1)}{\Gamma(\gamma_1)} \prod_{i \geq 2} \frac{\Gamma(\gamma_i+m_i)}{\Gamma(\gamma_i)}}{\frac{\Gamma(\gamma)}{\Gamma(\gamma+n)} \frac{\Gamma(\gamma_1+y)}{\Gamma(\gamma_1)} \prod_{i \geq 2} \frac{\Gamma(\gamma_i+m_i)}{\Gamma(\gamma_i)}} = \frac{\Gamma(\gamma+n)}{\Gamma(\gamma+n+1)} \frac{\Gamma(\gamma_1+y+1)}{\Gamma(\gamma_1+y)}$$

$$= \frac{\gamma_1 + y}{\gamma + n}$$

$$= \frac{\frac{(1-\theta)p_i}{\theta} + y}{\frac{1-\theta}{\theta} + n}$$

$$= \frac{y\theta + (1-\theta)p_i}{1 + (n-1)\theta}.$$

Hence, Equation (3.17) is obtained.

5. According to Equation (3.17), at locus THO1,

$$P(V = 6/6, S = 6/7) = 2P(6, 6, 6, 7)$$

$$= 2P(6)P(6|6)P(6|6, 6)P(7|6, 6, 6)$$

$$= 2p_6 \left[\frac{\theta + (1-\theta)p_6}{1 + (1-1)\theta} \right] \left[\frac{2\theta + (1-\theta)p_6}{1 + (2-1)\theta} \right] \left[\frac{(1-\theta)p_7}{1 + (3-1)\theta} \right]$$

$$= \frac{2p_6[\theta + (1-\theta)p_6][2\theta + (1-\theta)p_6](1-\theta)p_7}{(1+\theta)(1+2\theta)}$$

$$= \frac{2(1-\theta)p_6 p_7[\theta + (1-\theta)p_6][2\theta + (1-\theta)p_6]}{(1+\theta)(1+2\theta)}.$$

At locus TPOX,

$$P(V = 8/9, S = 9/10) = 4P(8, 9, 9, 10)$$

$$= 4P(8)P(9|8)P(9|8, 9)P(10|8, 9, 9)$$

$$= 4p_8 \left[\frac{(1-\theta)p_9}{1+(1-1)\theta} \right] \left[\frac{\theta+(1-\theta)p_9}{1+(2-1)\theta} \right] \left[\frac{(1-\theta)p_{10}}{1+(3-1)\theta} \right]$$

$$= \frac{4(1-\theta)^2 p_8 p_9 p_{10}[\theta+(1-\theta)p_9]}{(1+\theta)(1+2\theta)}.$$

6. Without loss of generality, assume that the genotypes of the father and the mother are A_1A_2 and A_3A_4, respectively. So there are a total of four kinds of genotypes for each offspring: A_1A_3, A_1A_4, A_2A_3 and A_2A_4, with an equal chance of $1/4$. For each pair of full siblings, all possible combinations of their genotypes are listed as follows:

Case	Genotype pair	Number of ibd alleles	Case	Genotype pair	Number of ibd alleles
1	(A_1A_3, A_1A_3)	2	9	(A_2A_3, A_1A_3)	1
2	(A_1A_3, A_1A_4)	1	10	(A_2A_3, A_1A_4)	0
3	(A_1A_3, A_2A_3)	1	11	(A_2A_3, A_2A_3)	2
4	(A_1A_3, A_2A_4)	0	12	(A_2A_3, A_2A_4)	1
5	(A_1A_4, A_1A_3)	1	13	(A_2A_4, A_1A_3)	0
6	(A_1A_4, A_1A_4)	2	14	(A_2A_4, A_1A_4)	1
7	(A_1A_4, A_2A_3)	0	15	(A_2A_4, A_2A_3)	1
8	(A_1A_4, A_2A_4)	1	16	(A_2A_4, A_2A_4)	2

Given parents' genotypes A_1A_2 and A_3A_4, the probability that each pair of genotypes as listed above occurs is $1/16$. So

$$k_0 = P(\text{no ibd alleles between the two full siblings})$$

$$= P(\text{cases } 4,\ 7,\ 10,\ 13)$$

$$= \frac{1}{16} + \frac{1}{16} + \frac{1}{16} + \frac{1}{16}$$

$$= \frac{1}{4},$$

$$k_2 = P(\text{cases } 1,\ 6,\ 11,\ 16)$$

$$= \frac{1}{4},$$

$$2k_1 = P(\text{cases } 2,\ 3,\ 5,\ 8,\ 9,\ 12,\ 14,\ 15)$$

$$= \frac{1}{2}.$$

7. Without loss of generality, we assume that the parent's genotype is A_1A_2 and the child's genotype is A_1A_3, where the allele A_1 in the parent and the allele A_1 in the child are ibd. Randomly choosing two alleles, one from the parent, the other one from the child, we have the following outcomes with an equal chance of $1/4$: (A_1, A_1), (A_1, A_2), (A_2, A_1) and (A_2, A_3). Only in case 1 are the two randomly chosen alleles ibd. So $F = 1/4$.

8. Let $X = ab$ and $Y = cd$ be two individuals' genotypes. Symbol '$\equiv$' is used to represent the ibd relationship between two alleles. From the definition in Equation (3.21) for the kinship coefficient, we have

$$F = \frac{1}{4}[P(a \equiv c) + P(a \equiv d) + P(b \equiv c) + P(b \equiv d)].$$

From the definition in Equation (3.18) for the relatedness coefficients, we have

$$k_2 = P(a \equiv c, b \equiv d) + P(a \equiv d, b \equiv c)$$

$$2k_1 = P(a \equiv c, b \not\equiv d) + P(a \equiv d, b \not\equiv c) + P(b \equiv c, a \not\equiv d) + P(b \equiv d, a \not\equiv c).$$

So

$$2k_1 + 2k_2 = P(a \equiv c, b \not\equiv d) + P(a \equiv c, b \equiv d) + P(a \equiv d, b \not\equiv c)$$

$$+ P(a \equiv d, b \equiv c) + P(b \equiv c, a \not\equiv d) + P(b \equiv c, a \equiv d)$$

$$+ P(b \equiv d, a \not\equiv c) + P(b \equiv d, a \equiv c)$$

$$= P(a \equiv c) + P(a \equiv d) + P(b \equiv c) + P(b \equiv d)$$

$$= 4F.$$

Thus, we have

$$2F = k_1 + k_2.$$

Particularly, if $k_2 = 0$, then $2F = k_1$.

9. Using a similar argument as in the derivation of Equations (3.19) and (3.23) and employing the recursive formula given in Equation (3.17), we obtain

$$P(A_i A_i | A_i A_i)$$

$$= \sum_{t=0}^{2} P(A_i A_i | A_i A_i, \ t \text{ ibd alleles}) P(t \text{ ibd alleles})$$

$$= P(A_i | A_i A_i) P(A_i | A_i A_i A_i) k_0$$

$$+ \left[(1/2) P(A_i | A_i A_i) + (1/2) P(A_i | A_i A_i) \right] (2k_1) + 1 \times k_2$$

$$= \left[\frac{2\theta + (1 - \theta) p_i}{1 + \theta} \right] \left[\frac{3\theta + (1 - \theta) p_i}{1 + 2\theta} \right] k_0 + \left[\frac{2\theta + (1 - \theta) p_i}{1 + \theta} \right] (2k_1) + k_2.$$

The required result is obtained after grouping of terms.

Solutions to Chapter 4

1. The paternity index, from Equation (4.4), is

$$PI = \frac{P(C | M, AF, H_p)}{P(C | M, H_d)}$$

$$= \frac{P(C = A_1 A_2 | M = A_1 A_2, AF = A_2 A_3, H_p)}{P(C = A_1 A_2 | M = A_1 A_2, H_d)}$$

$$= \frac{(1/2)(1/2)}{(1/2) p_2 + (1/2) p_1}$$

$$= \frac{1}{2(p_1 + p_2)}.$$

This result can also be obtained from Table 4.1. When $p_1 = 0.331$ and $p_2 = 0.326$,

$$PI = \frac{1}{2 \times (0.331 + 0.326)} = 0.76.$$

The software EasyDNA_Trio gives the same results; details are omitted.

2. Let C_P/C_M be the paternal/maternal allele of C. The likelihood ratio is

$$
\begin{aligned}
LR &= \frac{P(C|M, AF, H_p)}{P(C|M, AF, H_d)} \\
&= \frac{P(C = A_1 A_2 | M = A_1 A_3, AF = A_2 A_3, H_p)}{P(C = A_1 A_2 | M = A_1 A_3, AF = A_2 A_3, H_d)} \\
&= \frac{(1/2)(1/2)}{P(C_M = A_1 | M = A_1 A_3) P(C_P = A_2 | AF = A_2 A_3, H_d)} \\
&= \frac{(1/4)}{(1/2) \times (k_0 p_2 + k_1)} \\
&= \frac{1}{2 \times (p_2/2 + 1/4)} \\
&= \frac{2}{2p_2 + 1},
\end{aligned}
$$

where $(k_0, 2k_1, k_2)$ are the relatedness coefficients between child C and the alleged father AF (who is the uncle of C) under H_d, i.e. $k_0 = 1/2$, $2k_1 = 1/2$ and $k_2 = 0$. This LR can also be obtained from the penultimate row of Table 4.1 with $i = 1, j = 2, k = 2$, and the kinship coefficient $F = 1/4$ for full siblings.

3. Let C_P/C_M be the paternal/maternal allele of C. The likelihood ratio is

$$
\begin{aligned}
LR &= \frac{P(C|M, R, H_p)}{P(C|M, R, H_d)} \\
&= \frac{P(C = A_1 A_2 | M = A_1 A_2, R = A_2 A_3, H_p)}{P(C = A_1 A_2 | M = A_1 A_2, R = A_2 A_3, H_d)} \\
&= \frac{P(C_P = A_1, C_M = A_2 \text{ or } C_P = A_2, C_M = A_1 | M = A_1 A_2, R = A_2 A_3, H_p)}{P(C_P = A_1, C_M = A_2 \text{ or } C_P = A_2, C_M = A_1 | M = A_1 A_2, R = A_2 A_3, H_d)} \\
&= \frac{(1/2) P(C_P = A_1 | R = A_2 A_3, H_p) + (1/2) P(C_P = A_2 | R = A_2 A_3, H_p)}{(1/2) p_1 + (1/2) p_2} \\
&= \frac{(1/2) k_0 p_1 + (1/2) k_0 p_2 + k_1}{(1/2) p_1 + (1/2) p_2} \\
&= k_0 + \frac{k_1}{p_1 + p_2},
\end{aligned}
$$

where $(k_0, 2k_1, k_2)$ are the relatedness coefficients of the child and the relative R under H_p. Substituting $k_0 = 1/2$ and $k_1 = 1/4$ into the above equation, we have

$$LR = \frac{1}{2} + \frac{1}{4(p_1 + p_2)}.$$

4. In this situation, we have the genotypes of the child (C), the mother (M), and a relative (R) of the alleged father (AF), and three propositions about who the true father of the child is:

H_{p1} : R is the true father of the child;
H_{p2} : AF, a relative of R, is the true father of the child;
H_d : a random unrelated man is the true father of the child.

So

$$AI = \frac{P(C|M, R, H_{p2})}{P(C|M, R, H_d)}$$

$$PI = \frac{P(C|M, R, H_{p1})}{P(C|M, R, H_d)}.$$

Under H_{p2}, imagine that the true father's (i.e. AF under H_{p2}) genotype is the same as R's. When the TF (true father) and R share two ibd alleles, the relative R plays the same role as TF in the calculation of $P(C|M, R, H_{p2})$. When TF and R share only one ibd allele, R plays the role as TF and the role as a random man with equal probability $1/2$ in the calculation of $P(C|M, R, H_{p2})$. When TF and R share no ibd allele, R plays the same role as a random man in the calculation of $P(C|M, R, H_{p2})$. Considering the definition of the relatedness coefficients between two persons, we have

$$P(C|M, R, H_{p2}) = \left(k_2 + \frac{2k_1}{2}\right) P(C|M, R, H_{p1}) + \left(\frac{2k_1}{2} + k_0\right) P(C|M, R, H_d)$$

$$= (k_2 + k_1) P(C|M, R, H_{p1}) + (k_1 + k_0) P(C|M, R, H_d).$$

So, dividing by $P(C|M, R, H_d)$ on both sides, we obtain

$$AI = (k_1 + k_0) + (k_2 + k_1) PI$$

$$= (1 - 2F) + 2F \times PI.$$

Note $k_2 + k_1 = 2F$ is given in the solution to problem 8 of Chapter 3, where F is the kinship coefficient between the alleged father and the typed relative R.

5. For case (i),

$$PI = \frac{P(C|AF, H_p)}{P(C|H_d)}$$

$$= \frac{P(C = A_1 A_3 | AF = A_1 A_2, H_p)}{P(C = A_1 A_3 | H_d)}$$

$$= \frac{(1/2) \times p_3}{2 p_1 p_3}$$

$$= \frac{1}{4 p_1}.$$

For case (ii),

$$PI = \frac{P(C = A_1A_1|AF = A_1A_2, H_p)}{P(C = A_1A_1|H_d)} = \frac{(1/2) \times p_1}{p_1^2} = \frac{1}{2p_1}.$$

For case (iii),

$$PI = \frac{P(C = A_1A_1|AF = A_1A_1, H_p)}{P(C = A_1A_1|H_d)} = \frac{1 \times p_1}{p_1^2} = \frac{1}{p_1}.$$

These results can also be obtained from Table 4.5.

6. Let C_P/C_M be the paternal/maternal allele of C,

$$PI = \frac{P(C = A_1A_2|AF = A_2A_3, H_p)}{P(C = A_1A_2|AF = A_2A_3, H_d)}$$

$$= \frac{P(C_P = A_2, C_M = A_1|AF = A_2A_3, H_p)}{P(C_P = A_1, C_M = A_2 \text{ or } C_P = A_2, C_M = A_1|AF = A_2A_3, H_d)}$$

$$= \frac{(1/2) \times p_1}{p_2 \times k_0 p_1 + p_1(k_0 p_2 + k_1)}$$

$$= \frac{1}{4k_0 p_2 + 2k_1},$$

where $(k_0, 2k_1, k_2)$ are the relatedness coefficients between the child and the alleged father under H_d, i.e. $k_0 = 1/2, k_1 = 1/4, k_2 = 0$. So

$$PI = \frac{1}{2p_2 + 1/2} = \frac{2}{1 + 4p_2}.$$

7. Let C_P/C_M be the paternal/maternal allele of the child C,

$$PI = \frac{P(C = A_1A_2|R = A_1A_2, H_p)}{P(C = A_1A_2|R = A_1A_2, H_d)}$$

$$= \frac{P(C_P = A_1, C_M = A_2 \text{ or } C_P = A_2, C_M = A_1|R = A_1A_2, H_p)}{P(C_P = A_1A_2)}$$

$$= \frac{p_2 \times (k_0 p_1 + k_1) + p_1(k_0 p_2 + k_1)}{2p_1 p_2}$$

$$= \frac{2k_0 p_1 p_2 + k_1(p_1 + p_2)}{2p_1 p_2}$$

$$= k_0 + k_1 \frac{p_1 + p_2}{2p_1 p_2},$$

where $(k_0, 2k_1, k_2)$ are the relatedness coefficients between the child and the typed relative R under H_p, i.e. $k_0 = 1/2, k_1 = 1/4, k_2 = 0$. So

$$PI = \frac{1}{2} + \frac{p_1 + p_2}{8p_1 p_2}.$$

8. Let C and R denote the genotypes of the child and a relative of the alleged father. The corresponding hypotheses are:

H_{p1} : R is the true father of the child;
H_{p2} : AF, a relative of R, is the true father of the child;
H_d :   a random unrelated man is the true father of the child

The PI and AI can be expressed as

$$AI = \frac{P(C|R, H_{p2})}{P(C|R, H_d)},$$

$$PI = \frac{P(C|R, H_{p1})}{P(C|R, H_d)}.$$

Under H_{p2}, the relatedness coefficients between R and AF are $(k_0, 2k_1, k_2)$. Imagine that the true father's genotype is the same as R's. When the TF (true father) and R share two ibd alleles, the relative R plays the same role as TF in the calculation of $P(C|R, H_{p2})$. When TF and R share only one ibd allele, R plays the role as TF and the role as a random man with equal probability $1/2$ in the calculation of $P(C|R, H_{p2})$. When TF and R share no ibd allele, R plays the same role as a random man in the calculation of $P(C|R, H_{p2})$. So, by the law of total probability, we have

$$P(C|R, H_{p2}) = \left(k_2 + \frac{2k_1}{2}\right) P(C|R, H_{p1}) + \left(\frac{2k_1}{2} + k_0\right) P(C|R, H_d)$$

$$= (k_1 + k_2) P(C|R, H_{p1}) + (k_0 + k_1) P(C|R, H_d)$$

and dividing both sides by $P(C|R, H_d)$ gives

$$AI = (k_0 + k_1) + (k_1 + k_2) PI$$

$$= (1 - 2F) + 2F \times PI,$$

where $F = (k_1 + k_2)/2$ (see the solution to problem 8 of Chapter 3) is the kinship coefficient between the alleged father and the typed relative R.

9.

$$LR = \frac{P(C|AF, AM, H_p)}{P(C)}$$

$$= \frac{P(C = A_2 A_3 | AF = A_1 A_2, AM = A_3 A_3, H_p)}{P(C = A_2 A_3)}$$

$$= \frac{1/2 \times 1}{2 p_2 p_3}$$

$$= \frac{1}{4 p_2 p_3}.$$

10. Using the software EasyDNA_Motherless, the likelihood ratios, respectively, at loci D3S1358, vWA and FGA for H_p versus H_{d1} are 2.0921, 2.5023 and 2.2727, and for H_p versus H_{d2} are 1.3532, 1.429 and 1.3889.

Solutions to Chapter 5

1. The hypotheses are

   H_p : X and Y are first cousins;
   H_d : X and Y are unrelated

   The likelihood ratio is

   $$LR = \frac{P(X = A_1 A_2, Y = A_2 A_2 | H_p)}{P(X = A_1 A_2, Y = A_2 A_2 | H_d)}$$

   $$= \frac{k_0 P(X) P(Y) + 2k_1 p_1 p_2^2}{P(X) P(Y)}$$

   $$= k_0 + \frac{2k_1 p_1 p_2^2}{(2p_1 p_2)(p_2^2)}$$

   $$= k_0 + \frac{k_1}{p_2}$$

   $$= 0.5 + \frac{0.25}{0.37}$$

   $$= 1.18,$$

   where $(k_0, 2k_1, k_2) = (0.5, 0.5, 0)$ are the relatedness coefficients for first cousins. Note that the above LR can also be obtained from Table 5.2.

2. The two competing hypotheses about whether X and Y are in an uncle–nephew relationship can be expressed in the following forms:

   H_p : Y and Z are first cousins;
   H_d : Y and Z are unrelated

   The likelihood ratio is

   $$LR = \frac{P(Y = A_1 A_2, Z = A_1 A_3 | H_p)}{P(Y = A_1 A_2, Z = A_1 A_3 | H_d)}$$

   $$= \frac{(k_0) P(Y) P(Z) + (2k_1) P(A_1, A_2, A_3)}{P(X) P(Z)}$$

   $$= k_0 + \frac{2k_1 p_1 p_2 p_3}{(2p_1 p_2)(2p_1 p_3)}$$

   $$= k_0 + \frac{k_1}{2p_1}$$

   $$= \frac{1}{2} + \frac{1}{8p_1},$$

   where $(k_0, 2k_1, k_2) = (0.5, 0.5, 0)$ are the relatedness coefficients between the first cousins. Also, one can refer to Table 5.2 for derivation of the above LR.

3. The corresponding two competing hypotheses are

   H_p : X and Y are parent-child;
   H_d : X and Y are full siblings

So

$$LR = \frac{P(X = A_1 A_2, Y = A_1 A_2 | H_p)}{P(X = A_1 A_2, Y = A_1 A_2 | H_d)}$$

$$= \frac{P(A_1, A_2, A_2) + P(A_1, A_1, A_2)}{P(A_1, A_1, A_2, A_2) + \frac{1}{2} P(A_1, A_2, A_2) + \frac{1}{2} P(A_1, A_1, A_2) + \frac{1}{2} P(A_1, A_2)}$$

$$= \frac{P(A_2 | A_1, A_2) + P(A_1 | A_1, A_2)}{P(A_1, A_2 | A_1, A_2) + \frac{1}{2} P(A_2 | A_1, A_2) + \frac{1}{2} P(A_1 | A_1, A_2) + \frac{1}{2}}$$

$$= \frac{\frac{\theta + (1-\theta) p_2}{1 + (2-1)\theta} + \frac{\theta + (1-\theta) p_1}{1 + (2-1)\theta}}{\frac{\theta + (1-\theta) p_1}{1 + (2-1)\theta} \frac{\theta + (1-\theta) p_2}{1 + (3-1)\theta} + \frac{1}{2} \frac{\theta + (1-\theta) p_2}{1 + (2-1)\theta} + \frac{1}{2} \frac{\theta + (1-\theta) p_1}{1 + (2-1)\theta} + \frac{1}{2}}$$

$$= \frac{2(1 + 2\theta)[2\theta + (1 - \theta)(p_1 + p_2)]}{2[\theta + (1 - \theta) p_1][\theta + (1 - \theta) p_2] + (1 + 2\theta)[1 + 3\theta + (1 - \theta)(p_1 + p_2)]}.$$

When $p_1 = 0.18$, $p_2 = 0.43$ and $\theta = 0.03$, we have

$$LR = \frac{2 \times 1.06 \times (0.06 + 0.97 \times 0.61)}{2 \times (0.03 + 0.97 \times 0.18) \times (0.03 + 0.97 \times 0.43) + 1.06 \times (1.09 + 0.97 \times 0.61)}$$

$$= 0.7029.$$

4. The paternity index can be expressed as

$$PI = \frac{P(C = A_1 A_2 | M = A_1 A_1, AF = A_2 A_3, H_p)}{P(C = A_1 A_2 | M = A_1 A_1, AF = A_2 A_3, H_d)}.$$

Let C_P/C_M be the paternal/maternal allele of the child. It is concluded from $M = A_1 A_1$ that $C_P = A_2$ and $C_M = A_1$ under either hypothesis H_p or H_d. So

$$PI = \frac{P(C_M = A_1, C_P = A_2 | M = A_1 A_1, AF = A_2 A_3, H_p)}{P(C_M = A_1, C_P = A_2 | M = A_1 A_1, AF = A_2 A_3, H_d)}$$

$$= \frac{(1) \times (\frac{1}{2})}{(1) \times P(A_2 | A_1, A_1, A_2, A_3)}$$

$$= \frac{1 + 3\theta}{2[\theta + (1 - \theta) p_2]}.$$

This index can also be obtained from Table 5.12. When $p_2 = 0.23$ and $\theta = 0.03$, we have further

$$PI = \frac{1 + 3 \times 0.03}{2 \times [0.03 + (1 - 0.03) \times 0.23]} = \frac{1.09}{0.5062} = 2.15.$$

5. The paternity index can be expressed as

$$PI = \frac{P(C = A_1 A_1 | M = A_1 A_2, AF = A_1 A_3, H_p)}{P(C = A_1 A_1 | M = A_1 A_2, AF = A_1 A_3, H_d)}.$$

Let C_P/C_M be the paternal/maternal allele of the child C. Then $C_P = C_M = A_1$ and the numerator of the paternity index is

$$NUM = P(C_M = A_1, C_P = A_1 | M = A_1 A_2, AF = A_1 A_3, H_p)$$

$$= \frac{1}{2} \times \frac{1}{2}$$

$$= \frac{1}{4}.$$

The denominator of the paternity index is

$$DEN = P(C_M = A_1, C_P = A_1 | M = A_1A_2, AF = A_1A_3 | H_d)$$

$$= \frac{1}{2} \times P(C_P = A_1 | M = A_1A_2, AF = A_1A_3, H_d)$$

$$= \frac{1}{2} \left[\frac{1}{2} \times P(A_1 | A_1, A_1, A_2, A_3) + \frac{1}{4} \right]$$

$$= \frac{1}{8} \left\{ \frac{2[2\theta + (1-\theta)p_1]}{1 + (4-1)\theta} + 1 \right\}$$

$$= \frac{1 + 7\theta + 2(1-\theta)p_1}{8(1+3\theta)}.$$

Therefore

$$PI = \frac{2(1+3\theta)}{1 + 7\theta + 2(1-\theta)p_1}.$$

This index can also be obtained from Table 5.13. When $p_1 = 0.12$ and $\theta = 0.03$,

$$PI = \frac{2 \times (1 + 3 \times 0.03)}{1 + 7 \times 0.03 + 2 \times (1 - 0.03) \times 0.12}$$

$$= \frac{2.18}{1.2928}$$

$$= 1.69.$$

6. Let C, M and R, respectively, denote the genotypes of the child, the mother and the relative who is a full sibling of the alleged father. Then, the likelihood ratio

$$LR = \frac{P(C|M, R, H_p)}{P(C|M, R, H_d)}$$

$$= \frac{P(C = A_1A_1 | M = A_1A_1, R = A_1A_2, H_p)}{P(C = A_1A_1 | M = A_1A_1, R = A_1A_2, H_d)}$$

$$= \frac{P(C_M = A_1, C_P = A_1 | M = A_1A_1, R = A_1A_2, H_p)}{P(C_M = A_1, C_P = A_1 | M = A_1A_1, R = A_1A_2, H_d)}$$

$$= \frac{(\frac{1}{2})P(A_1 | A_1, A_1, A_1, A_2) + \frac{1}{4}}{P(A_1 | A_1, A_1, A_1, A_2)}$$

$$= \frac{1}{2} + \frac{1 + (4-1)\theta}{4[3\theta + (1-\theta)p_1]}$$

$$= \frac{1}{2} + \frac{1 + 3\theta}{4[3\theta + (1-\theta)p_1]},$$

where C_P/C_M are the paternal/maternal alleles of the child C.

7. Let $(k_0, 2k_1, k_2)$ be the relatedness coefficients between two individuals; then, for uncle–nephew and grandfather–child relationships, $(k_0, 2k_1, k_2) = (0.5, 0.5, 0)$. Denote Y_P/Y_M as the paternal/maternal allele of Y and the two competing hypotheses can be expressed as

$$H_p : \quad (X, Y) \sim (0.5, 0.5, 0) \text{ and } (Y, Z) \sim (0.5, 0.5, 0);$$
$$H_d : \quad (X, Y) \sim (1, 0, 0) \text{ and } (Y, Z) \sim (1, 0, 0).$$

The likelihood ratio is

$$LR = \frac{P(X = A_1A_1, Y = A_1A_2, Z = A_2A_3|H_p)}{P(X = A_1A_1, Y = A_1A_2, Z = A_2A_3|H_d)}.$$

The numerator of the LR can be further expressed as

$$NUM = P(X = A_1A_1, Y_P = A_1, Y_M = A_2, Z = A_2A_3|H_p)$$
$$+ P(X = A_1A_1, Y_P = A_2, Y_M = A_1, Z = A_2A_3|H_p)$$
$$= P(X = A_1A_1, Y_M = A_1|H_p)P(Y_P = A_2, Z = A_2A_3|H_p)$$
$$+ P(X = A_1A_1, Y_M = A_2|H_p)P(Y_P = A_1, Z = A_2A_3|H_p)$$
$$= \left[\left(\frac{1}{2}\right)(p_1)(p_1^2) + \left(2 \times \frac{1}{4}\right)p_1^2\right] \times \left[\left(\frac{1}{2}\right)(p_2)(2p_2p_3) + \left(2 \times \frac{1}{4}\right)p_2p_3\right]$$
$$+ \left[\left(\frac{1}{2}\right)(p_2)(p_1^2)\right] \times \left[\left(\frac{1}{2}\right)(p_1)(2p_2p_3)\right]$$
$$= \frac{1}{2}p_1^2(p_1 + 1) \times \frac{1}{2}p_2p_3(2p_2 + 1) + \frac{1}{2}p_1^2 \times \frac{1}{2}p_2p_3 \times 2p_1p_2$$
$$= \frac{1}{4}p_1^2p_2p_3[(1 + p_1)(1 + 2p_2) + 2p_1p_2]$$
$$= \frac{1}{4}p_1^2p_2p_3(1 + p_1 + 2p_2 + 4p_1p_2).$$

So, the likelihood ratio is

$$LR = \frac{\frac{1}{4}p_1^2p_2p_3(1 + p_1 + 2p_2 + 4p_1p_2)}{(p_1^2) \times (2p_1p_2) \times (2p_2p_3)}$$
$$= \frac{1 + p_1 + 2p_2 + 4p_1p_2}{16p_1p_2}.$$

8. From the figure, we have

$$P(X_1, X_2, X_3, X_4, X_5)$$
$$= P(X_1)P(X_2|X_1)P(X_3|X_1, X_2)P(X_4|X_1, X_2, X_3)P(X_5|X_1, X_2, X_3, X_4)$$
$$= P(X_1)P(X_2)P(X_3|X_1)P(X_4|X_2)P(X_5|X_3, X_4)$$
$$= P(X_1 = A_1A_2)P(X_2 = A_3A_3)P(X_3 = A_1A_4|X_1 = A_1A_2)$$
$$\times P(X_4 = A_2A_3|X_2 = A_3A_3)P(X_5 = A_1A_3|X_3 = A_1A_4, X_4 = A_2A_3)$$
$$= (2p_1p_2)(p_3^2)\left(\frac{1}{2}p_4\right)(p_2)\left(\frac{1}{2} \times \frac{1}{2}\right)$$

$$= \frac{1}{4} p_1 p_2^2 p_3^2.$$

If X_4 is not available, then we find that X_4 must carry allele A_3 because X_4's parent X_2 is homozygous $A_3 A_3$. So, we can express the genotype of X_4 as $A_3 A_x$, where $x = 1, 2, \ldots$. Therefore

$$P(X_1, X_2, X_3, X_5)$$

$$= \sum_{X_4} P(X_1, X_2, X_3, X_4, X_5)$$

$$= \sum_{X_4} P(X_1) P(X_2) P(X_3 | X_1) P(X_4 | X_2) P(X_5 | X_3, X_4)$$

$$= P(X_1) P(X_2) P(X_3 | X_1) \sum_{X_4} P(X_4 | X_2) P(X_5 | X_3, X_4)$$

$$= (2 p_1 p_2)(p_3^2) \left(\frac{1}{2} p_4 \right) \sum_x P(X_4 = A_3 A_x | X_2 = A_3 A_3)$$

$$\times P(X_5 = A_1 A_3 | X_3 = A_1 A_4, X_4 = A_2 A_x)$$

$$= p_1 p_2 p_3^2 p_4 \Big[P(X_4 = A_3 A_3 | X_2 = A_3 A_3) P(X_5 = A_1 A_3 | X_3 = A_1 A_4, X_4 = A_3 A_3)$$

$$+ \sum_{x \neq 3} P(X_4 = A_3 A_x | X_2 = A_3 A_3) P(X_5 = A_1 A_3 | X_3 = A_1 A_4, X_4 = A_3 A_x) \Big]$$

$$= p_1 p_2 p_3^2 p_4 \Big[(p_3) \left(\frac{1}{2} \times 1 \right) + \sum_{x \neq 3} (p_x) \left(\frac{1}{2} \times \frac{1}{2} \right) \Big]$$

$$= \frac{1}{4} p_1 p_2 p_3^2 p_4 \left(2 p_3 + \sum_{x \neq 3} p_x \right)$$

$$= \frac{1}{4} p_1 p_2 p_3^2 p_4 (1 + p_3).$$

Another solution: let X_{5P} and X_{5M} be, respectively, the paternal and maternal alleles of X_5; then

$$P(X_1, X_2, X_3, X_5)$$

$$= P(X_1 = A_1 A_2, X_3 = A_1 A_4, X_{5M} = A_1, X_{5P} = A_3, X_2 = A_3 A_3)$$

$$= P(X_1 = A_1 A_2, X_3 = A_1 A_4, X_{5M} = A_1) P(X_2 = A_3 A_3, X_{5P} = A_3)$$

$$= P(X_1 = A_1 A_2) P(X_3 = A_1 A_4 | X_1 = A_1 A_2) P(X_{5M} = A_1 | X_3 = A_1 A_4)$$

$$\times P(X_2 = A_3 A_3) P(X_{5P} = A_3 | X_2 = A_3 A_3)$$

$$= (2 p_1 p_2) \left(\frac{1}{2} p_4 \right) \left(\frac{1}{2} \right) (p_3^2) \left(\frac{1}{2} p_3 + 2 \times \frac{1}{4} \right)$$

$$= \frac{1}{4} p_1 p_2 p_3^2 p_4 (1 + p_3).$$

9. Using the computer program EasyDNA_2Persons, we obtain the following likelihood ratios:

	D3S1358	vWA	FGA
H_{p1} versus H_d			
$\theta = 0$	125.25	6.84	0.25
$\theta = 0.03$	4.53	5.76	0.25
H_{p2} versus H_d			
$\theta = 0$	125.50	2.08	0.5
$\theta = 0.03$	4.78	1.95	0.5

Solutions to Chapter 6

1. Under H_p, all the alleles in M are explained by V and S, so

$$P(M|K, H_p) = 1.$$

Under H_d, the allele A_2 must be present in the genotype G of the unknown contributor. So

$$P(M|K, H_d) = P(G = A_1 A_2) + P(G = A_2 A_2) + P(G = A_2 A_3)$$

$$= p_2(2p_1 + p_2 + 2p_3).$$

Therefore, $LR = 1/[p_2(2p_1 + p_2 + 2p_3)]$.

2. Under H_p, the unknown contributor G must carry allele A_1, so

$$P(M|K, H_p) = P(G = A_1 A_1) + P(G = A_1 A_2)$$

$$= p_1^2 + 2p_1 p_2.$$

Under H_d, the genotypes G_1 and G_2 of the two unknown contributors have seven kinds of combinations: $(A_1 A_1, A_1 A_2)$, $(A_1 A_1, A_2 A_2)$, $(A_1 A_2, A_1 A_1)$, $(A_1 A_2, A_1 A_2)$, $(A_1 A_2, A_2 A_2)$, $(A_2 A_2, A_1 A_1)$ and $(A_2 A_2, A_1 A_2)$. So

$$P(M|K, H_d) = P(G_1 = A_1 A_1, G_2 = A_1 A_2) + P(G_1 = A_1 A_1, G_2 = A_2 A_2)$$

$$+ P(G_1 = A_1 A_2, G_2 = A_1 A_1) + P(G_1 = A_1 A_2, G_2 = A_1 A_2)$$

$$+ P(G_1 = A_1 A_2, G_2 = A_2 A_2) + P(G_1 = A_2 A_2, G_2 = A_1 A_1)$$

$$+ P(G_1 = A_2 A_2, G_2 = A_1 A_2)$$

$$= 2p_1 p_2 (2p_1^2 + 3p_1 p_2 + 2p_2^2).$$

Finally, $LR = (p_1 + 2p_2)/[2p_2(2p_1^2 + 3p_1 p_2 + 2p_2^2)]$.

3. Under H_p, all three alleles in M are present in V or S, so

$$P(M|K, H_p) = 1.$$

Under H_d, the unknown contributor must carry allele A_1. So the genotype of the unknown can take $A_1 A_1$, $A_1 A_2$ or $A_1 A_3$. So

$$P(M|K, H_d) = P(G = A_1 A_1 | V = A_1 A_2, S = A_2 A_3)$$

$$+ P(G = A_1A_2|V = A_1A_2, S = A_2A_3)$$

$$+ P(G = A_1A_3|V = A_1A_2, S = A_2A_3)$$

$$= \frac{[\theta + (1-\theta)p_1][2\theta + (1-\theta)p_1]}{(1+3\theta)(1+4\theta)}$$

$$+2\frac{[\theta + (1-\theta)p_1][2\theta + (1-\theta)p_2]}{(1+3\theta)(1+4\theta)}$$

$$+2\frac{[\theta + (1-\theta)p_1][\theta + (1-\theta)p_3]}{(1+3\theta)(1+4\theta)}$$

$$= \frac{[\theta + (1-\theta)p_1][8\theta + (1-\theta)(p_1 + 2p_2 + 2p_3)]}{(1+3\theta)(1+4\theta)}.$$

The likelihood ratio is just the reciprocal of $P(M|K, H_d)$.

4. Under H_p, the genotype of X_1 must be A_1A_3, so

$$P(M|K, H_p) = P(X_1 = A_1A_3) = 2p_{a1}p_{a3}.$$

Under H_d, the genotypes of two unknown contributors X_1 and X_2 have six kinds of combinations, so

$$P(M|K, H_d) = P(X_1 = A_1A_2, X_2 = A_3A_4) + P(X_1 = A_1A_3, X_2 = A_2A_4)$$

$$+ P(X_1 = A_1A_4, X_2 = A_2A_3) + P(X_1 = A_2A_3, X_2 = A_1A_4)$$

$$+ P(X_1 = A_2A_4, X_2 = A_1A_3) + P(X_1 = A_3A_4, X_2 = A_1A_2)$$

$$= 4p_{a1}p_{a2}p_{b3}p_{b4} + 4p_{a1}p_{a3}p_{b2}p_{b4} + 4p_{a1}p_{a4}p_{b2}p_{b3}$$

$$+ 4p_{a2}p_{a3}p_{b1}p_{b4} + 4p_{a2}p_{a4}p_{b1}p_{b3} + 4p_{a3}p_{a4}p_{b1}p_{b2}.$$

The likelihood ratio follows immediately from the ratio of $P(M|K, H_p)$ to $P(M|K, H_d)$.

5. Under H_p, the four alleles in the mixture are explained by two contributors S_1 and S_2, so $P(M|K, H_p) = 1$. Under H_d, the genotypes of X_1 and X_2 must be one of the following six combinations: (A_1A_2, A_3A_4), (A_1A_3, A_2A_4), (A_1A_4, A_2A_3), (A_2A_3, A_1A_4), (A_2A_4, A_1A_3), (A_3A_4, A_1A_2).

(a) If the two unknowns and the suspect S_1 come from ethnic group a, and the suspect S_2 comes from ethnic group b, then

$$P(M|K, H_d) = P(X_1 = A_1A_2, X_2 = A_3A_4|S_1 = A_1A_2)$$

$$+ P(X_1 = A_1A_3, X_2 = A_2A_4|S_1 = A_1A_2)$$

$$+ P(X_1 = A_1A_4, X_2 = A_2A_3|S_1 = A_1A_2)$$

$$+ P(X_1 = A_2A_3, X_2 = A_1A_4|S_1 = A_1A_2)$$

$$+ P(X_1 = A_2A_4, X_2 = A_1A_3|S_1 = A_1A_2)$$

$$+ P(X_1 = A_3A_4, X_2 = A_1A_2|S_1 = A_1A_2)$$

$$= (6 \times 2 \times 2)P(A_1, A_2, A_3, A_4|S_1 = A_1A_2)$$

$$= 24P(A_1|A_1A_2)P(A_2|A_1^2A_2)P(A_3|A_1^2A_2^2)P(A_4|A_1^2A_2^2A_3)$$

$$= 24\frac{(1-\theta_a)^2 p_{a3} p_{a4}[\theta_a + (1-\theta_a) p_{a1}][\theta_a + (1-\theta_a) p_{a2}]}{(1+\theta_a)(1+2\theta_a)(1+3\theta_a)(1+4\theta_a)},$$

and $LR = 1/P(M|K, H_d)$.

(b) If the two unknowns come from ethnic group a, and the two suspects do not come from ethnic group a, then we have simply

$P(M|K, H_d)$

$$= P(X_1 = A_1A_2, X_2 = A_3A_4) + P(X_1 = A_1A_3, X_2 = A_2A_4)$$

$$+ P(X_1 = A_1A_4, X_2 = A_2A_3) + P(X_1 = A_2A_3, X_2 = A_1A_4)$$

$$+ P(X_1 = A_2A_4, X_2 = A_1A_3) + P(X_1 = A_3A_4, X_2 = A_1A_2)$$

$$= (6 \times 2 \times 2) P(A_1, A_2, A_3, A_4)$$

$$= 24 P(A_1) P(A_2|A_1) P(A_3|A_1, A_2) P(A_4|A_1, A_2, A_3)$$

$$= 24\frac{(1-\theta_a)^3 p_{a1} p_{a2} p_{a3} p_{a4}}{(1+\theta_a)(1+2\theta_a)}.$$

So the likelihood ratio is just $1/P(M|K, H_d)$.

(c) If the first unknown X_1 comes from ethnic group a, the second unknown X_2 comes from ethnic group b, and the two tested suspects come from ethnic group c, then we have

$P(M|K, H_d)$

$$= P(X_1 = A_1A_2) P(X_2 = A_3A_4) + P(X_1 = A_1A_3) P(X_2 = A_2A_4)$$

$$+ P(X_1 = A_1A_4) P(X_2 = A_2A_3) + P(X_1 = A_2A_3) P(X_2 = A_1A_4)$$

$$+ P(X_1 = A_2A_4) P(X_2 = A_1A_3) + P(X_1 = A_3A_4) P(X_2 = A_1A_2)$$

$$= 4(1-\theta_a)(1-\theta_b) p_{a1} p_{a2} p_{b3} p_{b4} + 4(1-\theta_a)(1-\theta_b) p_{a1} p_{a3} p_{b2} p_{b4}$$

$$+ 4(1-\theta_a)(1-\theta_b) p_{a1} p_{a4} p_{b2} p_{b3} + 4(1-\theta_a)(1-\theta_b) p_{a2} p_{a3} p_{b1} p_{b4}$$

$$+ 4(1-\theta_a)(1-\theta_b) p_{a2} p_{a4} p_{b1} p_{b3} + 4(1-\theta_a)(1-\theta_b) p_{a3} p_{a4} p_{b1} p_{b2}.$$

Again, the likelihood ratio is the reciprocal of $P(M|K, H_d)$.

6. Under H_p, the two contributors V and S explain the three alleles in M, so

$$P(M|K, H_p) = 1.$$

Under H_d, the unknown contributor must carry allele A_3, so

$$P(M|K, H_d) = P(G = A_1A_3) + P(G = A_2A_3) + P(G = A_3A_3)$$

$$= 2p_1 * p_3 + 2p_2 * p_3 + p_3 * p_3$$

$$= 2p_1 p_3 + 2p_2 p_3 + p_3^2 + \theta p_3(1 - p_3).$$

The likelihood ratio is just $1/P(M|K, H_d)$.

Solutions to Chapter 7

1. Under H_p, $P(M|K, H_p) = 1$. Under H_d, the relative's genotype G must be A_2A_4. So we have

$$P(M|K, H_d) = P(G = A_2A_4|S = A_2A_4)$$
$$= k_0 P(A_2A_4) + k_1 p_2 + k_1 p_4 + k_2$$
$$= 2k_0 p_2 p_4 + k_1(p_2 + p_4) + k_2,$$

and $LR = 1/[2k_0 p_2 p_4 + k_1(p_2 + p_4) + k_2]$.

2. Under H_p, $P(M|K, H_p) = 1$. Under H_d, let G_1 and G_2 denote, respectively, the genotypes of the two related unknowns; then, we have

$$P(M|K, H_d) = P(G_1 = A_1A_2, G_2 = A_3A_4) + P(G_1 = A_1A_3, G_2 = A_2A_4)$$
$$+ P(G_1 = A_1A_4, G_2 = A_2A_3) + P(G_1 = A_2A_3, G_2 = A_1A_4)$$
$$+ P(G_1 = A_2A_4, G_2 = A_1A_3) + P(G_1 = A_3A_4, G_2 = A_1A_2)$$
$$= 24k_0 p_1 p_2 p_3 p_4.$$

Note that in this situation, the two related unknown contributors to the mixed stain cannot share ibd allele and so $P(G_1 = A_iA_j, G_2 = A_kA_l) = 4k_0 p_i p_j p_k p_l$ for any permutation $ijkl$ of 1234. So $LR = 1/(24k_0 p_1 p_2 p_3 p_4)$.

3. Under H_p, $P(M|K, H_p) = 1$. Under H_d, it is concluded that the relative's genotype is of A_1A_4, so

$$P(M|K, H_d) = 2k_0 P(A_1, A_4|V = A_2A_3, S = A_1A_4)$$
$$+ k_1 P(A_4|V = A_2A_3, S = A_1A_4)$$
$$+ k_1 P(A_1|V = A_2A_3, S = A_1A_4) + k_2$$
$$= 2k_0 \frac{[\theta + (1 - \theta)p_1][\theta + (1 - \theta)p_4]}{(1 + 3\theta)(1 + 4\theta)}$$
$$+ k_1 \frac{\theta + (1 - \theta)p_4}{1 + 3\theta} + k_1 \frac{\theta + (1 - \theta)p_1}{1 + 3\theta} + k_2$$
$$= 2k_0 \frac{[\theta + (1 - \theta)p_1][\theta + (1 - \theta)p_4]}{(1 + 3\theta)(1 + 4\theta)}$$
$$+ k_1 \frac{2\theta + (1 - \theta)(p_1 + p_4)}{1 + 3\theta} + k_2.$$

Finally, the likelihood ratio is just the reciprocal of $P(M|K, H_d)$.

4. Under H_p, $P(M|M, H_p) = 1$. Under H_d, let G_1 and G_2 denote, respectively, the genotypes of the two related unknowns; then, we have

$$P(M|K, H_d) = P(G_1 = A_1A_2, G_2 = A_3A_4|V = A_1A_3, S = A_2A_4)$$
$$+ P(G_1 = A_1A_3, G_2 = A_2A_4|V = A_1A_3, S = A_2A_4)$$
$$+ P(G_1 = A_1A_4, G_2 = A_2A_3|V = A_1A_3, S = A_2A_4)$$

$$+ P(G_1 = A_2 A_3, G_2 = A_1 A_4 | V = A_1 A_3, S = A_2 A_4)$$

$$+ P(G_1 = A_2 A_4, G_2 = A_1 A_3 | V = A_1 A_3, S = A_2 A_4)$$

$$+ P(G_1 = A_3 A_4, G_2 = A_1 A_2 | V = A_1 A_3, S = A_2 A_4)$$

$$= 24 k_0 \frac{[\theta + (1 - \theta) p_i][\theta + (1 - \theta) p_j][\theta + (1 - \theta) p_k][\theta + (1 - \theta) p_l]}{(1 + 3\theta)(1 + 4\theta)(1 + 5\theta)(1 + 6\theta)}.$$

Note that in this situation, the two related unknown contributors to the mixed stain cannot share ibd allele and so

$$P(G_1 = A_i A_j, G_2 = A_k A_l | V = A_1 A_3, S = A_2 A_4)$$

$$= 4 k_0 P(A_i, A_j, A_k, A_l | A_1 A_2 A_3 A_4)$$

$$= 4 k_0 \left[\frac{\theta + (1 - \theta) p_i}{1 + 3\theta} \right] \left[\frac{\theta + (1 - \theta) p_j}{1 + 4\theta} \right] \left[\frac{\theta + (1 - \theta) p_k}{1 + 5\theta} \right] \left[\frac{\theta + (1 - \theta) p_l}{1 + 6\theta} \right]$$

for any permutation $ijkl$ of 1234. The likelihood ratio is just $1/P(M|K, H_d)$.

5. $M = \{A_1, A_2, A_3\}$, $P(M|K, H_p) = 1$. Under H_d, $x = 1$, $U = \{A_3\}$, the tested person $T = A_1 A_3$, i.e. $t_1 = A_1 \in M \setminus U$, $t_2 = A_3 \in U$, $K = A_1 A_2$ and $A_1 A_3$; so, from Equation (7.18), we have

$$P(M|K, H_d) = k_0 Q(2, U, \theta) + k_1 Q(1, U, \theta) + k_1 Q(1, \phi, \theta) + k_2 Q(0, \phi, \theta).$$

From Equations (7.15) and (7.16), $c_1 = 2$, $c_2 = 1$, $c_3 = 1$, $c = c_1 + c_2 + c_3 = 4$, we have

$$Q(2, U, \theta) = q(2, \{A_1, A_2, A_3\}, \theta) - q(2, \{A_1, A_2\}, \theta)$$

$$= \frac{(p_1 + p_2 + p_3)^{(2)}(c_1 + c_2 + c_3)}{1^{(2)}(c)} - \frac{(p_1 + p_2)^{(2)}(c_1 + c_2)}{1^{(2)}(c)}$$

$$= \frac{[4\theta + (1 - \theta)(p_1 + p_2 + p_3)][5\theta + (1 - \theta)(p_1 + p_2 + p_3)]}{(1 + 3\theta)(1 + 4\theta)}$$

$$- \frac{[3\theta + (1 - \theta)(p_1 + p_2)][4\theta + (1 - \theta)(p_1 + p_2)]}{(1 + 3\theta)(1 + 4\theta)}$$

$$= \frac{[\theta + (1 - \theta) p_3][8\theta + (1 - \theta)(2 p_1 + 2 p_2 + p_3)]}{(1 + 3\theta)(1 + 4\theta)},$$

$$Q(1, U, \theta) = q(1, \{A_1, A_2, A_3\}, \theta) - q(1, \{A_1, A_2\}, \theta)$$

$$= \frac{(p_1 + p_2 + p_3)^{(1)}(4)}{1^{(1)}(4)} - \frac{(p_1 + p_2)^{(1)}(3)}{1^{(1)}(4)}$$

$$= \frac{4\theta + (1 - \theta)(p_1 + p_2 + p_3)}{1 + 3\theta} - \frac{3\theta + (1 - \theta)(p_1 + p_2)}{1 + 3\theta}$$

$$= \frac{\theta + (1 - \theta) p_3}{1 + 3\theta},$$

$$Q(1, \phi, \theta) = q(1, \{A_1, A_2, A_3\}, \theta)$$

$$= \frac{4\theta + (1 - \theta)(p_1 + p_2 + p_3)}{1 + 3\theta},$$

$$Q(0, \phi, \theta) = 1.$$

So, we have

$$P(M|K, H_d) = k_0 \frac{[\theta + (1 - \theta)p_3][8\theta + (1 - \theta)(2p_1 + 2p_2 + p_3)]}{(1 + 3\theta)(1 + 4\theta)}$$

$$+ k_1 \frac{5\theta + (1 - \theta)(p_1 + p_2 + 2p_3)}{1 + 3\theta} + k_2.$$

Thus, the likelihood ratio, i.e. $1/P(M|K, H_d)$ is the same as that in Table 7.8 when $M = \{A_1, A_2, A_3\}$, $V = A_1 A_2$ and $S = A_1 A_3$.

Appendix A: The standard normal distribution

Areas under the standard normal curve

z	.00	.01	.02	.03	.04	.05	.06	.07	.08	.09
0.0	0.0000	0.0040	0.0080	0.0120	0.0160	0.0199	0.0239	0.0279	0.0319	0.0359
0.1	0.0398	0.0438	0.0478	0.0517	0.0557	0.0596	0.0636	0.0675	0.0714	0.0753
0.2	0.0793	0.0832	0.0871	0.0910	0.0948	0.0987	0.1026	0.1064	0.1103	0.1141
0.3	0.1179	0.1217	0.1255	0.1293	0.1331	0.1368	0.1406	0.1443	0.1480	0.1517
0.4	0.1554	0.1591	0.1628	0.1664	0.1700	0.1736	0.1772	0.1808	0.1844	0.1879
0.5	0.1915	0.1950	0.1985	0.2019	0.2054	0.2088	0.2123	0.2157	0.2190	0.2224
0.6	0.2257	0.2291	0.2324	0.2357	0.2389	0.2422	0.2454	0.2486	0.2517	0.2549
0.7	0.2580	0.2611	0.2642	0.2673	0.2704	0.2734	0.2764	0.2794	0.2823	0.2852
0.8	0.2881	0.2910	0.2939	0.2967	0.2995	0.3023	0.3051	0.3078	0.3106	0.3133
0.9	0.3159	0.3186	0.3212	0.3238	0.3264	0.3289	0.3315	0.3340	0.3365	0.3389
1.0	0.3413	0.3438	0.3461	0.3485	0.3508	0.3531	0.3554	0.3577	0.3599	0.3621
1.1	0.3643	0.3665	0.3686	0.3708	0.3729	0.3749	0.3770	0.3790	0.3810	0.3830
1.2	0.3849	0.3869	0.3888	0.3907	0.3925	0.3944	0.3962	0.3980	0.3997	0.4015
1.3	0.4032	0.4049	0.4066	0.4082	0.4099	0.4115	0.4131	0.4147	0.4162	0.4177
1.4	0.4192	0.4207	0.4222	0.4236	0.4251	0.4265	0.4279	0.4292	0.4306	0.4319
1.5	0.4332	0.4345	0.4357	0.4370	0.4382	0.4394	0.4406	0.4418	0.4429	0.4441
1.6	0.4452	0.4463	0.4474	0.4484	0.4495	0.4505	0.4515	0.4525	0.4535	0.4545
1.7	0.4554	0.4564	0.4573	0.4582	0.4591	0.4599	0.4608	0.4616	0.4625	0.4633
1.8	0.4641	0.4649	0.4656	0.4664	0.4671	0.4678	0.4686	0.4693	0.4699	0.4706
1.9	0.4713	0.4719	0.4726	0.4732	0.4738	0.4744	0.4750	0.4756	0.4761	0.4767
2.0	0.4772	0.4778	0.4783	0.4788	0.4793	0.4798	0.4803	0.4808	0.4812	0.4817

Statistical DNA Forensics: Theory, Methods and Computation   Wing Kam Fung and Yue-Qing Hu
© 2008 John Wiley & Sons, Ltd

z	.00	.01	.02	.03	.04	.05	.06	.07	.08	.09
2.1	0.4821	0.4826	0.4830	0.4834	0.4838	0.4842	0.4846	0.4850	0.4854	0.4857
2.2	0.4861	0.4864	0.4868	0.4871	0.4875	0.4878	0.4881	0.4884	0.4887	0.4890
2.3	0.4893	0.4896	0.4898	0.4901	0.4904	0.4906	0.4909	0.4911	0.4913	0.4916
2.4	0.4918	0.4920	0.4922	0.4925	0.4927	0.4929	0.4931	0.4932	0.4934	0.4936
2.5	0.4938	0.4940	0.4941	0.4943	0.4945	0.4946	0.4948	0.4949	0.4951	0.4952
2.6	0.4953	0.4955	0.4956	0.4957	0.4959	0.4960	0.4961	0.4962	0.4963	0.4964
2.7	0.4965	0.4966	0.4967	0.4968	0.4969	0.4970	0.4971	0.4972	0.4973	0.4974
2.8	0.4974	0.4975	0.4976	0.4977	0.4977	0.4978	0.4979	0.4979	0.4980	0.4981
2.9	0.4981	0.4982	0.4982	0.4983	0.4984	0.4984	0.4985	0.4985	0.4986	0.4986
3.0	0.4987	0.4987	0.4987	0.4988	0.4988	0.4989	0.4989	0.4989	0.4990	0.4990

Appendix B: Upper 1% and 5% points of χ^2 distributions

The value in the table corresponds to an upper tail probability α, for a χ^2 distribution with v degrees of freedom. The figure on the right is a χ^2 distribution with $v = 5$.

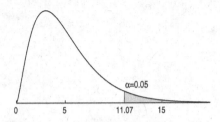

Degrees of freedom v	α 5%	α 1%	Degrees of freedom v	α 5%	α 1%
1	3.84	6.63	17	27.59	33.41
2	5.99	9.21	18	28.87	34.81
3	7.81	11.34	19	30.14	36.19
4	9.49	13.28	20	31.41	37.57
5	11.07	15.09	21	32.67	38.93
6	12.59	16.81	22	33.92	40.29
7	14.07	18.48	23	35.17	41.64
8	15.51	20.09	24	36.42	42.98
9	16.92	21.67	25	37.65	44.31
10	18.31	23.21	26	38.89	45.64
11	19.68	24.72	27	40.11	46.96
12	21.03	26.22	28	41.34	48.28
13	22.36	27.69	29	42.56	49.59
14	23.68	29.14	30	43.77	50.89
15	25.00	30.58	40	55.76	63.69
16	26.30	32.00	50	67.50	76.15

Statistical DNA Forensics: Theory, Methods and Computation   Wing Kam Fung and Yue-Qing Hu
© 2008 John Wiley & Sons, Ltd

Bibliography

Aitken C and Taroni F 2004 *Statistics and the Evaluation of Evidence for Forensic Scientists*, 2nd edn. John Wiley & Sons, Ltd, New York.

Aitken CGG, Taroni F and Garbolino P 2003 A graphical model for the evaluation of cross-transfer evidence in DNA profiles. *Theor Popul Biol* **63**, 179–190.

Ayres KL 2000 Relatedness testing in subdivided populations. *Forensic Sci Int* **114**, 107–115.

Ayres KL 2002 Paternal exclusion in the presence of substructure. *Forensic Sci Int* **129**, 142–144.

Balding DJ 1995 Estimating products in forensic identification using DNA profile. *J Am Stat Assoc* **90**, 839–844.

Balding DJ 2005 *Weight-of-evidence for Forensic DNA Profiles*. John Wiley & Sons, New York.

Balding DJ and Donnelly P 1994 How convincing is DNA evidence?. *Nature* **368**, 285–286.

Balding DJ and Donnelly P 1995 Inference in forensic identification. *J R Statist Soc A* **158**, 21–53.

Balding DJ and Donnelly P 1996 Evaluation DNA profile evidence when the suspect is identified through a database search. *J Forensic Sci* **41**, 603–607.

Balding DJ and Nichols RA 1994 DNA profile match probability calculation: how to allow for population stratification, relatedness, database selection and single bands. *Forensic Sci Int* **64**, 125–140.

Balding DJ and Nichols RA 1995 A method for quantifying differentiation between populations at multi-allelic loci and its implications for investigating identity and paternity. *Genetica* **96**, 3–12.

Balding DJ and Nichols RA 1997 Significant genetic correlations among Caucasians at forensic DNA loci. *Heredity* **78**, 583–589.

Ballantyne J 1997 Mass disaster genetics. *Nat Genet* **15**, 329–331.

Belin TR, Gjertson DW and Hu MY 1997 Summarizing DNA evidence when relatives are possible suspects. *J Am Stat Assoc* **92**, 706–716.

Box G 1980 Sampling and Bayes inference in scientific modeling and robustness. *J R Statist Soc B* **143**, 383–430.

Brenner CH 1997 Symbolic kinship program. *Genetics* **145**, 535–542.

Brenner CH and Weir BS 2003 Issues and strategies in the DNA identification of World Trade Center victims. *Theor Popul Biol* **63**, 173–178.

Brinkmann B, Klintschar M, Neuhuber F, Hühne J and Rolf B 1998 Mutation rate in human microsatellites: influence of the structure and length of the tandem repeat. *Am J Hum Genet* **62**, 1408–1415.

Brinkmann B, Pfeiffer H, Schürenkamp M and Hohoff C 2001 The evidential value of STRs: an analysis of exclusion cases. *Int J Legal Med* **114**, 173–177.

Brookfield FFY 1994 The effect of relatives on the likelihood ratio associated with DNA profile evidence in criminal cases. *J Forensic Sci Soc* **34**, 193–197.

Buckleton J and Triggs C 2005 Relatedness and DNA: are we taking it seriously enough? *Forensic Sci Int* **152**, 115–119.

Buckleton J, Triggs CM and Walsh SJ 2005 *Forensic DNA Evidence Interpretation.* CRC Press, London.

Budowle B and Chakraborty R 2001 Population variation at the CODIS core short tandem repeat loci in Europeans. *Legal Med* **3**, 29–33.

Budowle B, Giusti AM, Waye JS, Baechtel FS, Fourney RM, Adams DE, Presley LA, Deadman HA and Monson KL 1991a Fixed bin analysis for statistical evaluation of continuous distributions of allelic data from VNTR loci for use in forensic comparisons. *Am J Hum Genet* **48**, 841–855.

Budowle B, Monson KL, Anoe KS, Baechtel FS, Bergman DL, Buel E, Campbell PA, Clement ME, Corey HW, Davis LA, Dixon A, Fish P, Giusti AM, Grant TL, Gronert TM, Hoover DM, Jankowski L, Kilgore AJ, Kimoto W, Landrum WH, Leone H, Longwell CR, Maclaren DC, Medlin LE, Narveson SD, Pierson ML, Pollock JM, Raquel RJ, Reznicek JM, Rogers GS, Smerick JE and Thompson RM 1991b A preliminary report on binned general population data on six VNTR loci in Caucasians, Blacks, and Hispanics from the United States. *Crime Lab Dig* **18**, 9–26.

Budowle B, Shea B, Niezgoda S and Chakraborty R 2001 CODIS STR loci data from 41 sample populations. *J Forensic Sci* **46**, 453–489.

Carracedo A, Bär W, Lincoln P, Mayr W, Morling N, Olaisen B, Schneider P, Budowle B, Brinkmann B, Gill P, Holland M, Tully G and Wilson M 2000 DNA Commission of the International Society for Forensic Genetics: guidelines for mitochondrial DNA typing. *Forensic Sci Int* **110**, 79–85.

Chakraborty R and Stivers DN 1996 Paternity exclusion by DNA markers: effects of paternal mutations. *J Forensic Sci* **41**, 671–677.

Chakraborty R, Stivers DN, Su B, Zhong Y and Budowle B 1999 The utility of short tandem repeat loci beyond human identification: Implications for development of new DNA typing systems. *Electrophoresis* **20**, 1682–1696.

Clayton TM, Foreman LA and Carracedo A 2002 Letter to the editor: motherless case in paternity testing by Lee et al. *Forensic Sci Int* **125**, 284.

Conover WJ 1980 *Practical Nonparametric Statistics,* 2nd edn. John Wiley, New York.

Corradi F, Lago G and Stefanini FM 2003 The evaluation of DNA evidence in pedigrees requiring population inference. *J R Statist Soc A* **166**, 425–440.

Crow JF and Denniston C 1993 Population genetics as it relates to human identification. *Fourth International Symposium on Human Identification 1993: Proceedings*, pp. 31–36. Promega, Madison, WI.

Curran JM, Buckleton J and Triggs CM 2003 What is the magnitude of the subpopulation effect?. *J Forensic Sci* **135**, 1–8.

Curran JM, Triggs CM, Buckleton J and Weir BS 1999 Interpreting DNA mixtures in structured populations. *J Forensic Sci* **44**, 987–995.

Dawid AP 2001 Comment on Stockmarr (Likelihood ratios for evaluating DNA evidence when the suspect is found through a database search. *Biometrics*, 1999, **55**, 671-677). *Biometrics* **57**, 976–980.

Dawid AP and Mortera J 1996 Coherent analysis of forensic identification evidence. *J R Statist Soc B* **58**, 425–443.

Dawid AP, Mortera J and Pascali VL 2001 Non-fatherhood or mutation? A probabilistic approach to parental exclusion in paternity testing. *Forensic Sci Int* **124**, 55–61.

Dawid AP, Mortera J, Pascali VL and Van Boxel D 2002 Probabilistic expert systems for forensic inference from genetic markers. *Scand J Statist* **29**, 577–595.

Donnelly P 1995 Nonindependence of matches at different loci in DNA profiles: quantifying the effect of close relatives on the match probability. *Heredity* **75**, 26–34.

Dornheim MA 2002 Crash spurs revamp of China Airlines. *Aviation Week & Space Technology* **156**, 39.

Efron B and Tibshirani R 1993 *An Introduction to the Bootstrap Methods.* John Wiley, New York.

Egeland T, Dalen I and Mostad PF 2003 Estimating the number of contributors to a DNA profile. *Int J Legal Med* **117**, 271–275.

Egeland T, Mostad P and Olaisen B 1997 Computerized probability assessments of family relations. *Sci Justice* **37**, 269–274.

Egeland T, Mostad PF, Mevåg B and Stenersen M 2000 Beyond traditional paternity and identification cases: selecting the most probable pedigree. *Forensic Sci Int* **110**, 47–59.

Evett IW 1992 Evaluating DNA profiles in case where the defense is "It is my brother". *J Forensic Sci Soc* **32**, 5–14.

Evett IW and Weir BS 1998 *Interpreting DNA Evidence*. Sinauer Associates, Sunderland, Massachusetts.

Evett IW, Gill PD and Lambert JA 1998 Taking account of peak areas when interpreting mixed DNA profiles. *J Forensic Sci* **43**, 62–69.

Evett IW, Gill PD, Jackson G, Whitaker J and Champod C 2002 Interpreting small quantities of DNA: the hierarchy of propositions and the use of Bayesian networks. *J Forensic Sci* **47**, 520–530.

Fienberg SE 1979 The use of chi-squared statistics for categorical data problems. *J R Statist Soc B* **41**, 54–64.

Fimmer R, Henke L, Henke J and Baur MP 1992 How to deal with mutations in DNA-testing? In *Advances in Forensic Haemogenetics 4* (ed. Rittner C and Schneider PM), pp. 285–287. Springer-Verlag, Berlin.

Finkelstein MO and Levin B 2001 *Statistics for Lawyers*, 2nd edn. Springer, New York.

Fisher RA 1935 The logic of scientific inference. *J R Statist Soc* **98**, 39–54.

Foreman LA, Smith AFM and Evett IW 1997 Bayesian analysis of DNA profiling data in forensic identification applications (with discussion). *J R Statist Soc A* **160**, 429–469.

FSI Genetics 2007 Announcement: Launching Forensic Science International daughter journal in 2007. *Forensic Sci Int: Genetics* **1**, 1–2.

Fukshansky N and Bär W 1998 Interpreting forensic DNA evidence on the basis of hypotheses testing. *Int J Legal Med* **111**, 62–66.

Fukshansky N and Bär W 1999 Biostatistical evaluation of mixed stains with contributors of different ethnic origin. *Int J Legal Med* **112**, 383–387.

Fukshansky N and Bär W 2000 Biostatistics for mixed stain: the case of tested relatives of a non-tested suspect. *Int J Legal Med* **114**, 78–82.

Fukshansky N and Bär W 2005 DNA mixtures: biostatistics for mixed stains with haplotypic genetic markers. *Int J Legal Med* **119**, 285–290.

Fung WK 1996 10% or 5% match window in DNA profiling. *Forensic Sci Int* **78**, 111–118.

Fung WK 1997 Testing linkage equilibrium on allelic data between VNTR loci. *Am J Foren Med Path* **18**, 172–176.

Fung WK 2000 User friendly programs for paternity calculations. *Proceedings of the 11th International Symposium on Human Identification and Paternity Minisymposium*, pp. 1–10, Mississippi, USA. In http://www.promega.com/geneticidproc/ussymp11proc/paternity_minisymp/fung.pdf.

Fung WK 2003a Statistical analysis of forensic DNA: computational problems solved and to be solved (Keynote Speech). *ISI Satellite Meeting, International Conference on New Trends in Computational Statistics with Biometrical Applications*. A Special Volume in Journal of the Japanese Society of Computational Statistics. 2003, **15**, 15–26.

Fung WK 2003b User-friendly programs for easy calculations in paternity testing and kinship determinations. *Forensic Sci Int* **136**, 22–34.

Fung WK and Hu YQ 2000a Interpreting DNA mixtures based on the NRC-II recommendation 4.1. *Forensic Sci Commun* **2**. Available at http://www.fbi.gov/hq/lab/fsc/backissu/oct2000/fung.htm.

Fung WK and Hu YQ 2000b Interpreting forensic DNA mixtures: allowing for uncertainty in population substructure and dependence. *J R Statist Soc A* **163**, 241–254.

Fung WK and Hu YQ 2001 The evaluation of mixed stains from different ethnic origin: general result and common cases. *Int J Legal Med* **115**, 48–53.

Fung WK and Hu YQ 2002a Evaluating mixed stains with contributors of different ethnic groups under the NRC-II recommendation 4.1. *Statist Med* **21**, 3583–3593.

Fung WK and Hu YQ 2002b The statistical evaluation of DNA mixtures with contributors from different ethnic groups. *Int J Legal Med* **116**, 79–86.

Fung WK and Hu YQ 2004 Interpreting DNA mixtures with related contributors in subdivided populations. *Scand J Statist* **31**, 115–130.

Fung WK and Hu YQ 2005 Deoxyribonucleic acid: statistical analysis. In *Encyclopedia of Forensic and Legal Medicine* (ed. Payne-James J, Byard RW, Corey TS and Henderson C), vol. 2, pp. 184–189. Elsevier: Oxford.

Fung WK, Carracedo A and Hu YQ 2003a Testing for kinship in a subdivided population. *Forensic Sci Int* **135**, 105–109.

Fung WK, Chung YK and Wong DM 2002 Power of exclusion revisited: probability of excluding relatives of the true father from paternity. *Int J Legal Med* **116**, 64–67.

Fung WK, Hu YQ and Chung YK 2005 Statistical analysis of forensic DNA: theory, methods and computer programs (Keynote Speech). *17th World of the International Association of Forensic Sciences*, Hong Kong.

Fung WK, Hu YQ and Chung YK 2006 On statistical analysis of forensic DNA: theory, methods and computer programs. *Forensic Sci Int* **162**, 17–23.

Fung WK, Wong DM and Chung YK 2003b How well do serial tandem repeat loci perform in excluding paternity in relatives of the biological father among immigration cases?. *Transfusion* **43**, 982–983.

Fung WK, Wong DM and Hu YQ 2004 Full siblings impersonating parent/child prove most difficult to discredit with DNA profiling alone. *Transfusion* **44**, 1513–1515.

Fung WK, Wong DM and Tsui P 1996 Determination of both parents using DNA profiling. *Jurimet J Law Sci Techno* **36**, 337–342.

Garber RA and Morris JW 1983 General equations for the average power of exclusion for genetic systems of *n* codominant alleles in one-parent and in no-parent cases of disputed parentage. *Inclusion Probabilities in Parentage Testing*, pp. 277–280. American Association of Blood Banks, Arlington, VA.

Garbolino P and Taroni F 2002 Evaluation of scientific evidence using Bayesian networks. *Forensic Sci Int* **125**, 149–155.

Gastwirth JL 2000 *Statistical Science in the Courtroom*. Springer-Verlag, New York.

Gaytmenn R, Hildebrand DP, Sweet D and Pretty IA 2002 Determination of the sensitivity and specificity of sibship calculations using AmpF/STR Profiler Plus. *Int J Legal Med* **116**, 161–164.

Geisser S and Johnson W 1992 Testing Hardy-Weinberg equilibrium on allelic data from *VNTR* loci. *Am J Hum Genet* **51**, 1084–1088.

Geisser S and Johnson W 1995 Testing independence when the form of the bivariate distribution is unspecified. *Statist Med* **14**, 1621–1639.

Gill P, Brenner C, Brinkmann B, Budowle B, Carracedo A, Jobling MA, de Knijff P, Kayser M, Krawczak M, Mayr WR, Morling N, Olaisen B, Pascali V, Prinz M, Roewer L, Schneider PM, Sajantila A and Tyler-Smith C 2001 DNA Commission of the International Society of Forensic Genetics: recommendations on forensic analysis using Y-chromosome STRs. *Int J Legal Med* **114**, 305–309.

Gill P, Ivanov PL, Kimpton C, Piercy R, Benson N, Tully G, Evett I, Hagelberg E and Sullivan K 1994 Identification of the remains of the Romanov family by DNA analysis. *Nat Genet* **6**, 130–135.

Gill PD, Sparkes RL, Pinchin R, Clayton TM, Whitaker JP and Buckleton JS 1998 Interpreting simple STR mixtures using allelic peak areas. *Forensic Sci Int* **91**, 41–53.

Good PI 2001 *Applying Statistics in the Courtroom*. Chapman and Hall, London.

Goodwin W, Linacre A and Vanezis P 1999 The use of mitochondrial DNA and short tandem repeat typing in the identification of air crash victims. *Electrophoresis* **20**, 1707–1711.

Gorlin JB and Polesky HF 2000 The use and abuse of the full-sibling and half-sibling indices. *Transfusion* **40**, 1148.

Gunn PR, Trueman K, Stapleton P and Klarkowski DB 1997 DNA analysis in disputed parentage: the occurrence of two apparently false exclusions of paternity, both at short tandem repeat (STR) loci, in the one child. *Electrophoresis* **18**, 1650–1652.

Guo SW and Thompson EA 1992 Performing the exact test of Hardy-Weinberg proportion for multiple alleles. *Biometrics* **48**, 361–372.

Gusmão L, Butler JM, Carracedo A, Gill P, Kayser M, Mayr WR, Morling N, Prinz M, Roewer L, Tyler-Smith C and Schneider PM 2006 DNA Commission of the International Society of Forensic Genetics (ISFG): an update of the recommendations on the use of Y-STRs in forensic analysis. *Forensic Sci Int* **157**, 187–197.

Gusmão L, Sánchez-Diz P, Alves C, Lareu MV, Carracedo A and Amorim A 2000 Genetic diversity of nine STRs in two NW Iberian populations: Galicia and Northern Portugal. *Int J Legal Med* **114**, 109–113.

Hammer MF, Chamberlain VF, Kearney VF, Stover D, Zhang G, Karafet T, Walsh B and Redd AJ 2006 Population structure of Y chromosome SNP haplogroups in the United States and forensic implications for constructing Y chromosome STR databases. *Forensic Sci Int* **164**, 45–55.

Harbison SA and Buckleton JS 1998 Applications and extensions of subpopulation theory: a caseworkers guide. *Sci Justice* **38**, 249–254.

Hartl DL and Clark AG 1989 *Principles of Population Genetics*, 2nd edn. Sinauer, Sunderland, MA.

Heyer E, Puymirat J, Dieltjes P, Bakker E and de Knijff P 1997 Estimating Y-chromosome specific microsatellite mutation frequencies using deep rooting pedigrees. *Hum Mol Genet* **6**, 799–803.

Holland MM and Parsons TJ 1999 Mitochondrial DNA sequence analysis – validation and use for forensic casework. *Forensic Sci Rev* **11**, 21–50.

Hu YQ and Fung WK 2003a Evaluating forensic DNA mixtures with contributors of different structured ethnic origins: a computer software. *Int J Legal Med* **117**, 248–249.

Hu YQ and Fung WK 2003b Interpreting DNA mixtures with the presence of relatives. *Int J Legal Med* **117**, 39–45.

Hu YQ and Fung WK 2005a Evaluation of DNA mixtures involving two pairs of relatives. *Int J Legal Med* **119**, 251–259.

Hu YQ and Fung WK 2005b Power of excluding an elder brother of a child from paternity. *Forensic Sci Int* **152**, 321–322.

Hu YQ and Fung WK 2005c Power of excluding relatives of the child from paternity using X-linked markers. *Proceedings of the 5th IASC Asian Conference on Statistical Computing, December 15-17, Hong Kong*, pp. 57–60.

Hu YQ, Fung WK and Lu J 2005 Evaluating mixed DNA profiles with the presence of relatives: theory, method and computer software. *Forensic Sci Commun* **7**. Available: http://www.fbi.gov/hq/lab/fsc/backissu/april2005/research/2005_04_research01.htm.

Hu YQ, Fung WK and Yang CT 2004 On the power of excluding relatives of the true father from paternity. In *Progress in Forensic Genetics 10* (ed. Doutrempuich C and Morling N), pp. 514–516. Elsevier Science, Amsterdam.

Jamieson A and Taylor SS 1997 Comparisons of three probability formulae for parentage exclusion. *Anim Genet* **28**, 397–400.

Jeffreys AJ, Wilson V and Thein SL 1985 Individual-specific 'fingerprints' of human DNA. *Nature* **316**, 76–79.

Jobling MA, Hurles ME and Tyler-Smith C 2004 *Human Evolutionary Genetics: Origins, Peoples, and Disease*. Garland Science, New York.

Johnson NL and Kotz S 1972 *Distributions in Statistics: Continuous Multivariate Distributions*. John Wiley, New York.

Jones DA 1972 Blood samples: probabilities of discrimination. *J Forensic Sci Soc* **12**, 355–359.

Kaye DH 1989 The probability of an ultimate issue: the strange cases of paternity testing. *Iowa Law Rev* **75**, 75–109.

Kayser M, Brauer S, Willuweit S, Schadlich H, Batzer MA, Zawacki J, Prinz M, Roewer L and Stoneking M 2002 Online Y-chromosomal short tandem repeat haplotype reference database (YHRD) for US populations. *J Forensic Sci* **47**, 513–519.

Kayser M, Roewer L, Hedman M, Henke L, Henke J, Brauer S, Kruger C, Krawczak M, Nagy M, Dobosz T, Szibor R, de Knijff P, Stoneking M and Sajantila A 2000 Characteristics and frequency of germline mutations at microsatellite loci from the human Y chromosome, as revealed by direct observation in father/son pairs. *Am J Hum Genet* **66**, 1580–1588.

Lauritzen SL 1996 *Graphical Models*. Clarendon, Oxford.

Law MY, Wong DM, Fung WK, Chan KL, Li C, Lun TS, Lai KM, Cheung KY and Chiu CT 2001 Genetic polymorphism at three STR loci-CSF1PO, HUMTHO1 and TPOX, and the AMP-FLP locus D1S80 for the Chinese population in Hong Kong. *Forensic Sci Int* **115**, 103–105.

Leclair B, Freqeau CJ, Bowen KL, Borys SB, Elliott J and Fourney RM 2000 Enhanced kinship analysis and STR-based DNA typing for human identification in mass disasters. In *Progress in Forensic Genetics 8 (1193)* (ed. Sensabaugh GF, Lincoln PJ and Olaisen B), pp. 91–93. Elsevier Science, Netherlands.

Lee CL, Lebeck L and Pothiawala M 1980 Exclusion of paternity without testing the mother. *Am J Clin Path* **74**, 809–812.

Lee HS, Lee JW, Han GR and Hwang JJ 2000 Motherless case in paternity testing. *Forensic Sci Int* **114**, 57–65.

Lee JW, Lee HS, Park M and Hwang JJ 1999 Paternity probability when a relative of the father is an alleged father. *Sci Justice* **39**, 223–230.

Lempert R 1991 Some caveats concerning DNA as criminal identification evidence: with thanks to the reverend bayes. *Cardozo Law Rev* **13**, 303–341.

Li CC and Chakravarti A 1988 An expository review of 2 methods of calculating the paternity probability. *Am J Hum Genet* **43**, 197–205.

Li CC and Sacks L 1954 The derivation of joint distribution and correlation between relatives by the use of stochastic matrices. *Biometrics* **10**, 247–260.

Lidor D 2002 Be all that DNA can be. Available from http://www.wired.com/medtech/health/news/2002/09/54631 (accessed 25 May 2007).

Lindley DV 1990 The present position of Bayesian statistics. *Statist Sci* **5**, 44–89.

Lucy D 2005 *Introduction to Statistics for Forensic Scientists*. John Wiley & Sons, Chichester.

Meester R and Sjerps M 2003 The evidential value in the DNA database search controversy and the two-stain problem. *Biometrics* **59**, 727–732.

Melvin JR, Kateley JR, Oaks MK, Simson LR and Maldonado WE 1998 Paternity testing. In *Forensic Science Handbook* (ed. Saferstein R), vol. 2, pp. 273–346. Prentice-Hall, Englewood Cliffs, NJ.

Miller I and Miller M 2004 *John E. Freund's Mathematical Statistics with Applications,* 7th edn. Prentice Hall.

Morris JW, Garber RA, d'Autremont J and Brenner CH 1988 The avuncular index and the incest index. In *Advances in Forensic Haemogenetics 2* (ed. Mayr WR), pp. 607–611. Springer-Verlag, Berlin.

Mortera J, Dawid AP and Lauritzen SL 2003 Probabilistic expert systems for DNA mixture profiling. *Theor Popul Biol* **63**, 191–205.

Morton NE 1992 Genetic structure of forensic populations. *Proc Natl Acad Sci USA* **89**, 2556–2560.

National Research Council 1992 *DNA Technology in Forensic Science*. National Academy Press, Washington DC.

National Research Council 1996 *The Evaluation of Forensic DNA Evidence*. National Academy Press, Washington DC.

Nei M 1987 *Molecular Evolutionary Genetics*. Columbia University Press, New York.

Nei M and Roychoudhury AK 1974 Sampling variances of heterozygosity and genetic distance. *Genetics* **76**, 379–390.

Ohno Y, Sebetan IM and Akaishi S 1982 A simple method for calculating the probability of excluding paternity with any number of codominant alleles. *Forensic Sci Int* **19**, 93–98.

Perlin MW and Szabady B 2001 Linear mixture analysis: a mathematical approach to resolving mixed DNA samples. *J Forensic Sci* **46**, 1372–1378.

Pu CE, Hsieh CM, Chen MY, Wu FC and Sun CF 1999 Genetic variation at nine STR loci in populations from the Philippines and Thailand living in Taiwan. *Forensic Sci Int* **106**, 1–6.

Roeder K 1994 DNA fingerprinting: a review of the controversy. *Statist Sci* **9**, 222–278.

Roewer L, Kayser M, de Knijff P, Anslinger K, Betz A, Cagliá A, Corach D, Füredi S, Henke L, Hidding M, Kärgel HJ, Lessig R, Nagy M, Pascali VL, Parson W, Rolf B, Schmitt C, Szibor R, Teifel-Greding J and Krawczak M 2000 A new method for the evaluation of matches in non-recombining genomes: application to Y-chromosomal short tandem repeat (STR) haplotypes in European males. *Forensic Sci Int* **114**, 31–43.

Roewer L, Krawczak M, Willuweit S, Nagy M, Alves C, Amorim A, Anslinger K, Augustin C, Betz A, Bosch E, Cagliá A, Carracedo A, Corach D, Dekairelle AF, Dobosz T, Dupuy BM, Füredi S, Gehrig C, Gusmaõ L, Henke J, Henke L, Hidding M, Hohoff C, Hoste B, Jobling MA, Kärgel HJ, de Knijff P, Lessig R, Liebeherr E, Lorente M, Martínez-Jarreta B, Nievas P, Nowak M, Parson W, Pascali VL, Penacino G, Ploski R, Rolf B, Sala A, Schmidt U, Schmitt C, Schneider PM, Szibor R, Teifel-Greding J and Kayser M 2001 Online reference database of European Y-chromosomal short tandem repeat (STR) haplotypes. *Forensic Sci Int* **118**, 106–113.

Rolf B, Keil W, Brinkmann B, Roewer L and Fimmers R 2001 Paternity testing using Y-STR haplotypes: assigning a probability for paternity in cases of mutations. *Int J Legal Med* **115**, 12–15.

Sensabaugh GF 1982 Biochemical markers of individuality. In *Forensic Science Handbook* (ed. Saferstein R), pp. 338–415. Prentice-Hall, New York.

Shepard EM and Herrera RJ 2006 Iranian STR variation at the fringes of biogeographical demarcation. *Forensic Sci Int* **158**, 140–148.

Sjerps M and Kloosterman AD 1999 On the consequences of DNA profile mismatches for close relatives of an excluded suspect. *Int J Legal Med* **112**, 176–180.

Stockmarr A 1999 Likelihood ratios for evaluating DNA evidence when the suspect is found through a database search. *Biometrics* **55**, 671–677.

Stockmarr A 2000 The choice of hypotheses in the evaluation of DNA profile evidence In *Statistical Science in the Courtroom* (ed. Gastwirth JL), pp. 143–160. Springer, New York.

Thomson JA, Ayres KL, Pilotti V, Barrett MN, Walker JIH and Debenham PG 2001 Analysis of disputed single-parent/child and sibling relationships using 16 STR loci. *Int J Legal Med* **115**, 128–134.

Thomson JA, Pilotti V, Stevens P, Ayres KL and Debenham PG 1999 Validation of short tandem repeat analysis for the investigation of cases of disputed paternity. *Forensic Sci Int* **100**, 1–16.

Triggs CM, Harbison SA and Buckleton J 2000 The calculation of DNA match probabilities in mixed race populations. *Sci Justice* **40**, 33–38.

Tsokos M, Lessig R, Grundmann C, Benthaus S and Peschel O 2006 Experiences in tsunami victim identification. *Int J Legal Med* **120**, 185–187.

Tsui P and Wong DM 1996 Allele frequencies of four VNTR loci in the Chinese population in Hong Kong. *Forensic Sci Int* **79**, 175–185.

Tully G, Bär W, Brinkmann B, Carracedo A, Gill P, Morling N, Parson W and Schneider P 2001 Considerations by the European DNA profiling, (EDNAP) group on the working practices, nomenclature and interpretation of mitochondrial DNA profiles. *Forensic Sci Int* **12**, 83–91.

Valdes AM, Slatkin M and Freimer NB 1993 Allele frequencies at microsatellite loci: the stepwise mutation model revisited. *Genetics* **133**, 737–749.

Vastag B 2002 Out of tragedy, identification innovation. *J Am Med Asso* **288**, 1221–1223.

Wang T, Xue N and Birdwell JD 2006 Least-square deconvolution: a framework for interpreting short tandem repeat mixtures. *J Forensic Sci* **51**, 1284–1297.

Weir BS 1993 Independence tests for VNTR alleles defined as quantile bins. *Am J Hum Genet* **53**, 1107–1113.

Weir BS 1994 The effects of inbreeding on forensic calculations. *Annu Rev Genet* **28**, 597–621.

Weir BS 2003 Forensics. In *Handbook of Statistical Genetics, 2nd edn* (ed. Balding DJ, Bishop M and Cannings C), vol. 2, pp. 830–852. John Wiley & Sons.

Weir BS, Triggs CM, Starling L, Stowell LI, Walsh KAJ and Buckleton J 1997 Interpreting DNA mixtures. *J Forensic Sci* **42**, 213–222.

Wenk RE, Chiafari FA, Gorlin J and Polesky HF 2003 Better tools are needed for parentage and kinship studies. *Transfusion* **43**, 979–981.

Wiener ML, Lederer M and Polayes SH 1930 Studies in isohemagglutination IV: On the chances of proving non-paternity; with special reference to blood groups. *J Immunology* **19**, 259–282.

Wiuf C 2001 Recombination in human mitochondrial DNA? *Genetics* **159**, 749–756.

Wolf A, Caliebe A, Junge O and Krawczak M 2005 Forensic interpretation of Y-chromosomal DNA mixtures. *Forensic Sci Int* **152**, 209–213.

Wong DM, Law MY, Fung WK, Chan KL, Li C, Lun TS, Lai KM, Cheung KY and Chiu CT 2001 Population data for 12 STR loci in Hong Kong Chinese. *Int J Legal Med* **114**, 281–284.

Wright S 1951 The genetical structure of populations. *Ann Eugen* **15**, 323–354.

Zaykin D, Shivotovsky L and Weir BS 1995 Exact test for association between alleles at arbitrary numbers of loci. *Genetica* **96**, 169–178.

Index

STATISTICS IN PRACTICE

Human and Biological Sciences

Berger – Selection Bias and Covariate Imbalances in Randomized Clinical Trials
Brown and Prescott – Applied Mixed Models in Medicine, Second Edition
Chevret (Ed) – Statistical Methods for Dose-Finding Experiments
Ellenberg, Fleming and DeMets – Data Monitoring Committees in Clinical Trials: A Practical Perspective
Hauschke, Steinijans & Pigeot – Bioequivalence Studies in Drug Development: Methods and Applications
Lawson, Browne and Vidal Rodeiro – Disease Mapping with WinBUGS and MLwiN
Lui – Statistical Estimation of Epidemiological Risk
Marubini and Valsecchi – Analysing Survival Data from Clinical Trials and Observation Studies
Molenberghs and Kenward – Missing Data in Clinical Studies
O'Hagan, Buck, Daneshkhah, Eiser, Garthwaite, Jenkinson, Oakley & Rakow – Uncertain Judgements: Eliciting Expert's Probabilities
Parmigiani – Modeling in Medical Decision Making: A Bayesian Approach
Pintilie – Competing Risks: A Practical Perspective
Senn – Cross-over Trials in Clinical Research, Second Edition
Senn – Statistical Issues in Drug Development, Second Edition
Spiegelhalter, Abrams and Myles – Bayesian Approaches to Clinical Trials and Health-Care Evaluation
Whitehead – Design and Analysis of Sequential Clinical Trials, Revised Second Edition
Whitehead – Meta-Analysis of Controlled Clinical Trials
Willan and Briggs – Statistical Analysis of Cost Effectiveness Data
Winkel and Zhang – Statistical Development of Quality in Medicine

Earth and Environmental Sciences

Buck, Cavanagh and Litton – Bayesian Approach to Interpreting Archaeological Data
Glasbey and Horgan – Image Analysis in the Biological Sciences
Helsel – Nondetects and Data Analysis: Statistics for Censored Environmental Data
Illian, Penttinen, Stoyan, H and Stoyan D–Statistical Analysis and Modelling of Spatial Point Patterns
McBride – Using Statistical Methods for Water Quality Management
Webster and Oliver – Geostatistics for Environmental Scientists, Second Edition
Wymer (Ed) – Statistical Framework for Recreational Water Quality Criteria and Monitoring

Industry, Commerce and Finance

Aitken – Statistics and the Evaluation of Evidence for Forensic Scientists, Second Edition
Balding – Weight-of-evidence for Forensic DNA Profiles
Brandimarte – Numerical Methods in Finance and Economics: A MATLAB-Based Introduction, Second Edition

Brandimarte and Zotteri – Introduction to Distribution Logistics

Chan – Simulation Techniques in Financial Risk Management

Coleman, Greenfield, Stewardson and Montgomery (Eds) – Statistical Practice
in Business and Industry

Frisen (Ed) – Financial Surveillance

Fung and Hu – Statistical DNA Forensics

Lehtonen and Pahkinen – Practical Methods for Design and Analysis of Complex Surveys,
Second Edition

Ohser and Mücklich – Statistical Analysis of Microstructures in Materials Science

Taroni, Aitken, Garbolino and Biedermann – Bayesian Networks and Probabilistic Inference
in Forensic Science